T0383206

Handbook of Complications during Percutaneous Cardiovascular Interventions

Handbook of Complications during Percutaneous Cardiovascular Interventions

Eric Eeckhout MD PhD
Associate Professor of Cardiology
Service de Cardiologie
Centre Hospitalier Universitaire Vandois (CHUV) Lausanne
Switzerland

Amir Lerman MD
Professor of Medicine
Division of Cardiovascular Diseases and Internal Medicine
Mayo Clinic
Rochester, MN
USA

Stéphane Carlier MD
Director of Intravascular Imaging and Physiology
Columbia University Medical Center and the Cardiovascular Research Foundation
New York, NY
USA

Morton Kern MD
Pacific Cardiovascular Associates
Cosa Mesa, CA
USA

informa
healthcare

First published in the United Kingdom in 2007 by Informa Healthcare, Telephone House, 69-77 Paul Street, London EC2A 4LQ. Informa Healthcare is a trading division of Informa UK Ltd. Registered Office: 37/41 Mortimer Street, London W1T 3JH. Registered in England and Wales number 1072954.

Tel: +44 (0)20 7017 5000
Fax: +44 (0)20 7017 6699
Website: www.informahealthcare.com

Second printing, 2007

A CIP record for this book is available from the British Library.
Library of Congress Cataloging-in-Publication Data

Data available on application

ISBN-10: 1 84184 380 6
ISBN-13: 978 1 84184 380 3

Distributed in North and South America by
Taylor & Francis
6000 Broken Sound Parkway, NW, (Suite 300)
Boca Raton, FL 33487, USA

Within Continental USA
Tel: 1 (800) 272 7737; Fax: 1 (800) 374 3401
Outside Continental USA
Tel: (561) 994 0555; Fax: (561) 361 6018
Email: orders@crcpress.com

Distributed in the rest of the world by
Thomson Publishing Services
Cheriton House
North Way
Andover, Hampshire SP10 5BE, UK
Tel: +44 (0)1264 332424
Email: tps.tandfsalesorder@thomson.com

Composition by Phoenix Photosetting, Chatham, Kent, UK
Printed and bound in India by Replika Press Pvt Ltd

To my wife, Ann, and children Seline, Pauline and Tanguy and my parents for their indulgence, continuous support, and patience . . .

EE

Contents

List of Contributors

Alexandre Abizaid
Institute Dante Pazzanese de Cardiologia
Sao Paulo
Brazil

Carla Agatiello
Department of Cardiology
Hôpital Charles Nicolle
Rouen
France

David Antoniucci
Division of Cardiology
Careggi Hospital
Florence
Italy

Vasilis Babaliaros
Department of Cardiology
Hôpital Charles Nicolle
Rouen
France

Jean-Pierre Bassand
Department of Cardiology
Hôpital Jean Minjoz
Besançon
France

Malcolm R Bell
Department of Cardiovascular Diseases
    and Internal Medicine
Mayo Clinic
Rochester, MN
USA

Edouard Benit
Department of Cardiology
Hartcentrum Virga Jesseziekenhuis
Hasselt
Belgium

Alexandre Berger
Cardiology Clinic
Centre Hospitalier Universitaire
    Vaudois
Lausanne
Switzerland

Michel E Bertrand
Hôpital Cardiologique
Lille
France

Patricia J M Best
Department of Cardiovascular Diseases
Mayo Clinic
Rochester, MN
USA

François Beygui
Pitié – Salpétriére University Hospital
Institut de Cardiologie
Paris
France

Younes Boudjemline
Service de Cardiologie Pediatrique
Hôpital Necker Enfant Malades
Paris
France

Pedro Brugada
Cardiovascular Center
OLV Hospital
Aalst
Belgium

Stéphane Carlier
Cardiovascular Research Foundation
New York, NY
USA

Antonio Colombo
Department of Cardiology
Columbus Hospital
Milan
Italy

Jose de Ribamar Costa Jr
Institute Dante Pazzanese de Cardiologia
Sao Paulo
Brazil

Alain Cribier
Department of Cardiology
Hôpital Charles Nicolle
Rouen
France

Vinicius Daher
Institute Dante Pazzanese de Cardiologia
Sao Paulo
Brazil

Dariusz Dudek
Second Department of Cardiology
Institute of Cardiology
Jagiellonian University Medical College
Krakow
Poland

Raphaelle Dumaine
Pitié – Salpétriére University Hospital
Institut de Cardiologie
Paris
France

Eric Eeckhout
Service de Cardiologie
Centre Hospitalier Universitaire
   Vandois (CHUV)
Lausanne
Switzerland

Jean Fajadet
Unité de Cardiologie Interventionnelle
Clinique Pasteur
Toulouse
France

Bruno Farah
Unité de Cardiologie Interventionnelle
Clinique Pasteur
Toulouse
France

Ted Feldman
Evanston Northwestern Healthcare
   Cardiology Unit
Evanston, IL
USA

Kenichi Fujii
Cardiovascular Research Foundation
New York, NY
USA

Eulogio García
Interventional Cardiology Unit
Hospital Gregorio Marañón
Madrid
Spain

Peter Geelen
Cardiovascular Center
OLV Hospital
Aalst
Belgium

Richard J Gumina
Division of Cardiovascular and Internal
   Medicine
Mayo Clinic
Rochester, MN
USA

David R Holmes Jr
Division of Cardiovascular Diseases and
   Internal Medicine
Mayo Clinic
Rochester, MN
USA

Ioannis Iakovou
Interventional Cardiology
Army Hospital of Thessaloniki
Thessaloniki and Euromedica
Thessaloniki
Greece

Morton Kern
Pacific Cardiovascular Associates
Costa Mesa
California, CA
USA

Young-Hak Kim
Department of Medicine
University of Ulsan College of
   Medicine
Seoul
Korea

Georgios Kourgiannidis
Cardiovascular Center
OLV Hospital
Aalst
Belgium

Seung-Whan Lee
Department of Medicine
Soon Chun Hyang University Bucheon
   Hospital
Gyeonggi-do
Korea

Thierry Lefèvre
Institut Cardiovasculaire Paris Sud
Massy
France

Amir Lerman
Department of Cardiovascular
   Diseases
Mayo Clinic
Rochester, MN
USA

Xuebo Liu
Cardiovascular Research Foundation
New York, NY
USA

Yves Louvard
Institut Cardiovasculaire Paris Sud
Massy
France

Carlos Macaya
Cardiovascular Institute
Hospital Clínico San Carlos
Madrid
Spain

Jean Marco
Unité de Cardiologie Interventionnelle
Clinique Pasteur
Toulouse
France

Tetsuo Matsubara
Department of Cardiology
Toyohashi Heart Center
Toyohashi
Japan

Roxanna Mehran
Cardiovascular Research Foundation
New York, NY
USA

Bernhard Meier
Department of Cardiology
University Hospital
Bern
Switzerland

Nicolas Meneveau
Department of Cardiology
Hôpital Jean Minjoz
Besançon
France

Gilles Montalescot
Pitié-Salpétrière University Hospital
Institut de Cardiologie
Paris
France

Marie-Claude Morice
Institut Cardiovasculaire Paris Sud
Massy
France

Jeffrey Moses
Cardiovascular Research Foundation
New York, NY
USA

Seong-Wook Park
Department of Medicine
University of Ulsan College of Medicine
Asan Medical Center
Seoul
Korea

Seung-Jung Park
Department of Medicine
University of Ulsan College of Medicine
Asian Medical Center
Seoul
Korea

Guy S Reeder
Division of Cardiovascular Diseases and
    Internal Medicine
Mayo Clinic
Rochester, MN
USA

Charanjit S Rihal
Cardiac Catheterization Laboratory
Division of Cardiovascular Diseases and
    Internal Medicine
Mayo Clinic
Rochester, MN
USA

Manel Sabaté
Cardiology Department
Hospital de la Santa Creu i Sant Pau
Barcelona
Spain

Koichi Sano
Cardiovascular Research Foundation
New York, NY
USA

François Schiele
Department of Cardiology
Hôpital Jean Minjoz
Besançon
France

Horst Sievert
Cardiovascular Centre Bethanien
Frankfurt
Germany

Jose A Silva
Department of Cardiology
Ochsner Clinic Foundation
New Orleans, LA
USA

J Eduardo Sousa
Institute Dante Pazzanese de Cardiologia
Sao Paulo
Brazil

Gregg Stone
Cardiovascular Research Foundation
New York, NY
USA

Takahiko Suzuki
Department of Cardiology
Toyohashi Heart Center
Toyohashi
Japan

Etsuo Tsuchikane
Department of Cardiology
Toyohashi Heart Center
Toyohashi
Japan

Alec Vahanian
Service de Cardiologie
Hôpital Bichat
Paris
France

Pascal Vranckx
Hartcentrum Virga Jesseziekenhuis
Hasselt
Belgium

Christopher J White
Department of Cardiology
Ochsner Clinic Foundation
New Orleans, LA
USA

Stephan Windecker
Invasive Cardiology Department
University Hospital
Bern
Switzerland

Foreword

A few years ago, Eric Eeckhout and his team initiated in Lausanne a course of interventional cardiology focusing on complications. Rapidly this course became highly appreciated by an audience who were more interested in learning from complications rather than from successes. It was not surprising that Eric was also invited by the ESC and the Euro PCR to organize a focus session on complications – the following step was obviously to put into writing all this extremely valuable information. This has been achieved and the author has assembled a very competent panel of co-authors who have covered all the facets of interventional cardiology from one of the most critical points of view: the prevention and the treatment of complications.

People used to say that we have to be sadomasochist to report and analyse the cause and origin of complications. On the one hand we have to describe the consequences of our sometimes foolish interventional acts on our patients; death, stroke, MI, bleeding, pain, chronic suffering, the list goes on; and on the other hand we have to search within our behaviour and judgement, for the origin and cause of these complications which is a sobering experience in self criticism. As David Holmes once said 'complications, a rich emotional experience'.

Beyond the 'rich emotional experience' this is a fantastic opportunity to learn not at the expense of our patients. Richard Miller, a pioneer in interventional cardiology used to say, 'Good judgement is based on bad experience and bad experience results from poor judgement'. This is the essence of what Eric and his co-authors try to achieve: teach good judgement by learning from the bad experience. It has, and it will, spare our patients suffering and unnecessary disappointment.

Professor Patrick Serruys MD PhD
Chief Interventional Cardiology
Thoraxcenter-Erasmus University
Rotterdam
The Netherlands

Preface

Currently, the medical community considers interventional cardiology as a fascinating sub-speciality. It attracts young cardiologists all around the world who wish to embark in what they probably consider as a 'career with a future'. Indeed, over the past 30 years, interventional technology has progressed exponentially. A technologic revolution, resulting from collaboration between clinicians and engineers, currently provides outstanding material for percutaneous treatment of cardiovascular diseases in daily practice. These interventions often provide instant symptom relief for the patient. The particular setting of the catheterization laboratory allows direct contact between the operator and patient, who may, even as a layman, visually observe the obtained angiographic result. This situation is quite unique in medicine and can be particularly gratifying for the physician who is, for example, performing primary angioplasty for acute myocardial infarction. Furthermore, the interventional cardiologist is often invited to demonstrate his 'skills' on huge video screens which are transmitted live to thousands of colleagues during international congresses. Indeed, the interventional cardiologist is indulged by great professionalism and surrounded by a sort of 'stardom', chased by the medical and industrial community.

However, there isn't only the bright side of interventional cardiology. Percutaneous interventions may be very demanding, challenging, and complicated. Even in an apparently simple case, it still holds true that you know exactly when you start but never when you are done … Complications do occur; they might have been anticipated, but more often they are unexpected. Unfortunately, they can be a pitiful demonstration of lack of experience or illustrate a truly wrong strategy or lack of insight into the real problem of the patient. The latter, indeed, is not to be confounded with the angiographic images!

This textbook of interventional cardiology is the first to focus solely on complications during cardiovascular interventions. Together with Morton Kern, Stéphane Carlier and Amir Lerman, I launched this initiative a few years ago. Alan Burgess from Taylor & Francis Medical Publishers was associated with the concept and the result is currently lying in your hands. It is the effort of many cardiologists worldwide who have contributed to this work and we truly want to thank them for their engagement. Remarkably, we were able to gather authors from almost all continents, each known for their contribution in a particular field.

Jean Marco, one of my mentors, has repeatedly insisted on the role of education in interventional cardiology. This is the main objective of this book. We wish to provide a guide for the young and 'less young' interventional cardiologist in the prevention and treatment of complications during cardiovascular interventions. This book is especially practically oriented and includes many tips and tricks, most of which you will not find in the classic textbooks. We encourage you to organize morbidity and mortality conferences where you can interactively discuss your complications. Guided by experienced operators, you will discover the high educational value of such a meeting. A 'solved' complication is often a demonstration of human creativity. Discussing a complication is a catharsis for the presenters who can finally share their doubts and benefit from the input of other colleagues.

Interventional cardiology is a fascinating speciality with a bright future. May this book guide you in difficult times and remain a reference during more quiet moments.

Eric Eeckhout

Section A
Introduction

1

More than 25 years of percutaneous cardiovascular interventions: A historical perspective

Michel E Bertrand

First angioplasty in Zurich • Steerable catheters • The new devices • Coronary stenting • Conclusion

After the courageous experience of Werner Forssmann[1] in 1929, heart catheterization was really introduced into cardiology after the pioneering work of Cournand and collaborators in the 1950s.[2] However, it was initially limited to measurements of pressure and blood flow. This was particularly important for the evaluation of valvular diseases which, in the 1950s, were very frequent and mostly related to rheumatic fever which subsequently disappeared, at least in the western world. The great pandemic of industrialized countries, i.e. coronary atherosclerosis, started within the latter half of the 20th century. Selective coronary angiography, initiated by Mason Sones,[3] allowed an understanding of coronary atherosclerosis. But, in this area, like many others in medicine, major technical or procedural developments are linked to the therapeutic implications. Coronary bypass surgery, performed for the first time by René Favaloro,[4] was a major therapeutic advance and was responsible for considerable improvements in terms of quality and expectancy of life of patients suffering from coronary artery disease. However, this approach was very aggressive and many cardiologists were initially reluctant to recommend this operation.

FIRST ANGIOPLASTY IN ZURICH

In this context, the first percutaneous coronary angioplasty performed by Andreas Grüntzig[5-7] (Figure 1.1) was a true revolution since he proposed a less invasive approach as an alternative to a very aggressive operation.

Andreas Grüntzig was born in Dresden, Germany, in 1939. After his medical studies, he started a training period in radiology (1971–2) and worked with Eberhardt Zeitler who was applying a method of dilatation with stiff catheters of increasing diameter for percutaneous treatment of peripheral arteries. Andreas Grüntzig started to use the Dotter technique but he was looking for a better approach. He met a retired chemist from the technical University of Zurich who introduced him to polyvinyl compounds and together they built a crude, single-lumen balloon. At the end of 1973 Grüntzig treated a patient with a short occlusion of the superficial femoral artery. In spite of a superb result, the chief of general surgery was very

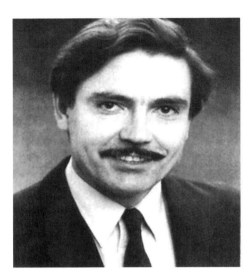

Figure 1.1   Andreas Grüntzig (1939–85).

concerned but, fortunately, Grüntzig was strongly supported by Dr Ake Senning, the chief of cardiac surgery. In the following years, Grüntzig struggled to build the double-lumen balloon catheter since no medical equipment manufacturers would produce this device.

Nevertheless, he continued his experiments and he did the first coronary canine angioplasty in October 1975, followed by several other dog experiments. Meanwhile, a double-lumen catheter had been produced by Schneider Medintag.

During the first quarter of 1977, four cases of intraoperative procedures during open heart surgery were successfully performed in San Francisco. Back in Zurich, Grüntzig identified a patient with a single discrete proximal left anterior descending (LAD) lesion. He proposed the new procedure to a 38-year-old engineer and the first human coronary angioplasty was successfully performed in September 1977. An angiogram performed one month later showed an excellent result. The second case was performed in Frankfurt with Martin Kaltenbach and they treated within the same procedure a left main tight narrowing and a lesion of the right coronary artery.

The report of the first five patients was published in *The Lancet* followed by a series of 50 cases published in the *New England Journal of Medicine*.[7]

From 1977 to 1981, coronary angioplasty was recommended for very select cases. The patients should be symptomatic, with stable angina and good left ventricular function, and be candidates for coronary artery bypass surgery. A careful analysis of the coronary angiogram and angioplasty was used in patients with single-vessel disease with significant discrete stenoses, proximal, concentric noncalcified, not located at bifurcations and in an angulated segment. Andreas Grüntzig himself stated in a meeting that the technique should be limited to a small number of patients presenting the above-mentioned criteria.

One of the major reasons for these limitations was the balloon catheter characteristics. There was a very small fixed guidewire at the tip of the balloon, precluding changes in the curvature after the balloon had been introduced into the coronary artery. The size (1.5–2.0 mm), the straightness, and the stiffness of the balloon did not allow it to pass some curvatures and in most cases it was only possible to push it into very straight coronary segments, mainly in the proximal left anterior descending coronary artery and the first segment of the right coronary artery. In addition, the guiding catheters (9 F) had a very thick wall and relatively small lumen; it was therefore difficult, with the bulky balloon material, to inject contrast medium and to recognize the position of the balloon inside the vessel. For example, it was very difficult to enter the circumflex artery.

This initial balloon catheter was manufactured by the Schneider company and it was necessary to prove attendance at the live course demonstration in Zurich before one could order the device. The connection to the pressure strain gauge, contrast medium, and the system for balloon inflation were very complex.

STEERABLE CATHETERS

The second revolution was the steerable guidewire. In 1979, a short wire, straight or with a J shape (DG or DJ), was attached at the distal tip of the catheter. When this small wire was manually profiled with an adapted curve, it was sometimes possible to cross curvatures and even to pass into angulated vessels.

A major advance was achieved when John Simpson proposed the steerable guidewire.[8] Simpson applied the Seldinger technique, used for several years in the peripheral vessels, to the coronary artery tree. Sven-Ivar Seldinger (1921–99) was a Swedish radiologist who in 1953 described a new technique to safely catheterize the arteries.

John Simpson designed an improved guidewire for use with coronary balloon dilatation catheters. The guidewire had a solid core wire which makes up the proximal end of the guidewire. The core wire was tapered toward the distal end to increase flexibility. The tapered distal end of the core wire was surrounded by a coil spring, which was made completely or partially from a highly radiopaque material. The tip of the small guidewire might also serve to predilate very tight stenoses, making it easier to cross the lesion with an angioplasty balloon. A removable handle for maneuvering the guidewire was also proposed. It was the co-axial over-the-wire technique.

After testing in animal and cadaver hearts, in 1982 Simpson reported the first human experiences with the new catheter system. He performed angioplasty in 53 patients with single-vessel disease and the success rate was 64%. Using a smaller balloon in the last 41 cases, he was able to increase the success rate to 73%.

The major advantages were the easy selection of the vessel to be treated, since it was possible to withdraw and to reshape the guidewire, and also avoiding the risk of dissection in pushing the balloon beneath the atherosclerotic plaque. Nevertheless, there was still a problem: treatment of a very tight stenosis implied a small balloon (2 mm) but to optimize the results a bigger balloon (3 or 3.5 mm) was needed. In the early stages, it was necessary to remove not only the balloon catheter but also the guidewire. The next step was to pass again through the stenosis disrupted by the first balloon inflation. In some cases, this new passage led to a dissection because during the second approach, the guidewire passed beneath the plaque.

To overcome this issue, the first solution was to extend the guidewire. Initially the length of these wires was 175 cm. To exchange the balloon catheter whilst the wire was still in place required a longer guidewire (aproximatively 300 cm). An extension was created and special devices to connect a standard coronary guidewire to an extension were proposed.

The connection between the two parts of the guidewire was not always very solid and in a number of cases, removal of the initial balloon was followed by the removal of the distal part of the small guidewire proximal to the lesion or by the disconnection between the two parts of the small wire. In these cases, all the benefit of an initially tedious procedure was lost with, in some cases, occlusive dissection of the vessel requesting emergency bypass surgery.

An alternative to the extension was the long guidewire technique described by M Kaltenbach.[9,10] Another important advance was the monorail system invented by Tassilio Bonzel in Freiburg.[11] This allowed rapid exchanges of the balloon catheter and, at least in Europe, the monorail technique rapidly replaced the co-axial method.

In the mid 1980s, these new technologic advances (steerable guidewire, monorail catheters) made angioplasty easier and easier. The number of procedures rapidly increased since the indications concerned more patients with double and even triple lesions. In this field Jeffrey Hartzler soon became a leader. Unfortunately, in 1985, Andreas Grüntzig died in an aircraft accident.

It also appeared that restenosis was becoming a crucial issue. Numerous clinical trials were launched to identify the 'magic bullet' or the 'magic device' able to prevent restenosis. Thus started the third revolution and the era of 'new devices'.

THE NEW DEVICES

Directional atherectomy (DCA) was one of the first 'new devices' to be proposed and the concept was introduced by John Simpson in 1985.[12] John Simpson's interest in DCA derived from a steadfast belief that the best treatment for coronary artery atherosclerosis was to remove the obstructing plaque.

The first atherectomy was performed in 1985 in a superficial femoral artery.[13] This initial experience led the FDA to approve the device for peripheral vessel disease in 1987. Three years later, DCA was approved by the FDA as the first nonballoon percutaneous coronary interventional device. Initially Simpson's atherotome was a very bulky device requiring very large guiding catheters (11 F). Later, the miniaturization of the device and thinner wall guiding catheter allowed the use of 9.5 and 10 F guiding catheters.

In spite of a number of complications – abrupt closure (3–5%), distal embolization, myocardial infarction (6–17%), perforations (~1%) – the device became very popular, in particular in North America. Several clinical trials (CAVEAT-I,[14] CCAT,[15] CAVEAT-II[16]) failed to show a clear advantage in terms of restenosis rate reduction when compared with balloon angioplasty. Optimal atherectomy trials (OARS,[17] BOAT,[18] START[19]) showed a small improvement but the rate of restenosis (16–29%) was judged to be higher than the rate after stent implantation. Initial enthusiasm markedly decreased; DCA was used for selected indications, proximal LAD lesions, and complex bifurcations and finally the device was more or less completely abandoned. There were some attempts to 'resuscitate' atherectomy with the Silver Hawk system, with encouraging results.

The transluminal extraction atherectomy catheter (TEC) was designed by Richard Stack.[20] The concept of this device was based upon cutting and aspiration of atheroma and debris. The TEC was a torque-controlled catheter that incorporated an aspiration device into a distal rotational cutter.

After experimental studies in normal animal segments and in atherosclerotic cadaver arteries, the TEC was used in peripheral vessels and later in native coronary arteries and saphenous vein grafts.[21] The device was approved by the FDA in 1989 for peripheral vascular disease and for revascularization of saphenous vein grafts in 1995.[22] The device was also used in acute myocardial infarction (MI) owing to the ability of fresh thrombus removal. Nevertheless, the device was in most cases reserved for the treatment of the complex, fragile, friable lesions of venous conduits. Several papers reported the results obtained with the TEC but this device has been completely abandoned.

High-speed rotational coronary atherectomy has a different and unique mechanism; it removes plaque by abrading the atherosclerotic material, producing millions of tiny particles that are dispersed into the distal coronary circulation. The concept was developed by David Auth, a biomedical engineer.[23-25]

David Auth mentioned that the Rotablator (as it is called) preferably ablated atherosclerotic plaque according to the theory of differential cutting. This is the ability of a device to selectively cut one material while maintaining the integrity of the adjacent tissues. Rotary ablation preferentially attacked hard and even calcified atherosclerotic plaque because of its selective differential cutting effect. The first rotational atherectomy in coronary arteries was performed in Lille by our group in 1988.[26]

Rotary atherectomy became very popular in the early 1990s. A number of trials were launched; the first proposed different strategies: Rotablator alone, burr-balloon strategy (STRATAS trial), and Rota-Stenting.[27] Other trials included the ERBAC trial,[28] the DART study, and the COBRA study. The Rotablator was also proposed to treat in-stent restenosis. The ARTIST[29] and ROSTER[30] trials showed uncertain results and it was thought at that time that rotary ablation could not compete with vascular brachytherapy which was then the 'gold standard' treatment for in-stent restenosis.

However, with the extensive use of stent implantation, the practice of rotary atherectomy has markedly declined. In 1999, the Rotablator was used in 3% of the procedures in France. In the USA, rotary ablation was performed in 7% of the procedures in 1997 but the rate is now less than 1%.

Rotational atherectomy, with its unique mechanism of action, appears to fulfill a role for some types of lesion but is now limited to the initial treatment of calcified lesions.

In the first years of coronary interventional cardiology, total chronic complete occlusion was a limiting factor of nonsurgical recanalization procedures. With conventional methods and traditional guidewires, recanalization had a very low success rate; Vallbracht and Kaltenbach[31] invented a new system which was specifically designed for chronic total occlusion. Basically, it was an electrically driven rotating catheter, consisting of four steel coil wires (0.2 mm each) with an inner lumen allowing an exchange of wires and the injection of contrast medium. The two pioneers started to work with this device in Frankfurt in 1984 in 16 post-mortem human femoral and popliteal arteries, of which eight were completely occluded. Seven of the eight occlusions were successfully reopened with low-speed rotation. Between December 1986 and October 1988, they treated 83 patients with chronic peripheral artery occlusions with this new technique.[32] Then, they started treating patients with total chronic coronary occlusion. In 1991, Kaltenbach and Vallbracht published their experience in 152 patients and the mean percentage of success was 55%. The angiographically determined long-term success was 72%. However, new wires and new techniques led to the abandonment of that method in the mid 1990s.

The interventional cardiology community was also excited by the introduction of laser angioplasty. Laser (Light Amplification by Stimulated Emission of Radiation) systems produce energy which has been used in several medical areas. They were introduced to interventional cardiology at the beginning of the 1980s. Choy and Stertzer performed the first laser angioplasty in animals.[33] They used an argon laser on the abdominal aorta of one rabbit and two femoral arteries of a dog. In March 1983, Jean Marco met Choy and Stertzer and they created a protocol of femoral artery debulking in animals.

The first recanalization of a chronic total femoral occlusion was performed by Choy at the Lennox Hill Hospital in May 1983. Four months later, the first animal experiments started in Toulouse (Purpan Hospital). From September 19 to 22 1983, Marco, Choy, and Stertzer performed laser recanalization of occluded coronary arteries in five patients during surgical interventions performed by Gerard Fournial. These preliminary results were presented during the first live course demonstration in Toulouse (September 22–23 1983) and later at the American College of Cardiology meeting in Dallas (March 25–29 1984).

After these preliminary experiences, laser radiation was applied extensively in interventional cardiology. The first generation used continuous-wave lasers with Nd-YAG lasers in Europe and argon in USA. However, it appeared that the thermal excess was creating important arterial damage, responsible for a high rate of restenosis, leading to discontinuation of the device.

The technique was revived when Grundfest proposed the delivery of excimer laser energy through optical fibers. Later, a second generation of pulsed-wave laser started, inducing a limited thermal injury to the surrounding tissue. Then excimer holmium or CO_2 devices were used.

A number of registries were opened. The Spectranetics excimer laser registry included 2432 patients. Another registry conducted by Litvack[34] enrolled 3000 patients, with 84% procedural success. However, several procedural complications were noted, with death, myocardial infarction and the need for emergency bypass surgery in 3.8% of cases. The restenosis rate was 58%.

Several randomized trials have compared laser angioplasty with other techniques of interventional cardiology (ERBAC trial,[28] AMRO study, LAVA study). All these trials showed a benefit of laser angioplasty over the comparative techniques. Laser techniques were applied for specific niche procedures: saphenous vein grafts, undilatable or uncrossable lesions, bifurcations, total occlusions, aorto-ostial lesions. Several technical modalities were proposed: smart laser, laser guidewire, etc.

The overall results were not convincing and laser angioplasty has been almost completely abandoned since the extensive use of coronary stenting. Several other devices have also been proposed, including laser balloon angioplasty, spark erosion, linear everting balloon, and therapeutic ultrasound, but they were abandoned after they failed to demonstrate a clear benefit.

CORONARY STENTING

The fourth revolution was coronary stenting. At the beginning of the 1980s, Dr Senning, a cardiac surgeon in Zurich, met a designer called Wallsten and explained that aortic dissection was a very serious acute disease; he described the concept of a mechanical scaffolding of the arterial wall using a latticed metallic tube. Wallsten decided to take over the problem of endocoronary prostheses. He created the

Wallstent but he had some difficulties in finding a solution for the percutaneous approach. This was eventually achieved by Christian Imbert, an engineer. The self-expandable stent which could be implanted via a percutaneous femoral approach was thus created.

The first stent implantation was performed on March 28 1986 in Toulouse by Jacques Puel. In the following weeks, seven other patients received a self-expandable Wallstent without any complications.

Initial results were promising and in particular, the risk of emergency bypass surgery was significantly decreased. As a consequence many centers started to perform coronary angioplasty without surgical back-up. However, for a while, stenting was performed only as a bail-out procedure. In fact, it appeared very quickly that with a single antithrombotic treatment based upon full doses of heparin, the risk of thrombosis was very high.

Later, Sigwart performed stent implantation under full anticoagulation with heparin followed by oral anticoagulation with warfarin. This medical treatment decreased the risk of stent thrombosis but it remained very high (between 5% and 10%).

These two clinical experiences,[35,36] conducted initially in Toulouse and later in Lausanne, proved the feasibility of the method and demonstrated the high potentially thrombogenic risk of this foreign body. Actually, at the beginning of the 1990s, coronary stenting was almost dying out owing to the risk of acute/subacute thrombosis. Ten years after the first stent implantation it was necessary to find the solution and to eliminate this risk with the use of dual antiplatelet treatment (aspirin + ticlopidine) and to prove the superiority of coronary stenting in comparison with other techniques for prevention of restenosis.

A number of new trials were launched. The BENESTENT I and II trials designed and conducted by Serruys[37,38] established that the rate of restenosis was decreased to 20% and the role of negative remodelling as the major factor of restenosis was demonstrated by intravenous ultrasound (G Mintz). Simultaneously, engineers and technicians were actively working on the concept of a stent as a platform to deliver drugs. A new approach was considered with two parts: the scaffolding device to avoid the negative remodelling of the artery and a polymer covering the struts but able to release a drug for prevention of neointimal hyperplasia.

The great breakthrough occurred in September during the ESC Congress of Vienna when Dr Marie Claude Morice[39] presented the results of the RAVEL study comparing a stent coated with sirolimus with a conventional bare metallic stent; no restenosis occurred in the sirolimus stent group. This was completely unbelievable and the interventional cardiology community was very excited, although some cardiologists remained sceptical and claimed that it was necessary to wait since there was a risk of delayed restenosis. However, as time goes by, this risk is decreasing and it is very unlikely that it might still occur.

Nowadays, millions of procedures have been performed with drug-eluting stents. Every day, new platforms and new compounds are proposed. Bioresorbable stents are studied. Stents releasing different compounds (anti-restenosis, anticoagulant) are involved in clinical trials.

CONCLUSION

Figure 1.2, which is a kind of fresco of interventional coronary cardiology, summarizes this period of very intense and exciting innovation.

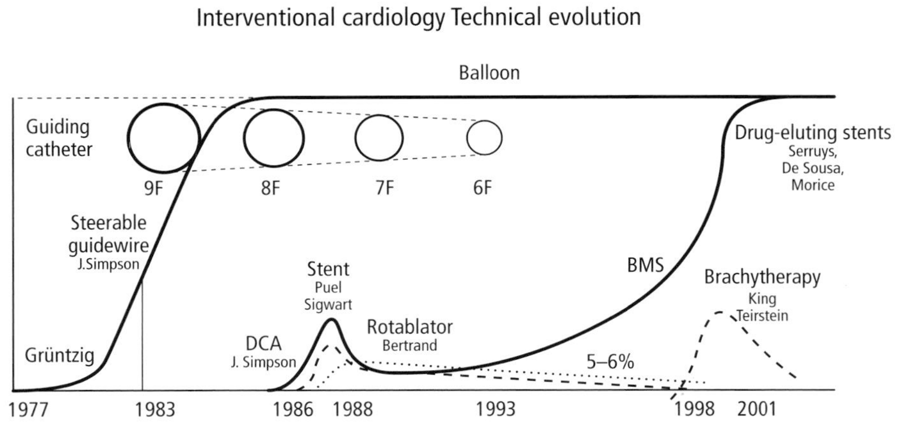

Interventional cardiology Technical evolution

Figure 1.2   A 'fresco' of 25 years of interventional cardiology.

The first five years of angioplasty were needed to convince the cardiology community that coronary angioplasty was a safe, noninvasive technique. The following years demonstrated that patients with single- and double-vessel disease have to be treated with percutaneous coronary interventions and not with surgery. The fight against restenosis was long and more than 100 randomized clinical trials failed to identify a pharmacologic agent preventing restenosis.

Since 2001, the rate of restenosis has been low (between 5% and 7%) and the ongoing randomized clinical trials conducted in diabetics and nondiabetics (FREEDOM and SYNTAX) and comparing modern surgery with modern angioplasty (with drug-eluting stents) will probably demonstrate that there is no longer a difference in the risk of subsequent intervention. This is an important complementary issue since it was demonstrated by the ARTS-I study that there was already no difference in terms of death and myocardial infarction between PCI and CABG.[40,41] The 'anti-balloonists' claimed that angioplasty is unable to improve survival in the long term but it has now been proved that angioplasty does improve survival. The study performed by the group of Zwolle[42] showed that in comparison to medical treatment of myocardial infarction, angioplasty was able to decrease the mortality rate in the long term. In the more recent RITA III trial,[43] the mortality rate at five-year follow-up is significantly lower after an invasive strategy than after a conservative medical strategy.

In 1997, the pioneers (Figure 1.3) met in Zurich on the 20th anniversary of the birth of percutaneous transluminal coronary angioplasty and observed that the first patient of Andreas Grüntzig was still in very good condition.

Nowadays, million of procedures are performed around the world and interventional cardiology has significantly expanded to include valvular disease, congenital heart disease, arrhythmias, etc.

Methodical research, innovative technology, and committed clinicians have combined to create a subspeciality which has had a major impact on public health care.

There is no doubt that with the development of interventional cardiology within the last 25 years, cardiology has made more progress than in all preceding centuries.

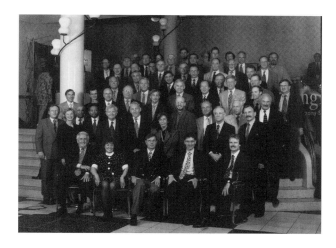

Figure 1.3 Pioneers of interventional cardiology.

REFERENCES

1. Forssmann W. Die Sondierung des Rechten Herzens. Klin Wochenschr. 1929;8:2085.
2. Cournand A. Some aspects of the pulmonary circulation in normal man and in chronic cardiopulmonary diseases. Circulation 1950;2:641–57.
3. Sones F, Shirey E, Proudfit W, Wescott R. Cine coronary arteriography. Circulation 1959;20:773–4.
4. Effler DB, Groves LK, Suarez EL, Favaloro RG. Direct coronary artery surgery with endarterotomy and patch-graft reconstruction. Clinical application and technical considerations. J Thorac Cardiovasc Surg 1967;53:93–101.
5. Gruntzig A, Schneider HJ. [The percutaneous dilatation of chronic coronary stenoses – experiments and morphology]. Schweiz Med Wochenschr 1977;107:1588.
6. Gruntzig A, Kumpe DA. Technique of percutaneous transluminal angioplasty with the Gruntzig balloon catheter. AJR Am J Roentgenol 1979;132:547–52.
7. Gruntzig AR, Senning A, Siegenthaler WE. Nonoperative dilatation of coronary-artery stenosis: percutaneous transluminal coronary angioplasty. N Engl J Med 1979;301:61–8.
8. Simpson JB, Baim DS, Robert EW, Harrison DC. A new catheter system for coronary angioplasty. Am J Cardiol 1982;49:1216–22.
9. Kaltenbach M. The long wire technique – a new technique for steerable balloon catheter dilatation of coronary artery stenoses. Eur Heart J 1984;5:1004–9.
10. Kaltenbach M. [New technic for guidable balloon dilatation of coronary vessel stenoses]. Z Kardiol 1984;73:669–73.
11. Bonzel T, Wollschlager H, Just H. [A new catheter system for the mechanical dilatation of coronary stenoses with exchangeable intracoronary catheters, fast flow of the contrast agent and improved control]. Biomed Tech (Berl) 1986;31:195–200.
12. Simpson J, Johnson D, Thapliyal HV et al. Transluminal atherectomy: a new approach to the treatment of atherosclerotic vascular disease. Circulation 1985;72 (suppl III):111.
13. Simpson JB, Selmon MR, Robertson GC et al. Transluminal atherectomy for occlusive peripheral vascular disease. Am J Cardiol 1988;61:96G–101G.
14. Topol EJ, Leya F, Pinkerton CA et al. A comparison of directional atherectomy with coronary angioplasty in patients with coronary artery disease. The CAVEAT Study Group. N Engl J Med 1993;329:221–7.

15. Adelman AG, Cohen EA, Kimball BP et al. A comparison of directional atherectomy with balloon angioplasty for lesions of the left anterior descending coronary artery. N Engl J Med 1993;329:228–33.
16. Holmes DR Jr, Topol EJ, Califf RM et al. A multicenter, randomized trial of coronary angioplasty versus directional atherectomy for patients with saphenous vein bypass graft lesions. CAVEAT-II Investigators. Circulation 1995;91:1966–74.
17. Simonton CA, Leon MB, Baim DS et al. 'Optimal' directional coronary atherectomy: final results of the Optimal Atherectomy Restenosis Study (OARS). Circulation 1998;97:332–9.
18. Baim DS, Cutlip DE, Sharma SK et al. Final results of the Balloon vs Optimal Atherectomy Trial (BOAT). Circulation 1998;97:322–31.
19. Tsuchikane E, Sumitsuji S, Awata N et al. Final results of the STent versus directional coronary Atherectomy Randomized Trial (START). J Am Coll Cardiol 1999;34:1050–7.
20. Sketch MH Jr, Phillips HR, Lee MM, Stack RS. Coronary transluminal extraction-endarterectomy. J Invasive Cardiol 1991;3:13–18.
21. Popma JJ, Leon MB, Mintz GS et al. Results of coronary angioplasty using the transluminal extraction catheter. Am J Cardiol 1992;70:1526–32.
22. Dooris M, Hoffmann M, Glazier S et al. Comparative results of transluminal extraction coronary atherectomy in saphenous vein graft lesions with and without thrombus. J Am Coll Cardiol 1995;25:1700–5.
23. Hansen DD, Auth DC, Hall M, Ritchie JL. Rotational endarterectomy in normal canine coronary arteries: preliminary report. J Am Coll Cardiol 1988;11:1073–7.
24. Hansen DD, Auth DC, Vracko R, Ritchie JL. Rotational atherectomy in atherosclerotic rabbit iliac arteries. Am Heart J 1988;115:160–5.
25. Ahn SS, Auth D, Marcus DR, Moore WS. Removal of focal atheromatous lesions by angioscopically guided high-speed rotary atherectomy. Preliminary experimental observations. J Vasc Surg 1988;7:292–300.
26. Fourrier JL, Bertrand ME, Auth DC, Lablanche JM, Gommeaux A, Brunetaud JM. Percutaneous coronary rotational angioplasty in humans: preliminary report. J Am Coll Cardiol 1989;14:1278–82.
27. Whitlow PL, Bass TA, Kipperman RM et al. Results of the study to determine rotablator and transluminal angioplasty strategy (STRATAS). Am J Cardiol 2001;87:699–705.
28. Reifart N, Vandormael M, Krajcar M et al. Randomized comparison of angioplasty of complex coronary lesions at a single center. Excimer Laser, Rotational Atherectomy, and Balloon Angioplasty Comparison (ERBAC) Study. Circulation 1997;96:91–8.
29. vom Dahl J, Radke PW, Haager PK et al. Clinical and angiographic predictors of recurrent restenosis after percutaneous transluminal rotational atherectomy for treatment of diffuse in-stent restenosis. Am J Cardiol 1999;83:862–7.
30. Sharma SK, Kini A, Mehran R, Lansky A, Kobayashi Y, Marmur JD. Randomized trial of Rotational Atherectomy Versus Balloon Angioplasty for Diffuse In-stent Restenosis (ROSTER). Am Heart J 2004;147:16–22.
31. Vallbracht C, Kress J, Schweitzer M et al. [Rotation angioplasty – a new procedure for reopening and dilating blood vessels. Experimental findings]. Z Kardiol 1987;76:608–11.
32. Vallbracht C, Liermann DD, Prignitz I et al. Low-speed rotational angioplasty in chronic peripheral artery occlusions: experience in 83 patients. Work in progress. Radiology 1989;172:327–30.
33. Choy DS, Stertzer SH, Rotterdam HZ, Bruno MS. Laser coronary angioplasty: experience with 9 cadaver hearts. Am J Cardiol 1982;50:1209–11.
34. Litvack F, Eigler N, Margolis J et al. Percutaneous excimer laser coronary angioplasty: results in the first consecutive 3,000 patients. The ELCA Investigators. J Am Coll Cardiol 1994;23:323–9.
35. Rousseau H, Puel J, Joffre F et al. Self-expanding endovascular prosthesis: an experimental study. Radiology 1987;164:709–14.
36. Sigwart U, Puel J, Mirkovitch V, Joffre F, Kappenberger L. Intravascular stents to prevent occlusion and restenosis after transluminal angioplasty. N Engl J Med 1987;316:701–6.

37. Serruys PW, van Hout B, Bonnier H et al. Randomised comparison of implantation of heparin-coated stents with balloon angioplasty in selected patients with coronary artery disease (Benestent II). Lancet 1998;352:673–81.
38. Serruys PW, de Jaegere P, Kiemeneij F et al. A comparison of balloon-expandable-stent implantation with balloon angioplasty in patients with coronary artery disease. Benestent Study Group. N Engl J Med 1994;331:489–95.
39. Morice MC, Serruys PW, Sousa JE et al. A randomized comparison of a sirolimus-eluting stent with a standard stent for coronary revascularization. N Engl J Med 2002;346:1773–80.
40. Serruys PW, Unger F, van Hout BA et al. The ARTS study (Arterial Revascularization Therapies Study). Semin Interv Cardiol 1999;4:209–19.
41. Serruys PW, Ong AT, van Herwerden LA et al. Five-year outcomes after coronary stenting versus bypass surgery for the treatment of multivessel disease: the final analysis of the Arterial Revascularization Therapies Study (ARTS) randomized trial. J Am Coll Cardiol 2005;46:575–81.
42. Zijlstra F, Hoorntje JC, de Boer MJ et al. Long-term benefit of primary angioplasty as compared with thrombolytic therapy for acute myocardial infarction. N Engl J Med 1999;341:1413–19.
43. Fox KA, Poole-Wilson P, Clayton TC et al. Five-year outcome of an interventional strategy in non-ST-elevation acute coronary syndrome: the British Heart Foundation RITA 3 randomised trial. Lancet 2005;366:914–20.

Section B
Patient preparation and selection

2

Optimal patient preparation and selection to avoid complications

Richard J Gumina and David R Holmes Jr

Clinical determinants of complications • **Angiographic/procedural determinants of complications** • **Global risk assessment** • **Post-procedure management** • **Conclusion**

If not for thoughtful patient preparation and selection, the first balloon angioplasty conducted by Andreas Grüntzig in 1977 could have easily met with a catastrophic outcome.[1] Indeed, report of the initial 50 coronary interventions made clear the possible complications and suggested clinical and anatomic parameters suitable for percutaneous cardiovascular intervention (PCI).[2] Now, with greater than 1 million percutaneous coronary interventions conducted yearly worldwide, the need for careful risk assessment and management to avoid complications remains imperative.

Patients in whom PCI is conducted should have a clear indication for the procedure as outlined in the American College of Cardiology/American Heart Association Guidelines for Percutaneous Coronary Intervention[3] or the Guidelines for Percutaneous Coronary Interventions issued by the Task Force for Percutaneous Coronary Interventions of the European Society of Cardiology.[4] Patients considered as candidates for PCI range in clinical presentation from asymptomatic and stable to severely symptomatic and unstable, therefore when considering a patient for PCI, the risk and benefits of the procedure must be weighed against the risks and benefits of surgical revascularization or medical therapy. Key areas for consideration prior to PCI include: assessment of the key clinical and angiographic/procedural variables, consideration of alternative therapies such as coronary artery bypass graft (CABG) surgery or medical therapy, availability of surgical standby and hemodynamic support.[3] Evaluation of a patient's suitability to undergo PCI can be viewed as an assessment of clinical and angiographic/procedural characteristics associated with adverse outcomes or complications. Appropriate selection and preparation of the patient dictates that the interventional cardiologist has an understanding of the clinical and angiographic/procedural factors associated with increased complications and adverse clinical outcomes following PCI.

CLINICAL DETERMINANTS OF COMPLICATIONS

Careful review of the patient's history and clinical data is required prior to any PCI. Patients at higher risk for complications can be identified by both clinical and angiographic variables reviewed here. Recognition of these variables allows for either pretreatment or implementation of measures to reduce the overall risk of complications or mortality.

Contrast reactions

In the general population, the incidence of contrast allergy is relatively low (0.01–0.5%). Patients should be adequately screened for prior exposure to x-ray contrast and any history of allergic reaction verified prior to undergoing PCI. Allergic reactions are classified as minor (hives/rash), moderate (urticaria, bronchospasm) or severe (anaphylactoid reaction with hemodynamic collapse). While anaphylactoid reactions are rare, in patients with a history of contrast reaction the risk for repeat anaphylactoid reaction is increased.[5]

For those patients who have suffered only minor urticarial reaction, pretreatment with diphenhydramine prior to procedure is sufficient. Patients with documented anaphylactoid reactions should receive more aggressive therapy, with oral steroids 24 hours prior to procedure (intravenous if administered at time of procedure) in addition to diphenhydramine.[6] Nursing and anesthesia staff should be alerted to the history of prior reactions and be diligent throughout the case to recognize any signs of a progressing reaction.

Diabetes

Diabetic patients have higher mortality after both percutaneous and surgical coronary revascularization than patients without diabetes.[7-13] Despite advances in interventional techniques, diabetes remains a significant independent predictor of adverse events after PCI.[14] Patients with diabetes consistently have been shown to have the highest risk for adverse procedural and clinical outcomes following either PCI or CABG surgery.[15]

In diabetic patients with multivessel disease, the BARI trial found an increased periprocedural risk of ischemic complications and increased five-year mortality in patients treated with percutaneous transluminal coronary angioplasty (PTCA) when compared to patients without diabetes or to patients with diabetes undergoing CABG surgery using internal thoracic arterial grafts.[16,17] However, it is important to note that the BARI trial did not employ stents, glycoprotein IIb/IIIa receptor antagonists or dual oral antiplatelet therapy with aspirin and clopidogrel. Indeed, the use of a glycoprotein IIb/IIIa receptor antagonist (abciximab) decreases the mortality of diabetic patients.[18,19] Despite a high angiographic success with multivessel stenting, diabetic patients have increased revascularization rates and lower one-year survival than nondiabetic patients;[20] thus, current guidelines suggest CABG surgery in diabetic patients with left main disease or three-vessel disease.[3] Evolving data on the use of drug-eluting stents in patients with multivessel disease and/or diabetes mellitus may change this situation. A recent analysis of randomized control trials suggests that earlier mortality advantages and decreased rates of revascularization observed in patients undergoing CABG surgery may not be applicable in the era of drug-eluting stents.[15]

Periprocedural management of diabetic patients should include adjusting the insulin dose to half of the normal dose administered the morning of procedure to avoid hypoglycemic episodes in the fasting patient. While no studies have shown that strict glycemic control affects immediate procedural outcomes, there is a reduction in long-term restenosis in patients who maintain tight glycemic control.[21] Use of metformin, a common therapy for diabetes, does not itself cause renal dysfunction but may lead to fatal lactic acidosis. Therefore it should be discontinued at the time of or prior to angiographic procedure and withheld for at least 48 hours after procedure, and only restarted after a recheck of serum creatinine is found to be at baseline.[22] Diabetics with impaired renal function are at increased risk for contrast nephropathy.[23,24]

Left ventricular dysfunction and shock

Left ventricular dysfunction is one of the most important predictors of immediate and long-term clinical outcomes in patients with coronary artery disease. Analysis of the NHLBI Dynamic Registry from 1997 to 1998 reveals that the rates of in-hospital death and post-PCI myocardial infarction were significantly associated with left ventricular ejection fraction (Table 2.1).[25] Numerous studies also have demonstrated that patients presenting with an acute myocardial infarction complicated by cardiogenic shock represent a subgroup at high risk for mortality, who benefit from PCI.[26–29]

The factors associated with increased risk for significant cardiovascular collapse during PTCA include:

- percentage of myocardium at risk (e.g. >50% viable myocardium at risk and LV ejection fraction of <25%)
- pre-angioplasty percent diameter stenosis
- multivessel CAD
- diffuse disease in the dilated segment.[6,30,31]

Patients with higher preprocedural myocardial jeopardy scores also have a greater likelihood of cardiovascular collapse when abrupt vessel closure occurs during PTCA.[32,33]

In those patients with LV dysfunction or shock, use of a pulmonary artery catheter for pressure monitoring and use of inotropic support is often warranted. In patients with hemodynamic compromise, ischemia or cardiogenic shock, use of an intra-aortic balloon prior to coronary intervention has been associated with improved outcomes.[34,35] Earlier studies of high-risk PTCA using percutaneous cardiopulmonary support demonstrated good procedural success but a high incidence of vascular complications.[36,37] Alternatively, with the advent of newer techniques such as percutaneous left ventricular assist devices (PLVADs), effective hemodynamic support can be achieved during higher risk procedures.[38,39] Comparison of intra-aortic

Table 2.1 Incidence of in-hospital complications following PCI (left ventricular ejection fraction)

Outcome	EF ≤40% (n=166) (%)	EF 41–49% (n=126) (%)	EF ≥50% (n=866) (%)	*P*-value
Death	3	1.6	0.1	≤0.001
Death/MI	6	5.6	2.9	0.024
CABG	1.2	0.8	1.2	0.956

Modified from Keelan et al, reference 133.

balloon pump (IABP) to LVAD suggested that hemodynamic and metabolic parameters can be managed more effectively with the use of a ventricular assist device than by standard treatment with IABP, albeit with more complications.[40]

Acuity of presentation

The acuity of presentation necessitating PCI clearly influences short-term outcomes.[41] Post-PCI myocardial infarction, CABG and death are increased in patients undergoing PCI for acute myocardial infarction when compared to stable or unstable angina (Table 2.2). Those patients presenting with cardiogenic shock complicating an acute myocardial infarction have a higher morbidity and mortality.[27–29]

Renal insufficiency

Renal insufficiency increases the risk of short-term and long-term morbidity and mortality following PCI.[24,42–45] Patients with impaired renal function also are at increased risk for contrast-induced nephropathy (CIN).[23,24]

The incidence of CIN, defined as an increase in the postprocedural serum creatinine of >0.5 mg/dL, ranges from ~2% to 40% in low- to high-risk patients.[24] Several risk scores have been developed to predict the relative risk of developing CIN.[45,46] Common to these analyses are congestive heart failure, age, intra-aortic balloon pump use, renal function (creatinine >1.5 g/dL or creatinine clearance <60 mL/min), diabetes, and contrast volume. Development of CIN not only results in increased morbidity but there is also an increased in-hospital mortality in those patients requiring dialysis.[47] Patients with pre-existing renal dysfunction, especially diabetic patients, are at higher risk for CIN.[24]

Therapies that have been evaluated to prevent CIN include adequate hydration preprocedure, low ionic contrast, hydration with sodium bicarbonate,[48] and n-acetylcysteine.[49–53] However, these have met with limited success. Diuretic therapy, fenoldapam, and dopamine are not routinely employed. The use of iso-osmolar contrast appears to cause less renal dysfunction than high osmolar contrast in high-risk patients.[47] Nephrotoxic drugs such as certain antibiotics, nonsteroidal anti-inflammatory agents, and ciclosporin should be held for 24–48 hours prior to performing PCI and for 48 hours afterwards when possible. Intravenous hydration with 0.9% or 0.45% saline for 12–18 hours before contrast administration is recommended in those patients with renal insufficiency. A formula has been developed and externally validated for calculating the maximum radiographic contrast dose (MRCD = 5 mL × body weight (kg)/serum creatinine (mg/dL)).[54]

Table 2.2   In-hospital complications following PCI (acuity of presentation)

Outcome	Stable angina (n=32,516) (%)	Unstable angina (n=53,386) (%)	Acute MI (n=53,386) (%)	*P*-value
Post-PCI MI	0.4	0.5	0.6	0.0055
CABG	1.4	1.7	4.5	<0.0001
Death	1.1	1.0	5.2	<0.0001

Modified from Anderson et al, reference 41.

Patients in whom the MRCD is exceeded have a higher incidence of CIN. Additionally, imaging with biplane, eliminating unnecessary left ventriculograms, and the use of intravascular ultrasound (IVUS) can also reduce the amount of contrast used.

Peripheral vascular disease

Several studies demonstrate that patients with documented peripheral vascular disease are at higher risk for periprocedural complications and mortality.[55,56] The presence of peripheral vascular disease may also influence the choice of vascular access sites and incidence of vascular complications.[55,57]

Choice of vascular access and site care during and post procedure are critical. Options for vascular access include femoral artery, radial artery, brachial artery, and translumbar approach. The factors associated with vascular complications include use of warfarin, thrombolytic or platelet inhibitor therapy, co-existing peripheral vascular disease, female gender, obesity, postprocedural prolonged heparin use, delayed sheath removal, and older age.[58–60] Discontinuation of heparin immediately post procedure does not compromise procedural outcomes and allows for earlier sheath removal, decreased bleeding, and reduced vascular complications. Several reports have demonstrated that in uncomplicated cases, administration of protamine to reverse the unfractionated heparin-mediated anticoagulation does not pose an increased risk of target vessel closure and may decrease the incidence of hemorrhagic complications, especially in patients in whom a GP IIb/IIIa receptor antagonist is administered.[61–63]

Hematoma incidence ranges from 1% to 3%, with an increased incidence associated with increased sheath sizes, anticoagulation use, antiplatelet therapy use, and obesity.[64] Major hemorrhagic complications, defined as blood loss causing a decrease in hemoglobin >3.0 g/dL or need for a blood transfusion, are usually obvious. However, occult hematomas or retroperitoneal bleeding should always be suspected in patients with hypotension or flank/lower quadrant pain post PCI. Computed tomography confirms the diagnosis. Prompt transfusion is often necessary, with surgery consultation required in some cases.

Pseudoaneurysms and arteriovenous (AV) fistulas are associated with cannulation of the femoral artery below the bifurcation. Pseudoaneurysms often present as a mass over the puncture site (painless or painful). Those less than 2 cm often close spontaneously, while those >2 cm often require ultrasound-guided compression, injection of thrombin or surgical repair. A continuous murmur over the puncture site is characteristic of an AV fistula. Vascular insufficiency and high-output failure can develop. Prolonged compression, surgery or coiling may be necessary to close an AV fistula if symptoms develop.

Acute arterial thrombosis is a rare complication. The incidence is increased in females with small arteries, with the use of an intra-aortic balloon pump or in patients where the superficial saphenous artery is cannulated.

Percutaneous closure devices have become popular because they reduce bed rest and minimize medical personnel monitoring.[65] The overall incidence of vascular complication is comparable to or better than that of manual compression. However, the incidence of specific complications differs with device[66] and higher rates of infection and vessel occlusion have been reported.[67–70] Therefore, care should be exercised regarding the choice of patient in whom these devices are deployed.

ANGIOGRAPHIC/PROCEDURAL DETERMINANTS OF COMPLICATIONS

Acute procedural complications include compromise of the target vessel or branch vessel lumen or vessel integrity or unsuccessful procedure. A number of angiographic criteria are predictive of procedural success and clinical success.

Lesion characteristics

Numerous studies have identified angiographic features that influence angiographic and procedural outcomes. These data have led to a progression of lesion classification schemes with predictive value for angiographic and procedural success. The original ACC/AHA lesion classification scheme was proposed in 1986 as a mechanism by which the interventional cardiologist could predict procedural results.[71] It was subsequently modified in 1990 (Table 2.3).[72] The classification schemes require analysis of 11 angiographically determined variables of each lesion to predict the likelihood of procedural success. While these issues are beyond the scope of the

---

Table 2.3   ACC/AHA lesion classification system

Type A
  Discrete (<10 mm)
  Concentric
  Readily accessible
  Nonangulated segment <45°
  Smooth contour
  Little or no calcification
  Less than totally occlusive
  Not ostial in location
  No major branch involvement
  Absence of thrombus

Type B1
  Tubular (10–20 mm)
  Eccentric
  Moderate tortuosity of proximal segment
  Moderately angulated 45–90°
  Irregular contour
  Moderate to heavy calcification
  Ostial in location
  Bifurcation lesion requiring double guidewires
  Some thrombus present
  Total occlusion <3 months old

Type B2
  Two or more 'B1' characteristics

Type C
  Diffuse (>2 cm)
  Excessive tortuosity of proximal segment
  Extremely angulated segments >90°
  Inability to protect major side branches
  Degenerated vein grafts with friable lesions
  Total occlusion >3 months

Modified from Ellis et al, reference 134.

current discussion, lesion characteristics clearly influence the choice of guide selection, wire selection and the use of additional devices such as rotational atherectomy, thrombectomy devices, and cutting balloons, and also influence the decision to predilate rather than directly stent a lesion.

Current techniques which capitalize on the ability of stents to manage initial and subsequent complications of PCI have altered outcomes and the significance of prior classification schemes.[73] The Society for Cardiac Angiography and Interventions (SCAI) proposed a classification system collapsing the ACC/AHA lesions A, B1, and B2 into a non-C category and then stratifying the lesion by patency (Table 2.4). Analysis of the ACC–National Cardiovascular Data Registry revealed that the simpler SCAI lesion classification provided better discrimination for success and complications than the ACC/AHA lesion classification system, original or modified.[74]

Acute vessel closure

In the majority of patients undergoing elective PCI, death as a result of PCI is related to the occurrence of acute vessel closure precipitating LV failure and hemodynamic instability.[30,33] The risk of acute vessel closure is increased with lesion complexity. Procedure-related variables of persistent dissection, total stent length, number of stents placed, and final lumen diameter have been shown to be associated with the probability of stent thrombosis.[75,76] As discussed earlier, those patients at higher risk of developing hemodynamic compromise with acute occlusion of target vessel have a

---

Table 2.4   SCAI lesion classification system

Type I
   Does not meet the criteria for AHA/ACC Type C lesion
   Patent vessel

Type II
   Meets any of the following criteria for AHA/ACC Type C lesion:
      Diffuse (>2 cm)
      Excessive tortuosity of proximal segment
      Extremely angulated segments >90°
      Inability to protect major side branches
      Degenerated vein grafts with friable lesions
   Patent vessel

Type III
   Does not meet the criteria for AHA/ACC Type C lesion
   Occluded vessel

Type IV
   Meets any of the following criteria for AHA/ACC Type C lesion:
      Diffuse (>2 cm)
      Excessive tortuosity of proximal segment
      Extremely angulated segments >90°
      Inability to protect major side branches
      Degenerated vein grafts with friable lesions
      Total occlusion >3 months
   Occluded vessel

Modified from Krone et al, reference 133.

low LV ejection fraction, a target vessel that supplies greater than 50% of the viable myocardium or a high jeopardy score.

Prior to the stent era, the incidence of acute vessel closure was higher with increased adverse outcomes.[77-79] Unrestricted access to stent use has reduced acute closure and the need for emergent CABG surgery.[80-83]

Adjunctive pharmacotherapy

Use of adjunctive pharmacotherapy is associated with a reduced incidence of acute vessel closure and with improved procedural and clinical outcomes following PCI.

Based upon studies conducted in the pre-stent era, it is recommended that all patients receive aspirin therapy (80–325 mg) at least two hours prior to undergoing PCI.[3]

Clopidogrel, a thienopyridine, provides additional antiplatelet efficacy to that of aspirin. Clopidogrel pretreatment reduced PCI-related ischemic complications with greatest efficacy if administered more than six hours prior to PCI.[84,85] However, because of the increased risk of bleeding in patients who go on to CABG surgery, physicians are reluctant to pretreat with clopidogrel until the coronary anatomy is defined angiographically. In patients in whom CABG surgery could be performed within 5–7 days, pretreatment with clopidogrel is not currently recommended until the coronary anatomy has been defined and the decision for PCI has been made.[3]

Platelet glycoprotein IIb/IIIa receptor antagonists prevent the cross-linking of platelets by fibrinogen. GP IIb/IIIa receptor antagonists administered before or at the time of PCI decrease ischemic-related complications in patients undergoing elective PCI and in those patients presenting with an acute coronary syndrome.[86,87] As stated earlier, the use of a glycoprotein IIb/IIIa receptor antagonist decreases the complications in diabetic patients.[18,19] Thrombocytopenia occurs in 0.1–3% of patients; therefore platelet counts should be monitored. In the event of acute bleeding, platelet transfusion will counteract the effects of abciximab but not eptifibatide or tirofiban; however, the latter two agents clear within four hours and require renal dose adjustment.

Indirect thrombin inhibitors such as unfractionated heparin (UFH) and low molecular weight heparin (LMWH) are used for antithrombotic efficacy during PCI. The addition of heparin to aspirin therapy reduces the incidence of myocardial infarction and death in patients with unstable angina.[88] Weight-adjusted bolus of heparin (70–100 iu per kg) can be used to avoid excessive anticoagulation. In patients not treated with a glycoprotein IIb/IIIa receptor antagonist, UFH should be adjusted to obtain an activated clotting time (ACT) of 250–300 seconds with the HemoTec device (300–350 seconds with the Hemochron device). In those patients receiving a GP IIb/IIIa receptor antagonist, the UFH bolus should be reduced to 50–70 iu per kg with a goal ACT of 200–300 seconds using either the HemoTec or Hemochron device. It should be recognized that co-administration of a GP IIb/IIIa receptor antagonist will increase the ACT slightly. The ACT has been correlated inversely with acute vessel closure.[59] Discontinuation of heparin immediately post-procedure does not appear to compromise outcomes and allows for earlier sheath removal and decreased bleeding and vascular complications. LMWH offers a simple dosing regimen without the need for monitoring. In patients who present with unstable angina, LMWH offers equal or slightly superior efficacy compared to unfractionated heparin but with increased bleeding. However, it should be noted that the effects of LMWH cannot be completely reversed with protamine.

Direct thrombin inhibitors such as bivalirudin and argatroban inhibit fibrin-bound thrombin and platelet-mediated thrombosis. Comparison of unfractionated heparin infusion to bivalirudin administration, both with concomitant GP IIb/IIIa receptor antagonist use, revealed comparable short-term outcomes; however, the use of bivalirudin was associated with decreased major bleeding events.[89] Argatroban can be used as an alternative anticoagulant in patients with heparin-induced thrombocytopenia.[90]

Special considerations

Multivessel disease

In patients with multivessel coronary artery disease and many high-risk clinical and anatomic variables, multivessel coronary stent placement was associated with an excellent procedural success rate and a low rate of death or MI during follow-up.[91] However, CABG surgery was associated with better survival than multivessel PCI, after adjustment for risk profile.[92] However, at 10–12 years of follow-up, the early differences in cost and quality of life between CABG and PCI were no longer significant in patients with multivessel disease.[93] Three-year survival rates without stroke and myocardial infarction are identical in both groups, and the cost/benefit ratio of PCI is driven primarily by an increased need for revascularization in the PCI group.[94] The decision to perform either culprit vessel or complete revascularization can be made on an individual basis.[95]

Percutaneous cardiovascular intervention after coronary artery bypass surgery

When approaching PCI of a saphenous vein graft (SVG), the interventional cardiologist must consider the age and extent of disease within the graft and the potential for distal embolization.[96] GP IIb/IIIa receptor antagonists have not been shown to improve results of angioplasty or stenting in vein grafts.[97] However, the use of distal protection devices has been shown to decrease the incidence of periprocedural MI and complications.[98,99] A number of patients with SVG disease have anatomy that precludes the use of currently available distal protection devices.[100] If treatment of a SVG lesion is deemed too high risk for complications, treatment of the native vessels could be considered.

Unprotected left main disease

Left main (LM) coronary artery stenosis still represents an anatomic subset in which CABG surgery is recommended.[3] Stenting an unprotected LM should be considered in the absence of other revascularization options when bypass surgery has a very high perioperative risk.[101] The use of drug-eluting stents and newer percutaneous left ventricular assist devices in unprotected LM disease may alter how interventional cardiologists approach these patients in the future.[102–106]

Chronic total occlusions

Chronic total occlusion (CTO) represents the anatomic subset associated with the lowest technical success rates with PCI.[107,108] While stent implantation allows for

Table 2.5　Comparison of the variables included in currently available risk score for predicting post-PCI complications

	ACC-NCDR	NY State	NNE	Michigan	Beaumont	Cleveland Clinic	Mayo Clinic	Brigham and Women's
Risk studied	Mortality	Mortality	Mortality	Mortality	Mortality	Mortality, QWMI, emergent CABG	Mortality, QWMI, emergent CABG, stroke	Mortality, QWMI, CABG
Study period	01/1998–09/2000	01/1991–12/1994	01/1994–12/1996	07/1997–09/1999	01/1996–12/1998	01/1996–12/1998	01/1996–12/1999	01/1997–02/1999
Sample size	50,123	62,670	15,331	10,729	9954	19,985	5463	1877
Simplified scoring tool	No	No	No	Yes	Yes	No	Yes	Yes
Variables:	Odds ratios from logistic regression models							
Age								
By decade	–	1.83	–	–	–	24.9	1.37	–
Logarithm	–	–	–	–	–	–	–	1.35
≥75 y	–	–	–	–	–	–	–	–
>65 y	–	–	–	–	1.65	–	–	–
50–59 y	2.61	–	0.93	1.00	–	–	–	–
60–69 y	3.75	–	1.63	1.00	–	–	–	–
70–79 y	6.44	–	3.32	2.24	–	–	–	–
≥80 y	11.3	–	3.72	2.65	–	–	–	–
LV function (EF)								
0.50–0.59	1.00	1.00	2.53	1.00	–	–	–	–
0.40–0.49	0.87	1.00	3.32	1.66	–	–	–	–
0.30–0.39	0.99	1.49	5.16	1.66	–	–	–	–
0.20–0.29	2.04	1.49	5.16	1.66	–	–	–	–
0.10–0.19	3.43	3.68	5.16	1.66	–	–	–	–
<0.10	3.93	3.68	5.16	1.66	–	–	–	–
CHF	–	2.38	3.01	–	–	–	2.11*	3.76*

Acuity of presentation								
Urgent PCI	1.78	–	2.19	–	–	–	2.13	–
Emergent PCI	5.75	–	7.71	–	–	–	2.13	1.44
AMI 1–7 d	–	2.10	1.85	–	2.14 (<14 d)	–	–	3.15
AMI 6–23 h	1.31	3.67	Primary therapy	2.80	–	4.75	–	3.15
AMI <6 h	1.31	5.22	–	2.80	–	4.75	–	3.15
Cardiogenic shock	8.49	18.3	6.10	11.5	–	12.7	4.95	3.47
IABP use	1.68	2.39	3.91	–	–	–	–	–
High-risk angiographic features								
2-VD	–	1.82 (Multivessel intervention)	–	1.54	2.20	1.32	1.86	–
3-VD	–	–	–	2.37	2.20	1.74	1.86	–
LM disease	2.04	–	–	–	–	–	4.34	2.40
Thrombus	–	–	–	1.67	–	–	1.90	–
ACC/AHA B2	–	–	–	–	–	1.63	–	2.58
ACC/AHA C	–	–	1.94	–	–	2.66	–	2.58
SCAI II	1.64	–	–	–	–	–	–	–
SCAI III	1.87	–	–	–	–	–	–	–
SCAI IV	2.11	–	–	–	–	–	–	–
Other high-risk conditions								
Renal failure	3.04	3.51	2.32	5.5	20.06	–	2.41	1.54
PVD	–	1.78	2.12	1.57	3.21	–	–	–
Diabetes mellitus	1.41	1.41	–	–	1.54	–	–	–
Female sex	–	1.31	–	1.82	3.57	1.82	–	–

Modified from Singh et al, reference 110.

*(≥NYHA III).

angiographic success in those lesions successfully crossed, the long-term clinical outcomes have been limited by a higher restenosis rate. Drug-eluting stents appear to reduce restenosis and may provide for longer clinical success.[109] However, when approaching a chronic total occlusion, the interventional cardiologist should recognize the increased risk of side branch occlusion or perforation.

GLOBAL RISK ASSESSMENT

Identification of the multiple risk factors for angiographic, procedural, and clinical complications with PCI has led to attempts at risk stratification of patients.[110] Predictors of mortality have received much attention, with several models developed to study the risk factors associated with periprocedural mortality[111–116] (Table 2.5). While many of these risk analyses have been developed from data on patients undergoing percutaneous transluminal angioplasty, several have been validated in patients undergoing stent implantation.[117–119]

Co-existent clinical conditions can increase the complication rates for any given anatomic risk factor. Therefore, global assessment of the risk of the procedure to the patient should include anatomic/lesion characteristics in conjunction with clinical characteristics. Indeed, several analyses have attempted to develop a risk score for in-hospital complications following PCI[30,111,120–122] (Table 2.5). One simplified multivariable model for predicting in-hospital complications following PCI uses integer scores assigned to clinical and angiographic variables[122] (Table 2.6; Figure 2.1). The cumulative score predicts the combined event rate for death, myocardial infarction, emergent CABG surgery, and stroke. This model has been externally validated in patients undergoing PCI from the NHLBI Dynamic Registry[119] and offers better predictive value of cardiovascular complications than the AHA/ACC classification scheme.[123]

POST-PROCEDURE MANAGEMENT

Patient preparation, risk stratification, and management do not end with the completion of the PCI procedure. Following PCI, in-hospital care should focus on monitoring the patient for recurrent myocardial ischemia, achieving hemostasis at the catheter insertion site, and detecting and preventing contrast-induced nephropathy. Implementation of appropriate secondary prevention pharmacotherapy and lifestyle

Table 2.6   Multivariate predictors of procedural complications after PCI

Variable	Integer score	Odds estimate	95% CI	P- value
Cardiogenic shock	5	4.95	3.4–7.2	<0.001
Left main coronary artery disease	5	4.34	2.5–7.6	<0.001
Serum creatinine level >3 mg/dL	3	2.41	1.4–4.2	0.001
Urgent or emergent procedure	2	2.13	1.5–3.1	<0.001
NHYA classification >/= III	2	2.11	1.4–3.1	<0.001
Thrombus	2	1.90	1.4–2.6	<0.001
Multivessel disease	2	1.86	1.3–2.6	<0.001
Age, no. of decades after 30 y	1	1.37	1.2–1.6	<0.001

Modified from Singh et al, reference 122.

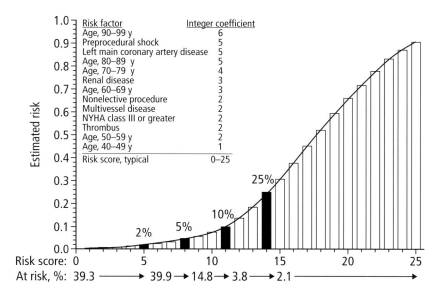

Figure 2.1 Estimated rates of procedural complications for the integer scoring system. Percentages at risk are shown for each of the five risk categories: ≤2% is very low risk for complications with coronary angioplasty; >2% to 5%, low risk; >5% to 10%, moderate risk; >10% to 25%, high risk; and >25%, very high risk. NYHA = New York Heart Association classification From Singh et al,[122] with permission.

modifications with formal education of the patient is imperative to the patient's understanding and adherence to recommended therapies to reduce subsequent morbidity and mortality from coronary heart disease.

Stent thrombosis occurs in ~1% of patients and usually manifests as chest pain and ST elevation. Persistent dissection, total stent length, bifurcation lesions, final lumen diameter, renal failure, diabetes, low ejection fraction, and premature antiplatelet therapy discontinuation have all been associated with acute stent thombosis.[75,76,124] Dual antiplatelet therapy with aspirin and clopidogrel is necessary for at least four weeks following bare metal stent placement and at least 3–6 months following placement of a drug-eluting stent. Earlier discontinuation of antiplatelet therapy has been associated with acute stent thrombosis.[124,125] In the era before drug-eluting stents, restenosis represented a major problem following stent placement[126–129] and methods to identify variables associated with restenosis had lower predictive value.[130] With the advent of drug-eluting stents, restenosis rates have dramatically decreased.[131,132]

CONCLUSION

Clinical characteristics associated with increased complications include age, diabetes, renal insufficiency, peripheral vascular disease, and depressed left ventricular ejection fraction. Angiographic characteristics associated with adverse outcomes include left main lesions, calcified lesions, angulation >45°, and bifurcation lesions.

Identification of these factors allows for proper and complete risk assessment and for the implementation of measures to reduce the risk of periprocedural complications. A number of risk scores have been proposed to assess the risk of complications using combined clinical and angiographic data. With careful analysis of the clinical and lesion characteristics, the interventional cardiologist can identify those patients at higher risk for complications and take appropriate preprocedural and intraprocedural measures to reduce those risks with a well-planned approach.

Despite best efforts to carefully select patients for PCI, the interventional cardiologist must accept, at times, that the patient has no other alternatives and proceed with PCI as long as there is a clear indication for the procedure and the factors associated with higher risks of complications have been identified and minimized, when possible.

REFERENCES

1. Gruntzig A. Transluminal dilatation of coronary-artery stenosis. Lancet 1978;1:263.
2. Gruntzig AR, Senning A, Siegenthaler WE. Nonoperative dilatation of coronary-artery stenosis: percutaneous transluminal coronary angioplasty. N Engl J Med 1979;301:61–8.
3. Smith SC Jr, Dove JT, Jacobs AK et al. ACC/AHA Guidelines for percutaneous coronary intervention (revision of the 1993 PTCA Guidelines) – executive summary. A Report of Am College of Cardiol/American Heart Association Task Force on Practice Guidelines (Committee to Revise the 1993 Guidelines for Percutaneous Transluminal Coronary Angioplasty) Endorsed by the Society for Cardiac Angiography and Interventions. Circulation 2001;103:3019–41.
4. Silber S, Albertsson P, Aviles FF et al. Guidelines for percutaneous coronary interventions: The Task Force for Percutaneous Coronary Interventions of the European Society of Cardiology. Eur Heart J 2005;26:804–47.
5. Goss JE, Chambers CE, Heupler FA Jnr. Systemic anaphylactoid reactions to iodinated contrast media during cardiac catheterization procedures: guidelines for prevention, diagnosis, and treatment. Laboratory Performance Standards Committee of the Society for Cardiac Angiography and Interventions. Cathet Cardiovasc Diagn 1995;34:99–104.
6. Lasser E, Berry C, Talner L et al. Pretreatment with corticosteroids to alleviate reactions to intravenous contrast material. N Engl J Med 1987;317:845–9.
7. Haffner SM, Lehto S, Ronnemaa T, Pyorala K, Laakso M. Mortality from coronary heart disease in subjects with type 2 diabetes and in nondiabetic subjects with and without prior myocardial infarction. N Engl J Med 1998;339:229–34.
8. Cohen Y, Raz I, Merin G, Mozes B. Comparison of factors associated with 30-day mortality after coronary artery bypass grafting in patients with versus without diabetes mellitus. Am J Cardiol 1998;81:7.
9. Gowda MS, Vacek JL, Hallas D. One-year outcomes of diabetic versus nondiabetic patients with non-Q-wave acute myocardial infarction treated with percutaneous transluminal coronary angioplasty. Am J Cardiol 1998;81:1067.
10. Barsness GW, Peterson ED, Ohman EM et al. Relationship between diabetes mellitus and long-term survival after coronary bypass and angioplasty. Circulation 1997;96:2551.
11. Aronson D, Rayfield EJ, Chesebro JH. Mechanisms determining course and outcome of diabetic patients who have had acute myocardial infarction. Ann Intern Med 1997;126:296.
12. Ellis SG, Narins CR. Problem of angioplasty in diabetics. Circulation 1997;96:1707.
13. Mak KH, Moliterno DJ, Granger CB, Miller DP. Influence of diabetes mellitus on clinical outcome in the thrombolytic era of acute myocardial infarction. J Am Coll Cardiol 1997;30:171–9.
14. Mathew V, Gersh BJ, Williams BA et al. Outcomes in patients with diabetes mellitus undergoing percutaneous coronary intervention in the current era: a report from the

Prevention of REStenosis with Tranilast and its Outcomes (PRESTO) Trial. Circulation 2004;109:476–80.

15. Flaherty JD, Davidson CJ. Diabetes and coronary revascularization. JAMA 2005;293:1501–8.

16. The Bypass Angioplasty Revascularization Investigation I. Comparison of coronary bypass surgery with angioplasty in patients with multivessel disease. N Engl J Med 1996;335:217–25.

17. Feit F, Brooks MM, Sopko G et al. Long-term clinical outcome in the Bypass Angioplasty Revascularization Investigation Registry: comparison with the randomized trial. Circulation 2000;101:2795–802.

18. Marso SP, Lincoff AM, Ellis SG et al. Optimizing the percutaneous interventional outcomes for patients with diabetes mellitus: results of the EPISTENT (Evaluation of Platelet IIb/IIIa Inhibitor for Stenting Trial) Diabetic Substudy. Circulation 1999;100:2477–84.

19. Bhatt DL, Marso SP, Lincoff AM et al. Abciximab reduces mortality in diabetics following percutaneous coronary intervention. J Am Coll Cardiol 2000;35:922.

20. Mehran R, Dangas GD, Kobayashi Y et al. Short- and long-term results after multivessel stenting in diabetic patients. J Am Coll Cardiol 2004;43:1348.

21. Corpus RA, George PB, House JA et al. Optimal glycemic control is associated with a lower rate of target vessel revascularization in treated type II diabetic patients undergoing elective percutaneous coronary intervention. J Am Coll Cardiol 2004;43:8.

22. Frederick AH Jr. Guidelines for performing angiography in patients taking metformin. Cathet Cardiovasc Diagn 1998;43:121–3.

23. Taliercio CP, Vlietstra RE, Fisher LD, Burnett JC. Risks for renal dysfunction with cardiac angiography. Ann Intern Med 1986;104:501–4.

24. Rihal CS, Textor SC, Grill DE et al. Incidence and prognostic importance of acute renal failure after percutaneous coronary intervention. Circulation 2002;105:2259–64.

25. Keelan PC, Johnston JM, Koru-Sengul T et al. Comparison of in-hospital and one-year outcomes in patients with left ventricular ejection fractions ≤40%, 41% to 49%, and ≥50% having percutaneous coronary revascularization. Am J Cardiol 2003;91:1168–72.

26. Holmes DR Jr, Berger PB, Hochman JS et al. Cardiogenic shock in patients with acute ischemic syndromes with and without ST-segment elevation. Circulation 1999;100:2067–73.

27. Hochman JS, Sleeper LA, Webb JG et al. Early revascularization in acute myocardial infarction complicated by cardiogenic shock. SHOCK Investigators. Should We Emergently Revascularize Occluded Coronaries for Cardiogenic Shock? N Engl J Med 1999;341:625–34.

28. Webb JG, Sanborn TA, Sleeper LA et al. Percutaneous coronary intervention for cardiogenic shock in the SHOCK Trial Registry. Am Heart J 2001;141:964.

29. Babaev A, Frederick PD, Pasta DJ et al. Trends in management and outcomes of patients with acute myocardial infarction complicated by cardiogenic shock. JAMA 2005;294:448–54.

30. Block PC, Peterson EC, Krone R et al. Identification of variables needed to risk adjust outcomes of coronary interventions: evidence-based guidelines for efficient data collection. J Am Coll Cardiol 1998;32:275.

31. Bergelson B, Jacobs A, Cupples L et al. Prediction of risk for hemodynamic compromise during percutaneous transluminal coronary angioplasty. Am J Cardiol 1992;70(20):1540–5.

32. Califf RM, Hindman MC, Phillips HR 3rd et al. Prognostic value of a coronary artery jeopardy score. J Am Coll Cardiol 1985;5:1055–63.

33. Ellis S, Myler R, King S et al. Causes and correlates of death after unsupported coronary angioplasty: implications for use of angioplasty and advanced support techniques in high-risk settings. Am J Cardiol 1991;68:1447–51.

34. Anwar A, Mooney MR, Stertzer SH et al. Intra-aortic balloon counterpulsation support for elective coronary angioplasty in the setting of poor left ventricular function: a two center experience. J Invasive Cardiol 1990;2:175–80.

35. Kreidieh I, Davies D, Lim R et al. High-risk coronary angioplasty with elective intra-aortic balloon pump support. Int J Cardiol 1992;35:147–52.
36. Vogel R, Tommaso C, Gundry S. Initial experience with coronary angioplasty and aortic valvuloplasty using elective semipercutaneous cardiopulmonary support. Am J Cardiol 1988;62:811–13.
37. Shawl F, Domanski M, Punja S, Hernandez T. Percutaneous cardiopulmonary bypass support in high-risk patients undergoing percutaneous transluminal coronary angioplasty. Am J Cardiol 1989;64:1258–63.
38. Lemos PA, Cummins P, Lee CH et al. Usefulness of percutaneous left ventricular assistance to support high-risk percutaneous coronary interventions. Am J Cardiol 2003;91:479–81.
39. Aragon J, Lee MS, Kar S, Makkar RR. Percutaneous left ventricular assist device: 'TandemHeart' for high-risk coronary intervention. Cathet Cardiovasc Interv 2005;65:346–52.
40. Thiele H, Sick P, Boudriot E et al. Randomized comparison of intra-aortic balloon support with a percutaneous left ventricular assist device in patients with revascularized acute myocardial infarction complicated by cardiogenic shock. Eur Heart J 2005;26:1276–83.
41. Anderson HV, Shaw RE, Brindis RG et al. A contemporary overview of percutaneous coronary interventions. Am Coll Cardiol-National Cardiovascular Data Registry (ACC-NCDR). J Am Coll Cardiol 2002;39:1096–103.
42. McCullough MPHPA, Wolyn R, Rocher LL et al. Acute renal failure after coronary intervention: incidence, risk factors, and relationship to mortality. Am J Med 1997;103:368.
43. Ting HH, Tahirkheli NK, Berger PB et al. Evaluation of long-term survival after successful percutaneous coronary intervention among patients with chronic renal failure. Am J Cardiol 2001;87:630–3, A9.
44. Best PJ, Lennon R, Ting HH et al. The impact of renal insufficiency on clinical outcomes in patients undergoing percutaneous coronary interventions. J Am Coll Cardiol 2002;39:1113–19.
45. Bartholomew BA, Harjai KJ, Dukkipati S et al. Impact of nephropathy after percutaneous coronary intervention and a method for risk stratification. Am J Cardiol 2004;93:1515.
46. Mehran R, Aymong ED, Nikolsky E et al. A simple risk score for prediction of contrast-induced nephropathy after percutaneous coronary intervention: development and initial validation. J Am Coll Cardiol 2004;44:1393.
47. Aspelin P, Aubry P, Fransson S-G et al. Nephrotoxic effects in high-risk patients undergoing angiography. N Engl J Med 2003;348:491–9.
48. Merten GJ, Burgess WP, Gray LV et al. Prevention of contrast-induced nephropathy with sodium bicarbonate: a randomized controlled trial. JAMA 2004;291:2328–34.
49. Tepel M, van der Giet M, Schwarzfeld C et al. Prevention of radiographic-contrast-agent-induced reductions in renal function by acetylcysteine. N Engl J Med 2000;343:180–4.
50. Miner SES, Dzavik V, Nguyen-Ho P et al. N-acetylcysteine reduces contrast-associated nephropathy but not clinical events during long-term follow-up. Am Heart J 2004;148:690.
51. Kay J, Chow WH, Chan TM et al. Acetylcysteine for prevention of acute deterioration of renal function following elective coronary angiography and intervention: a randomized controlled trial. JAMA 2003;289:553–8.
52. Birck R, Krzossok S, Markowetz F et al. Acetylcysteine for prevention of contrast nephropathy: meta-analysis. Lancet 2003;362:598.
53. Pannu N, Manns B, Lee H, Tonelli M. Systematic review of the impact of N-acetylcysteine on contrast nephropathy. Kidney Int 2004;65:1366–74.
54. Freeman RV, O'Donnell M, Share D et al. Nephropathy requiring dialysis after percutaneous coronary intervention and the critical role of an adjusted contrast dose. Am J Cardiol 2002;90:1068–73.
55. Singh M, Lennon R, Darbar D et al. Effect of peripheral arterial disease in patients undergoing percutaneous coronary intervention with intracoronary stents. Mayo Clin Proc 2004;79:1113–18.

56. Nikolsky E, Mehran R, Mintz GS et al. Impact of symptomatic peripheral arterial disease on 1-year mortality in patients undergoing percutaneous coronary interventions. J Endovasc Ther 2004;11:60–70.

57. Rihal CS, Sutton-Tyrrell K, Guo P et al. Increased incidence of periprocedural complications among patients with peripheral vascular disease undergoing myocardial revascularization in the bypass angioplasty revascularization investigation. Circulation 1999;100:171–7.

58. Davis C, Van Riper S, Longstreet J, Moscucci M. Vascular complications of coronary interventions. Heart Lung 1997;26:118–27.

59. Popma JJ, Prpic R, Lansky AJ, Piana R. Heparin dosing in patients undergoing coronary intervention. Am J Cardiol 1998;82:19P–24P.

60. Piper WD, Malenka DJ, Ryan TJ Jr et al. Predicting vascular complications in percutaneous coronary interventions. Am Heart J 2003;145:1022–9.

61. Kereiakes DJ, Broderick TM, Whang DD, Anderson L, Fye D. Partial reversal of heparin anticoagulation by intravenous protamine in abciximab-treated patients undergoing percutaneous intervention. Am J Cardiol 1997;80:633–4.

62. Pan M, Suarez de Lezo J, Medina A et al. In-laboratory removal of femoral sheath following protamine administration in patients having intracoronary stent implantation. Am J Cardiol 1997;80:1336–8.

63. Ducas J, Chan MC, Miller A, Kashour T. Immediate protamine administration and sheath removal following percutaneous coronary intervention: a prospective study of 429 patients. Cathet Cardiovasc Interv 2002;56:196–9.

64. Andersen K, Bregendahl M, Kaestel H, Skriver M, Ravkilde J. Haematoma after coronary angiography and percutaneous coronary intervention via the femoral artery frequency and risk factors. Eur J Cardiovasc Nurs 2005;4:123.

65. Crocker CH, Cragun KT, Timimi FK et al. Immediate ambulation following diagnostic coronary angiography procedures utilizing a vascular closure device (The Closer). J Invasive Cardiol 2002;14:728–32.

66. Vaitkus PT. A meta-analysis of percutaneous vascular closure devices after diagnostic catheterization and percutaneous coronary intervention. J Invasive Cardiol 2004;16:243–6.

67. Toursarkissian B, Mejia A, Smilanich RP, Shireman PK, Sykes MT. Changing patterns of access site complications with the use of percutaneous closure devices. Vasc Surg 2001;35:203–6.

68. Sprouse LR 2nd, Botta DM Jr, Hamilton IN Jr. The management of peripheral vascular complications associated with the use of percutaneous suture-mediated closure devices. J Vasc Surg 2001;33:688–93.

69. Lewis-Carey MB, Kee ST. Complications of arterial closure devices. Tech Vasc Interv Radiol 2003;6:103–6.

70. Hoffer EK, Bloch RD. Percutaneous arterial closure devices. J Vasc Interv Radiol 2003;14:865–85.

71. Ryan TJ, Faxon DP, Gunnar RM et al. Guidelines for percutaneous transluminal coronary angioplasty. A report of Am Coll Cardiol/American Heart Association Task Force on Assessment of Diagnostic and Therapeutic Cardiovascular Procedures (Subcommittee on Percutaneous Transluminal Coronary Angioplasty). Circulation 1988;78:486–502.

72. Ellis SG, Vandormael MG, Cowley MJ et al. Coronary morphologic and clinical determinants of procedural outcome with angioplasty for multivessel coronary disease. Implications for patient selection. Multivessel Angioplasty Prognosis Study Group. Circulation 1990;82:1193–202.

73. Kastrati A, Schomig A, Elezi S et al. Prognostic value of the modified American College Cardiology/American Heart Association stenosis morphology classification for long-term angiographic and clinical outcome after coronary stent placement. Circulation 1999;100:1285–90.

74. Krone RJ, Shaw RE, Klein LW et al. Evaluation of Am Coll Cardiol/American Heart Association and the Society for Coronary Angiography and Interventions lesion

classification system in the current 'stent era' of coronary interventions (from the ACC-National Cardiovascular Data Registry). Am J Cardiol 2003;92:389.

75. Orford JL, Lennon R, Melby S et al. Frequency and correlates of coronary stent thrombosis in the modern era: analysis of a single center registry. J Am Coll Cardiol 2002;40:1567–72.

76. Cutlip DE, Baim DS, Ho KK et al. Stent thrombosis in the modern era: a pooled analysis of multicenter coronary stent clinical trials. Circulation 2001;103:1967–71.

77. Simpfendorfer C, Belardi J, Bellamy G et al. Frequency, management and follow-up of patients with acute coronary occlusions after percutaneous transluminal coronary angioplasty. Am J Cardiol 1987;59:267–9.

78. Kuntz R, Piana R, Pomerantz R et al. Changing incidence and management of abrupt closure following coronary intervention in the new device era. Cathet Cardiovasc Diagn 1992;3:183–90.

79. de Feyter PJ, de Jaegrere PP, Serruys PW. Incidence, predictors, and management of acute coronary occlusion after coronary angioplasty. Am Heart J 1994;127:643–51.

80. Hearn J, King S, Douglas JJ et al. Clinical and angiographic outcomes after coronary artery stenting for acute or threatened closure after percutaneous transluminal coronary angioplasty. Initial results with a balloon-expandable, stainless steel design. Circulation 1993;88:2086–96.

81. Rankin JM, Spinelli JJ, Carere RG et al. Improved clinical outcome after widespread use of coronary-artery stenting in Canada. N Engl J Med 1999;341:1957–65.

82. Kimmel SE, Localio AR, Krone RJ, Laskey WK. The effects of contemporary use of coronary stents on in-hospital mortality. Registry Committee of the Society for Cardiac Angiography and Interventions. J Am Coll Cardiol 2001;37:499–504.

83. Suh WW, Grill DE, Rihal CS et al. Unrestricted availability of intracoronary stents is associated with decreased abrupt vascular closure rates and improved early clinical outcomes. Cathet Cardiovasc Interv 2002;55:294–302.

84. Mehta SR, Yusuf S, Peters RJ et al. Effects of pretreatment with clopidogrel and aspirin followed by long-term therapy in patients undergoing percutaneous coronary intervention: the PCI-CURE study. Lancet 2001;358:527–33.

85. Steinhubl SR, Berger PB, Mann JT 3rd et al. Early and sustained dual oral antiplatelet therapy following percutaneous coronary intervention: a randomized controlled trial. JAMA 2002;288:2411–20.

86. The EPISTENT Investigators. Randomised placebo-controlled and balloon-angioplasty-controlled trial to assess safety of coronary stenting with use of platelet glycoprotein-IIb/IIIa blockade. Evaluation of Platelet IIb/IIIa Inhibitor for Stenting. Lancet 1998;352:87–92.

87. Karvouni E, Katritsis DG, Ioannidis JPA. Intravenous glycoprotein IIb/IIIa receptor antagonists reduce mortality after percutaneous coronary interventions. J Am Coll Cardiol 2003;41:26.

88. Oler A, Whooley M, Oler J et al. Adding heparin to aspirin reduces the incidence of myocardial infarction and death in patients with unstable angina: a meta-analysis. JAMA 1996;276:811–15.

89. Lincoff AM, Bittl JA, Harrington RA et al. Bivalirudin and provisional glycoprotein IIb/IIIa blockade compared with heparin and planned glycoprotein IIb/IIIa blockade during percutaneous coronary intervention: REPLACE-2 randomized trial. JAMA 2003;289:853–63.

90. Lewis BE, Matthai WH Jr, Cohen M et al. Argatroban anticoagulation during percutaneous coronary intervention in patients with heparin-induced thrombocytopenia. Cathet Cardiovasc Interv 2002;57:177–84.

91. Mathew V, Rihal CS, Berger PB et al. Clinical outcome of patients undergoing multivessel coronary stent implantation. Int J Cardiol 1998;64:1–7.

92. Brener SJ, Lytle BW, Casserly IP et al. Propensity analysis of long-term survival after surgical or percutaneous revascularization in patients with multivessel coronary artery disease and high-risk features. Circulation 2004;109:2290–5.

93. Hlatky MA, Boothroyd DB, Melsop KA et al. Medical costs and quality of life 10 to 12 years after randomization to angioplasty or bypass surgery for multivessel coronary artery disease. Circulation 2004;110:1960–6.

94. Legrand VMG, Serruys PW, Unger F et al. Three-year outcome after coronary stenting versus bypass surgery for the treatment of multivessel disease. Circulation 2004;109:1114–20.

95. Ijsselmuiden AJJ, Ezechiels J, Westendorp ICD et al. Complete versus culprit vessel percutaneous coronary intervention in multivessel disease: a randomized comparison. Am Heart J 2004;148:467.

96. Hong MK, Mehran R, Dangas G et al. Creatine kinase-MB enzyme elevation following successful saphenous vein graft intervention is associated with late mortality. Circulation 1999;100:2400–5.

97. Roffi M, Mukherjee D, Chew DP et al. Lack of benefit from intravenous platelet glycoprotein IIb/IIIa receptor inhibition as adjunctive treatment for percutaneous interventions of aortocoronary bypass grafts: a pooled analysis of five randomized clinical trials. Circulation 2002;106:3063–7.

98. Baim DS, Wahr D, George B et al. Randomized trial of a distal embolic protection device during percutaneous intervention of saphenous vein aorto-coronary bypass grafts. Circulation 2002;105:1285–90.

99. Stone GW, Rogers C, Hermiller J et al. Randomized comparison of distal protection with a filter-based catheter and a balloon occlusion and aspiration system during percutaneous intervention of diseased saphenous vein aorto-coronary bypass grafts. Circulation 2003;108:548–53.

100. Verghese M Jr. Applicability of distal protection for aortocoronary vein graft interventions in clinical practice. Cathet Cardiovasc Interv 2004;63:148–51.

101. Kelley MP, Klugherz BD, Hashemi SM et al. One-year clinical outcomes of protected and unprotected left main coronary artery stenting. Eur Heart J 2003;24:1554–9.

102. Arampatzis CA, Lemos PA, Tanabe K et al. Effectiveness of sirolimus-eluting stent for treatment of left main coronary artery disease. Am J Cardiol 2003;92:327.

103. de Lezo JS, Medina A, Pan M et al. Rapamycin-eluting stents for the treatment of unprotected left main coronary disease. Am Heart J 2004;148:481.

104. Naidu SS, Rohatgi S, Herrmann HC, Glaser R. Unprotected left main 'kissing' stent implantation with a percutaneous ventricular assist device. J Invasive Cardiol 2004;16:683–4.

105. Bonvini RF, Hendiri T, Camenzind E, Verin V. High-risk left main coronary stenting supported by percutaneous left ventricular assist device. Cathet Cardiovasc Interv 2005;66:209–12.

106. Chieffo A, Stankovic G, Bonizzoni E et al. Early and mid-term results of drug-eluting stent implantation in unprotected left main. Circulation 2005;111:791–5.

107. Kandzari DE. The challenges of chronic total coronary occlusions: an old problem in a new perspective. J Interv Cardiol 2004;17:259–67.

108. Abbas AE, Brewington SD, Dixon SR et al. Success, safety, and mechanisms of failure of percutaneous coronary intervention for occlusive non-drug-eluting in-stent restenosis versus native artery total occlusion. Am J Cardiol 2005;95:1462–6.

109. Ge L, Iakovou I, Cosgrave J et al. Immediate and mid-term outcomes of sirolimus-eluting stent implantation for chronic total occlusions. Eur Heart J 2005;26:1056–62.

110. Singh M, Rihal CS, Lennon RJ, Garratt KN, Holmes DR Jr. A critical appraisal of current models of risk stratification for percutaneous coronary interventions. Am Heart J 2005;149:753–60.

111. Ellis SG, Weintraub W, Holmes D et al. Relation of operator volume and experience to procedural outcome of percutaneous coronary revascularization at hospitals with high interventional volumes. Circulation 1997;95:2479–84.

112. Moscucci M, Kline-Rogers E, Share D et al. Simple bedside additive tool for prediction of in-hospital mortality after percutaneous coronary interventions. Circulation 2001;104:263–8.

113. Hannan EL, Racz M, Ryan TJ et al. Coronary angioplasty volume–outcome relationships for hospitals and cardiologists. JAMA 1997;277:892–8.
114. O'Connor GT, Malenka DJ, Quinton H et al. Multivariate prediction of in-hospital mortality after percutaneous coronary interventions in 1994–1996. Northern New England Cardiovascular Disease Study Group. J Am Coll Cardiol 1999;34:681–91.
115. Qureshi MA, Safian RD, Grines CL et al. Simplified scoring system for predicting mortality after percutaneous coronary intervention. J Am Coll Cardiol 2003;42:1890.
116. Shaw RE, Anderson HV, Brindis RG et al. Updated risk adjustment mortality model using the complete 1.1 dataset from the American College of Cardiology National Cardiovascular Data Registry (ACC-NCDR). J Invasive Cardiol 2003;15:578–80.
117. Moscucci M, O'Connor GT, Ellis SG et al. Validation of risk adjustment models for in-hospital percutaneous transluminal coronary angioplasty mortality on an independent data set. J Am Coll Cardiol 1999;34:692–7.
118. Holmes DR Jr, Berger PB, Garratt KN et al. Application of the New York State PTCA mortality model in patients undergoing stent implantation. Circulation 2000;102:517–22.
119. Singh M, Rihal CS, Selzer F et al. Validation of Mayo Clinic risk adjustment model for in-hospital complications after percutaneous coronary interventions, using the National Heart, Lung, and Blood Institute dynamic registry. J Am Coll Cardiol 2003;42:1722–8.
120. Kimmel SE, Berlin JA, Strom BL, Laskey WK. Development and validation of simplified predictive index for major complications in contemporary percutaneous transluminal coronary angioplasty practice. The Registry Committee of the Society for Cardiac Angiography and Interventions. J Am Coll Cardiol 1995;26:931–8.
121. Resnic FS, Ohno-Machado L, Selwyn A, Simon DI, Popma JJ. Simplified risk score models accurately predict the risk of major in-hospital complications following percutaneous coronary intervention. Am J Cardiol 2001;88:5.
122. Singh M, Lennon RJ, Holmes DR Jr, Bell MR, Rihal CS. Correlates of procedural complications and a simple integer risk score for percutaneous coronary intervention. J Am Coll Cardiol 2002;40:387–93.
123. Singh M, Rihal CS, Lennon RJ, Garratt KN, Holmes DR Jr. Comparison of Mayo Clinic risk score and American College of Cardiology/American Heart Association lesion classification in the prediction of adverse cardiovascular outcome following percutaneous coronary interventions. J Am Coll Cardiol 2004;44:357–61.
124. Iakovou I, Schmidt T, Bonizzoni E et al. Incidence, predictors, and outcome of thrombosis after successful implantation of drug-eluting stents. JAMA 2005;293:2126–30.
125. Jeremias A, Sylvia B, Bridges J et al. Stent thrombosis after successful sirolimus-eluting stent implantation. Circulation 2004;109:1930–2.
126. Holmes DR Jr, Vlietstra RE, Smith HC et al. Restenosis after percutaneous transluminal coronary angioplasty (PTCA): a report from the PTCA Registry of the National Heart, Lung, and Blood Institute. Am J Cardiol 1984;53:77C–81C.
127. Vlietstra RE, Holmes DR Jr, Rodeheffer RJ, Bailey KR. Consequences of restenosis after coronary angioplasty. Int J Cardiol 1991;31:143–7.
128. Holmes DR Jr. In-stent restenosis. Rev Cardiovasc Med 2001;2:115–19.
129. Cutlip DE, Chauhan MS, Baim DS et al. Clinical restenosis after coronary stenting: perspectives from multicenter clinical trials. J Am Coll Cardiol 2002;40:2082–9.
130. Singh M, Gersh BJ, McClelland RL et al. Clinical and angiographic predictors of restenosis after percutaneous coronary intervention: insights from the Prevention of Restenosis With Tranilast and Its Outcomes (PRESTO) trial. Circulation 2004;109:2727–31.
131. Moses JW, Leon MB, Popma JJ et al. Sirolimus-eluting stents versus standard stents in patients with stenosis in a native coronary artery. N Engl J Med 2003;349:1315–23.
132. Holmes DR Jr, Leon MB, Moses JW et al. Analysis of 1-year clinical outcomes in the SIRIUS trial: a randomized trial of a sirolimus-eluting stent versus a standard stent in patients at high risk for coronary restenosis. Circulation 2004;109:634–40.

133. Sohail MR, Khan AH, Holmes DR Jr et al. Infectious complications of percutaneous vascular closure devices. Mayo Clin Proc 2005;80:1011–15.
134. Ellis SG, Guetta V, Miller D, Whitlow PL, Topol EJ. Relation between lesion characteristics and risk with percutaneous intervention in the stent and glycoprotein IIb/IIIa era: an analysis of results from 10,907 lesions and proposal for new classification scheme. Circulation 1999;100:1971–6.

3

Optimal antiplatelet and anticoagulation therapy, prevention and management of thrombotic complications

Raphaelle Dumaine, François Beygui and Gilles Montalescot

Antiplatelet therapy in percutaneous cardiovascular interventions • **Anticoagulation therapy in percutaneous cardiovascular interventions** • **Conclusion**

Endothelial denudation, plaque disruption, and implantation of stents during percutaneous coronary interventions (PCI) are systematically followed by platelet activation and deposition, and mural thrombus formation. Such phenomena may lead to acute or subacute stent thrombosis, distal embolization, and vessel occlusion. Since the very beginning of coronary angioplasty in the late 1970s, the key role of antiplatelet and anticoagulation therapy in this setting as well as the setting of acute coronary syndromes has been obvious. The improvement in guidewires and angioplasty balloons and the development of new coronary devices have generalized the use of PCI not only in patients with simple coronary lesions and stable coronary artery disease but also in complex, high thrombotic risk situations such as urgent or early PCI for acute coronary syndromes, multivessel PCI and complex lesions – bifurcations, long lesions, small vessels, etc. The development of highly active combinations of antithrombotic drugs has allowed the dramatic increase in the use of PCI. Nevertheless, such combinations may be associated with significantly higher risk of bleeding complications, especially in some patient subgroups such as the elderly or those with renal failure.

Hence optimal antiplatelet and anticoagulation regimens, safe and well adapted to the clinical and anatomic presentation of the coronary artery disease, should be used in various PCI patient subsets.

ANTIPLATELET THERAPY IN PERCUTANEOUS CARDIOVASCULAR INTERVENTIONS

Antiplatelet drugs (Table 3.1)

Aspirin

Aspirin partially inhibits platelet aggregation by irreversibly inactivating the cyclo-oxygenase activity of prostaglandin H synthase 1 and 2, thereby blocking the platelet production of thromboxane A2.

Significant long-lasting (up to seven days) inhibition of the platelet function occurs within an hour after a single oral dose of aspirin and within <5 minutes after an

Table 3.1 Antiplatelet drugs

Class	Drug	Antiplatelet action	Administration	Loading dose	First dose to effect time	Regimen after PCI	Dose adjustment in renal failure
Aspirin	Aspirin	Irreversible	Oral/IV*	75–325 mg/ 250–500 mg*	<1 hour	75–100 mg daily	No
Thienopyridines	Ticlopidine	Irreversible	Oral	1000 mg	24–48 hours	500 mg daily	No
	Clopidogrel	Irreversible	Oral	300 600/900 mg**	6–24 hours 2–6 hours	75 mg daily	No
GP IIb/IIIa inhibitors	Abciximab	Irreversible	IV	0.25 mg/kg	Minutes	0.125 µg/kg/min for 12 hours	No (not recommended if severe RF)
	Eptifibatide	Reversible	IV	Two 180 µg/kg bolus, 10 minutes apart	Minutes	2 µg/kg/min for 18 hours	No (not recommended if severe RF)
	Tirofiban	Reversible	IV	0.4 µg/kg/min for 30 minutes	Minutes	0.1 µg/kg/min for 12 hours	Yes, half dose if CrCl < 30 mL/min

* In some countries
** In untreated patients undergoing urgent PCI
RF: renal failure

intravenous bolus. Aspirin given 24–48 hours prior to PCI reduces the risk of acute coronary occlusion by 50–75% and its long-term administration after PCI is unequivocally associated with a reduced risk of major cardiovascular events.[1] These effects have been demonstrated for doses as low as 30 mg and as high as 1500 mg. There are no demonstrated advantages of doses higher than 75–100 mg daily while higher doses are associated with more gastrointestinal side effects, especially in patients treated by combination antiplatelet therapy. The recommended daily dose is 75–325 mg in different settings of coronary artery disease. Aspirin pretreatment (>24 hours) is recommended in patients undergoing elective PCI. An initial 162–325 mg loading dose of aspirin could be recommended in untreated patients undergoing urgent PCI.[2,3] In some European countries an intravenous loading dose of 250–500 mg of aspirin is used in the previous situation because of its fast effect.

Thienopyridines

Thienopyridines irreversibly inhibit the platelet ADP P2Y12 receptor, leading to an attenuated platelet aggregation in response to ADP stimuli. The mechanism of action of thienopyridines is complementary to that of aspirin.

The use of thienopyridines increased dramatically after ticlopidine, in combination with aspirin, was reported to reduce the risks of both subacute stent thrombosis and bleeding after stent placement compared to aspirin combined to warfarin.[4] The use of ticlopidine was nevertheless restricted in time to the first 15–28 days after stent placement because of the potentially lethal, up to 2.4%, risk of neutropenia associated with its use.

Clopidogrel

Clopidogrel is a thienopyridine derivative, structurally related to ticlopidine with less serious side effects, reported rates of neutropenia comparable to those of placebo, and faster and longer duration of action compared to ticlopidine. Clopidogrel in combination with aspirin has shown similar efficacy in reducing rates of subacute stent thrombosis compared to the combination of ticlopidine and aspirin.[5,6] Moreover, pretreatment and prolonged therapy (9–12 months) with clopidogrel have been reported to be associated with lower incidence of acute atherothrombotic events after PCI.[7,8] The increase in the use of potentially more thrombogenic drug-eluting stents has also contributed to the recommendation of prolonged clopidogrel therapy (3–6 months) after placement of such stents.[3]

Clopidogrel is a pro-drug, needing *in vivo* hepatic transformation for its antiplatelet effect. Significant platelet function inhibition is detected within two hours after a single oral dose of clopidogrel. With repeated daily doses of 75 mg, a steady state with 50–60% inhibition of platelet aggregation is reached in 4–7 days. An initial standard loading dose of 300 mg is usually used to achieve the platelet inhibition effects more rapidly. Recent data show that more significant inhibitory effects can be achieved even faster with higher loading doses of 600 or 900 mg.[9,10]

Glycoprotein IIb/IIIa inhibitors

GP IIb/IIIa inhibitors block the ligation of fibrinogen and von Willebrand factor by platelet GP IIb/IIIa receptors, consequently blocking the final common pathway of platelet aggregation. Unlike aspirin and thienopyridine derivatives, GP IIb/IIIa blockade results in platelet inhibition regardless of the initial aggregation stimuli.

Three intravenous (IV) inhibitors of platelet GP IIb/IIIa receptors – abciximab, eptifibatide, and tirofiban – are commercially available. All three agents provide significant antiplatelet action within minutes after an IV bolus. An IV continuous infusion is needed to maintain the antiplatelet effect of the drugs 12–18 hours after the procedure.

GP IIb/IIIa inhibitors have demonstrated variable degrees of efficacy in the setting of acute coronary syndromes and PCI. There is general consensus that GP IIb/IIIa agents, particularly abciximab, are recommended in patients undergoing primary PCI for ST-segment elevation myocardial infarction (STEMI); non ST-segment elevation myocardial infarction (NSTEMI) or planned PCI in high-risk patients such as diabetics. A meta-analysis of 20 studies, including 20,137 patients, reported a significant and sustained reduction in the risk of death and acute myocardial infarction (MI) after PCI by the use of GP IIb/IIIa inhibitors, with an increase in the risk of major bleeding only in patients with continued postprocedure heparin therapy.[11] The degree of evidence is best established for abciximab, especially in the setting of PCI for STEMI, less for eptifibatide and least for tirofiban.

There is still some controversy over the beneficial effect of such therapy in low-risk elective PCI, in the era of thienopyridine pre-PCI therapy. The randomized ISAR-REACT and ISAR-SWEET trials, using a 600 mg loading dose of clopidogrel prior to elective PCI, did not show any additional benefit of per-procedure GP IIb/IIIa inhibitors compared to placebo in reducing the rates of the 30-day primary thrombotic end-points in patients with low- to intermediate-risk levels and in diabetics.[12,13] Given the high cost of GP IIb/IIIa inhibitors, their systematic use in all cases of elective PCI is not recommended.

Other antiplatelet agents

Other agents with some antiplatelet activity such as dipyridamole, reversible COX-1 inhibitors (sulfinpyrazone, indobufen, triflusal, etc.) and oral GP IIb/IIIa inhibitors have been studied in clinical trials. There is no established evidence that these drugs may have a clinically relevant activity, comparable to aspirin or thienopyridines. Therefore, their use in the setting of PCI is not recommended.

Newer antiplatelet agents such as prasugrel, a thienopyridine derivative with potentially faster action and fewer non-responders (TRITON trial), and other P2Y12 receptor antagonists are being investigated and may improve antiplatelet therapy in the near future.

Indications for antiplatelet therapy in the setting of percutaneous cardiovascular intervention

Different antiplatelet regimens are recommended depending on the clinical presentation. These recommendations are summarized in Table 3.2.

Antiplatelets for thrombotic complications

Bail-out situations during PCI, due to extensive coronary dissection, abrupt vessel closure, acute stent thrombosis or distal embolization, are rare but potentially

Table 3.2 Use of antiplatelet drugs in the setting of PCI

Clinical presentation		Therapy prior to PCI	Therapy during PCI	Therapy after PCI
Elective PCI	Low risk	Aspirin 75–325 mg Clopidogrel, 300 mg if >6 hours or 600–900 mg if <6 hours before PCI	Abciximab or eptifibatide if high angiographic risk	Aspirin 75–100 mg daily Clopidogrel 75 mg daily at least 3–4 weeks, up to 9–12 months*
	High risk (diabetics, multivessel PCI, thrombus, complex lesions)	Aspirin 75–325 mg Clopidogrel, 300 mg >6 hours before or 600–900 mg <6 hours before PCI	Abciximab or eptifibatide	Aspirin 75–100 mg daily Clopidogrel 75 mg daily at least 3–4 weeks, up to 9–12 months* GP IIb/IIIa inhibitors for 12–18 hours
UA/NSTEMI	Nonurgent PCI	Aspirin 75–325 mg Clopidogrel, 300 mg >6 hours before or 600–900 mg <6 hours before PCI	Upstream eptifibatide or tirofiban	Aspirin 75–100 mg daily Clopidogrel 75 mg daily 9–12 months* GP IIb/IIIa inhibitors for 12–18 hours
	Urgent PCI	Aspirin 250–325 mg Clopidogrel 600–900 mg Abciximab or eptifibatide	Abciximab or eptifibatide	Aspirin 75–100 mg daily Clopidogrel 75 mg daily 9–12 months* GP IIb/IIIa inhibitors for 12–18 hours
STEMI	Urgent PCI	Aspirin 250–325 mg Clopidogrel 600–900 mg Abciximab as soon as possible	Abciximab	Aspirin 75–100 mg daily Clopidogrel 75 mg daily at least 3–4 weeks, up to 9–12 months* Abciximab for 12 hours

* In patients with sirolimus/paclitaxel-eluting stents: at least 3/6 months clopidogrel therapy is recommended

life-threatening complications that could occur despite optimal antithrombotic therapy. The pre-PCI therapy by aspirin, thienopyridines, and GP IIb/IIIa inhibitors reduces the risk of such complications. Bail-out situations are usually treated by coronary stents, mechanical assistance devices such as aortic balloon pumps or emergency coronary artery bypass. There is no established evidence on the medical treatment of these complications. Nevertheless, in patients untreated by GP IIb/IIIa inhibitors during the PCI, the use of abciximab is recommended in bail-out situations. The use of abciximab as a substitute for other GP IIb/IIIa inhibitors in patients already treated with such drugs could be considered in cases of extensive coronary thrombus formation. A supplementary loading dose of aspirin and/or clopidogrel could also be considered based on the hypothesis of a resistance to usual doses of such drugs.

Aspirin intolerance

Hypersensitivity reactions to aspirin, such as angioedema, urticaria, asthma, and anaphylactoid shock, have been reported. In aspirin-intolerant patients, thienopyridines or GP IIb/IIIa inhibitors could be used before and during the PCI procedure. The use of drug-eluting coronary stents in such patients should be avoided and surgical revascularization may be considered in some situations as a substitute for PCI. In patients showing aspirin intolerance after PCI, rapid oral challenge-desensitization to aspirin may be performed.[14]

ANTICOAGULATION THERAPY IN PERCUTANEOUS CARDIOVASCULAR INTERVENTIONS

Anticoagulation therapy in the setting of PCI aims to inhibit thrombin formation. Thrombin controls the conversion of fluid-phase fibrinogen into fibrin, which polymerizes into cross-linked fibrin polymers, the basis of the clot. Furthermore, thrombin sustains the clotting process by two mechanisms: amplification of its own production by activating the intrinsic pathway, and platelet activation.

Unfractionated heparin

Thrombin has an active site and two exosites, one of which – exosite 1 – binds to its fibrin substrate, orientating it towards the active site. Unfractionated heparin (UFH) binds thrombin's exosite 2 and antithrombin. Formation of this ternary complex catalyzes inhibition of thrombin by antithrombin. UFH also inhibits factor Xa but, unlike thrombin inhibition, inactivation of factor Xa does not require the formation of a ternary complex with antithrombin. UFH inhibits in the same proportion thrombin and factor Xa (the ratio anti-Xa/IIa activity equals 1). UFH also binds thrombin-bound fibrin, creating a heparin–thrombin–fibrin complex, rendering the bound thrombin resistant to inhibition by the heparin–antithrombin complex.

UFH has long been the only thrombin inhibitor used during PCI (see contemporary guidelines for UFH use in Table 3.3), but several pharmacologic limitations of variable efficacy and stability, poor bioavailability, nonspecific protein binding, neutralization by platelet factor-4 (PF-4) and poor control of von Willebrand factor release, associated with the necessity of close monitoring of anticoagulant activity, as well as a high incidence of heparin-induced thrombocytopenia, have encouraged the development of alternative antithrombin strategies.

Table 3.3   Contemporary guidelines for unfractionated heparin (UFH) use in patients undergoing PCI

	No concomitant GP IIb/IIIa inhibitor use	Concomitant GP IIb/IIIa inhibitor use
IV bolus	70–100 U/kg	50–70 U/kg
Activated clotting time (ACT) to achieve	250–300 s (HemoTec device) 300–350 s (Hemochron device)	<300 s
Additionnal bolus if target ACT not achieved	2000–5000 U	
Sheath removal	When ACT <180 s	

Low molecular weight heparins

Whilst the antithrombin activity of LMWH is also antithrombin dependent, their action is primarily against factor Xa. Furthermore, LMWH have reduced nonspecific protein binding, reduced neutralization by PF-4, lack of platelet activation, induce less von Willebrand factor release and have a more predictable pharmacologic profile than UFH, removing the need for therapeutic drug monitoring. Heparin-induced thrombocytopenia is also much less common with LMWH than UFH.

Enoxaparin is the most extensively studied LMWH in the setting of PCI.

Low molecular weight heparin for percutaneous cardiovascular intervention in the setting of acute coronary syndrome (ACS)

Current recommendations for antithrombin management in patients being treated with subcutaneous (SC) LMWH undergoing PCI suggest a transition to UFH as anticoagulant during coronary procedures.[15] In the setting of ACS, such strategy remains controversial as the use of enoxaparin as sole anticoagulant during PCI in ACS patients appears to be at least as safe and efficient as UFH.[16–18]

However, there are new data regarding anticoagulation using LMWH during PCI instead of UFH, in order to avoid anticoagulant agent switch when transferring the patient to the catheter lab.

Collet et al examined the safety and efficacy of performing PCI in the setting of ACS on LMWH therapy without interruption of or addition of anticoagulation for PCI. The only rule was to perform PCI within eight hours after the last SC enoxaparin injection (when anti-Xa levels are close to the peak of activity). Four hundred and fifty one consecutive patients with ACS received at least 48 hours treatment with enoxaparin 1 mg/kg/12 hours SC in the coronary care unit, and 65% underwent coronary angiography. PCI was performed in 28% of the patients, with no further anticoagulation. Mean anti-Xa activity at the time of catheterization was 0.98±0.03 iu/mL and the anti-Xa activity was > 0.5 iu/mL in 97.6% of patients. No in-hospital acute vessel closure or urgent revascularization following PCI was observed. Death/MI at 30 days occurred in 3.0% of the PCI patients and 10.8% of patients not undergoing catheterization. The 30-day major bleeding rate was 0.8% in the PCI group, versus 1.3% in patients managed medically.[19]

In the NICE-3 study,[20] 661 ACS patients were treated with enoxaparin SC 1 mg/kg plus abciximab, eptifibatide or tirofiban at standard doses and both strategies were combined for the transition from the ward to the catheter laboratory. There was no interruption and no addition of enoxaparin for PCI within eight hours of the last SC injection and an additive IV bolus of 0.3 mg/kg when PCI was performed at between eight and 12 hours after the last SC injection. The major bleeding rate was 4.5% and the in-hospital death/MI/urgent TVR rate 5.7%.

The SYNERGY randomized trial[21] compared enoxaparin and UFH among 10,027 high-risk patients with non-ST segment elevation ACS to be treated with an intended early invasive strategy. The incidence of death/MI at 30 days was similar between the two groups. The primary safety outcome was major bleeding or stroke. The incidence of major bleeding was increased in the enoxaparin group when using the TIMI classification (9.1% vs 7.6%, $P=0.008$) but not when using the GUSTO classification (2.7% vs 2.2%, $P=0.08$). When stratifying by prerandomization therapy, the benefit of enoxaparin was the highest among patients receiving either enoxaparin only or no antithrombin therapy before randomization. The authors stated that 'as a first-line agent in the absence of changing antithrombin therapy during treatment, enoxaparin appears to be superior to UFH without an increased bleeding risk'.[21]

Data from these various trials are becoming integrated into current recommendations. A recent expert consensus concluded that patients receiving SC LMWH in the management of ACS can safely undergo cardiac catheterization and PCI.[22] It was, furthermore, concluded that LMWH and GP IIb/IIIa antagonists can be safely used in combination without any apparent increase in the risk of major bleeding. A proposal for anticoagulation by enoxaparin as an alternative to UFH is displayed in Table 3.4.

Low molecular weight heparin for elective percutaneous cardiovascular intervention

There are increasing data regarding the comparison of UFH and IV LMWH as procedural anticoagulants for elective PCI, and the safety and efficacy *per se* of LMWH. In a meta-analysis of randomized trials comparing a single IV LMWH bolus and UFH, there was a nonsignificant trend favoring LMWH with regard to both a combined efficacy (death/MI/urgent revascularization) and hemorrhagic end-points.[23] When a further pooled analysis was performed, including data from all randomized trials and seven additional nonrandomized trials/registries, the composite efficacy end-point rates favored LMWH.[23] In this meta-analysis, the best outcome data were obtained with the 0.5 mg/kg IV dose of enoxaparin.

These results were confirmed in the recent STEEPLE trial[24] which randomized 3528 patients undergoing elective PCI to either enoxaparin (0.5 or 0.75 mg/kg) or an activated clotting time (ACT)-adjusted UFH regimen. The primary end-point was the incidence of noncoronary artery bypass graft (CABG)-related major and minor bleeding. Enoxaparin 0.5 mg/kg was associated with a significant 31% reduction in the primary end-point compared with UFH (6.0% vs 8.7%, $P=0.014$), and the 0.75 mg/kg dose was associated with a 24% reduction (6.6% vs 8.7%, $P=0.052$), meeting the criteria for noninferiority. There was a significant 57% reduction of major bleeding in both enoxaparin groups compared with UFH.

The incidence of the composite end-point death/MI/urgent target revascularization/major bleeding at 30 days was similar between the three groups.

Table 3.4 Proposal for enoxaparin use as an alternative to UFH during PCI

	Before cath	During PCI		After successful PCI	Sheath removal
		PCI performed within 8 hours after the last SC injection	PCI performed between 8–12 hours after the last SC injection		
ACS	Enoxaparin SC: 1 mg/kg/12 h if CrCl >60 mL/min 0.8 mg/kg/12 h if CrCl <60 mL/min 0.65 mg/kg/12 h if CrCl <30 mL/min 20 mg/12 h in hemodialysis patients (no enoxaparin on dialysis days)	0	Enoxaparin IV bolus: 0.25–0.30 mg/kg	0	Immediate
Elective PCI	0	Enoxaparin IV bolus : 0.5 mg/kg		0	Immediate

Direct thrombin inhibitors

Bivalirudin is to date the only direct thrombin inhibitor (DTI) indicated for use as an anticoagulant in patients undergoing PCI.

Bivalirudin binds thrombin's active site and exosite 1 and removes it from its fibrin substrate. DTIs do not bind to plasma proteins, providing a more predictable pharmacologic response than UFH. They are not affected by platelet factor-4, have a low immunogenic propensity and thus are very unlikely to induce thrombocytopenia. Furthermore, bivalirudin blocks thrombin signaling to the platelet's protease-activated receptors, limiting platelet activation. DTIs are also active against fibrin-bound thrombin.

Bivalirudin (or hirulog)

In the Bivalirudin Angioplasty Trial,[25] 4098 patients undergoing PCI were randomly allocated to UFH or bivalirudin as a procedural anticoagulant. The primary end-point of death/MI/abrupt vessel closure or clinical deterioration of cardiac origin was similar between the two groups on treatment analysis. The incidence of major bleeding was significantly reduced with bivalirudin (3.8% vs 9.8%, $P<0.001$).

Reanalysis of the Bivalirudin Angioplasty Trial including the entire intention-to-treat cohort (4312 patients) indicated a significant benefit of bivalirudin regarding the end-point of death/MI/repeat revascularization at seven days and 90 days (6.2% vs 7.9%, $P=0.04$ and 15.7% vs 18.5%, respectively, $P<0.05$). Major bleeding was again less frequent with bivalirudin than UFH (3.5% vs 9.3%, $P<0.001$).[26]

On the basis of these trials, bivalirudin does appear to be more effective and safer than UFH in ACS patients undergoing PCI. However, the high dose of heparin described above resulted in a median ACT of 383 seconds in the UFH group (as compared to 346 seconds in the bivalirudin group, $P<0.001$) which is higher than the recommended ACT, and this might have handicapped the UFH arm.

Bivalirudin+ GP IIb/IIIa inhibitors

The Randomised Evaluation in PCI Linking Angiomax to Reduced Clinical Events (REPLACE)-1 trial was designed to test the safety and efficacy of bivalirudin with or without GP IIb/IIIa antagonist, compared with low-dose weight-adjusted heparin plus GP IIb/IIIa antagonist. There was a nonsignificant reduction in the composite end-point of death/MI/revascularization in the bivalirudin arm as compared with heparin (5.6% vs 6.9%, $P=$NS). The incidence of major bleeding was similar in the two groups (2.1% vs 2.7%, $P=$NS).[27]

In the CACHET trial,[28] patients undergoing elective PCI were randomly allocated to a control group of low-dose UFH and abciximab or one of three bivalirudin arms (Table 3.5). In arms B and C abciximab was used 'provisionally' in 24% of patients. The composite end-point of death/MI/repeat revascularization or major bleeding at seven days occurred in 10.6% of the control group versus 3.3%, 5.9%, and 0% for the bivalirudin groups A, B and C respectively ($P=0.018$ for the pooled bivalirudin groups vs heparin). On the basis of these pilot studies, it appears that the safety benefits of bivalirudin may potentially be extended to contemporary practice with planned or provisional GP IIb/IIIa blockade.

Table 3.5 Doses of bivalirudin used in different settings of PCI

Trials	PCI setting	Bivalirudin dosage	Concomitant antithrombotic therapy
Bivalirudin Angioplasty Trial[24]	Unstable or postinfarction angina	1.0 mg/kg IV bolus 2.5 mg/kg/h IV 4 h infusion 0.2 mg/kg/h infusion up to 20 h, if needed	Aspirin
REPLACE–1[27]	Urgent/elective PCI (mainly elective)	0.75 mg/kg IV bolus 1.75 mg/kg/h IV infusion during procedure*	Aspirin/clopidogrel/provisional GP IIb/IIIa inhibitors
REPLACE–2[29]			
CACHET[28]	Elective PCI	Arm A: 1 mg/kg IV bolus + 2.5 mg/kg/h 4 h infusion Arm B: 0.5 mg/kg IV bolus +1.75 mg/kg/h infusion Arm C: 0.75 mg bolus + 1.75 mg/kg/h infusion	Aspirin/abciximab (only provisional in arms B and C)

* Corresponds to the actual recommended dosage (Angiomax® package insert per June 2005), in which infusion can be continued up to 4 hours. After 4 hours, an additional IV infusion, 0.2 mg/kg/h, may be initiated, if needed, for up to 20 hours.

The REPLACE-2 trial[29] aimed to determine whether bivalirudin, with GP IIb/IIIa blockade used on a provisional basis, was not inferior to what was taken as the standard of care of low-dose unfractionated heparin with planned GP IIb/IIIa blockade. The incidence of the primary composite end-point of death/MI/urgent repeat revascularization or in-hospital major bleeding at 30 days was similar in both groups while only 7.2% of patients in the bivalirudin group received GP IIb/IIIa inhibitors. In-hospital major bleeding rates were significantly reduced with bivalirudin (2.4% vs 4.1%, $P<0.001$). However, the median peak ACT for the heparin plus GP IIb/IIIa antagonist group in REPLACE-2 was 320 seconds, which is higher than recommended by the official ACC/AHA guidelines, and than seen in modern GP IIb/IIIa antagonist studies.

The results of the ongoing ACUITY trial comparing bivalirudin with or without GP IIb/IIIa inhibitors with enoxaparin + GP IIb/IIIa inhibitors among more than 13,000 patients undergoing early invasive management for non-ST elevation ACS should provide more definitive conclusions.

Usual doses of bivalirudin in different settings of PCI are reported in Table 3.5.

Other anticoagulants

Other strategies for anticoagulation are under investigation, including inhibitors of factor Xa. The development of fondaparinux, a synthetic factor Xa inhibitor, is to date the most advanced. The preliminary results of the OASIS-5 trial were presented at the 2005 European Society of Cardiology annual meeting. In this trial, 20,000 patients with NSTE-ACS were randomized to receive either fondaparinux or enoxaparin on top of other antithrombotic therapies as per local practice. The primary efficacy end-point of death/MI/recurrent ischemia at nine days was similar in fondaparinux- and enoxaparin-treated patients. The primary safety end-point of major bleeding at nine days occurred significantly more often in the enoxaparin group (4% vs 2.1% in the fondaparinux group, $P<0.00001$). Also, the composite risk/benefit end-point of death/MI/recurrent ischemia/major bleeding at nine days was significantly more frequent in enoxaparin-allocated patients (HR 0.82, 95% CI 0.74–0.90). If these results are confirmed by further studies, fondaparinux might be an interesting anticoagulation regimen in the setting of PCI for ACS.

CONCLUSION

The development of antithrombotic combination therapy, controlling both platelet aggregation and coagulation, has increased the safety and efficacy of PCI. Antithrombotic combinations should be adapted in each patient considering both thrombotic and hemorrhagic risk. Hence the spectrum of such combinations could go from simple aspirin–clopidogrel–LMWH in low-risk patients undergoing elective PCI to highly active aspirin–high loading dose of clopidogrel–LMWH–GP IIb/IIIa inhibitor in the setting of primary PCI for acute MI. Such highly active antithrombotic combinations are more securely used with 6 or 5 F guiding catheters, the transradial approach or the use of femoral closure devices.

The past ten years have dramatically changed antithrombotic therapy during PCI. Several new antithrombotic drugs with various efficacy and safety profiles are being investigated in different clinical settings, promising interesting changes in the management of PCI patients.

REFERENCES

1. Antithrombotic Trialists' Collaboration. Collaborative meta-analysis of randomised trials of antiplatelet therapy for prevention of death, myocardial infarction, and stroke in high risk patients. BMJ 2002;324:71–86.
2. Silber S, Albertsson P, Aviles FF et al. Task Force for Percutaneous Coronary Interventions of the European Society of Cardiology. Guidelines for percutaneous coronary interventions. The Task Force for Percutaneous Coronary Interventions of the European Society of Cardiology. Eur Heart J 2005;26:804–7.
3. Popma JJ, Berger P, Ohman EM, Harrington RA, Grines C, Weitz JI. Antithrombotic therapy during percutaneous coronary intervention: the Seventh ACCP Conference on Antithrombotic and Thrombolytic Therapy. Chest 2004;126(3 Suppl):576S–599S.
4. Schomig A, Neumann FJ, Kastrati A et al. A randomized comparison of antiplatelet and anticoagulant therapy after the placement of coronary-artery stents. N Engl J Med 1996;334:1084–9.
5. Bertrand ME, Rupprecht HJ, Urban P et al. Double-blind study of the safety of clopidogrel with and without a loading dose in combination with aspirin compared with ticlopidine in combination with aspirin after coronary stenting: the Clopidogrel Aspirin Stent International Cooperative study (CLASSICS). Circulation 2000;102:624–9.
6. Bhatt DL, Bertrand ME, Berger PB et al. Meta-analysis of randomized and registry comparisons of ticlopidine with clopidogrel after stenting. J Am Coll Cardiol 2002;39(1):9–14.
7. Mehta SR, Yusuf S, Peters RJ et al. Clopidogrel in Unstable angina to prevent Recurrent Events (CURE) Trial Investigators. Effects of pretreatment with clopidogrel and aspirin followed by long-term therapy in patients undergoing percutaneous coronary intervention: the PCI-CURE study. Lancet 2001;358:527–33.
8. Steinhubl SR, Berger PB, Mann JT 3rd et al; CREDO Investigators. Clopidogrel for the Reduction of Events During Observation. Early and sustained dual oral antiplatelet therapy following percutaneous coronary intervention: a randomized controlled trial. JAMA 2002;288:2411–20.
9. Kandzari DE, Berger PB, Kastrati A et al. ISAR-REACT Study Investigators. Influence of treatment duration with a 600-mg dose of clopidogrel before percutaneous coronary revascularization. J Am Coll Cardiol 2004;44:2133–6.
10. Montalescot G. Assessment of the Best Loading Dose of Clopidogrel to Blunt Platelet Activation, Inflammation, and Ongoing Necrosis (ALBION) Trial. Results presented at EuroPCR, May 24 2005, Paris, France.
11. Karvouni E, Katritsis DG, Ioannidis JP. Intravenous glycoprotein IIb/IIIa receptor antagonists reduce mortality after percutaneous coronary interventions. J Am Coll Cardiol 2003;41:26–32.
12. Kastrati A, Mehilli J, Schuhlen H et al. Intracoronary Stenting and Antithrombotic Regimen-Rapid Early Action for Coronary Treatment Study Investigators. A clinical trial of abciximab in elective percutaneous coronary intervention after pretreatment with clopidogrel. N Engl J Med 2004;350:232–8.
13. Mehilli J, Kastrati A, Schuhlen H et al. Intracoronary Stenting and Antithrombotic Regimen: Is Abciximab a Superior Way to Eliminate Elevated Thrombotic Risk in Diabetics (ISAR-SWEET) Study Investigators. Randomized clinical trial of abciximab in diabetic patients undergoing elective percutaneous coronary interventions after treatment with a high loading dose of clopidogrel. Circulation 2004;110:3627–35.
14. Gollapudi RR, Teirstein PS, Stevenson DD, Simon RA. Aspirin sensitivity: implications for patients with coronary artery disease. JAMA 2004;292:3017–23.
15. Smith SC Jr, Dove JT, Jacobs AK et al. ACC/AHA guidelines of percutaneous coronary interventions (revision of the 1993 PTCA guidelines) – executive summary. A report of the American College of Cardiology/American Heart Association Task Force on Practice Guidelines (Committee to Revise the 1993 Guidelines for Percutaneous Transluminal Coronary Angioplasty). J Am Coll Cardiol 2001;37:2215–39.

16. Cohen M, Theroux P, Borzak S et al. Randomized double-blind safety study of enoxaparin versus unfractionated heparin in patients with non-ST-segment elevation acute coronary syndromes treated with tirofiban and aspirin: the ACUTE II study. The Antithrombotic Combination Using Tirofiban and Enoxaparin. Am Heart J 2002;144:470–7.

17. Blazing MA, de Lemos JA, White HD et al. Safety and efficacy of enoxaparin vs unfractionated heparin in patients with non-ST-segment elevation acute coronary syndromes who receive tirofiban and aspirin: a randomized controlled trial. JAMA 2004;292:55–64.

18. Goodman SG, Fitchett D, Armstrong PW, Tan M, Langer A. Randomized evaluation of the safety and efficacy of enoxaparin versus unfractionated heparin in high-risk patients with non-ST-segment elevation acute coronary syndromes receiving the glycoprotein IIb/IIIa inhibitor eptifibatide. Circulation 2003;107:238–44.

19. Collet JP, Montalescot G, Lison L et al. Percutaneous coronary intervention after subcutaneous enoxaparin pretreatment in patients with unstable angina pectoris. Circulation 2001;103:658–63.

20. Ferguson JJ, Antman EM, Bates ER et al. Combining enoxaparin and glycoprotein IIb/IIIa antagonists for the treatment of acute coronary syndromes: final results of the National Investigators Collaborating on Enoxaparin–3 (NICE–3) study. Am Heart J 2003;146:628–34.

21. Ferguson JJ, Califf RM, Antman EM et al. Enoxaparin vs unfractionated heparin in high-risk patients with non-ST-segment elevation acute coronary syndromes managed with an intended early invasive strategy: primary results of the SYNERGY randomized trial. JAMA 2004;292:45–54.

22. Kereiakes DJ, Montalescot G, Antman EM et al. Low-molecular-weight heparin therapy for non-ST-elevation acute coronary syndromes and during percutaneous coronary intervention: an expert consensus. Am Heart J 2002;144:615–24.

23. Borentain M, Montalescot G, Bouzamondo A, Choussat R, Hulot JS, Lechat P. Low-molecular-weight heparin vs. unfractionated heparin in percutaneous coronary intervention: a combined analysis. Cathet Cardiovasc Interv 2005;65:212–21.

24. Montalescot GM, for the STEEPLE Investigators. Safety and efficacy of intravenous enoxaparin in elective percutaneous coronary intervention: an international randomized evaluation. Results presented at the European Society of Cardiology Congress, Stockholm, 2005.

25. Bittl JA, Strony J, Brinker JA et al. Treatment with bivalirudin (Hirulog) as compared with heparin during coronary angioplasty for unstable or postinfarction angina. Hirulog Angioplasty Study Investigators. N Engl J Med 1995;333:764–9.

26. Bittl JA, Chaitman BR, Feit F, Kimball W, Topol EJ. Bivalirudin versus heparin during coronary angioplasty for unstable or postinfarction angina: final report reanalysis of the Bivalirudin Angioplasty Study. Am Heart J 2001;142:952–9.

27. Lincoff AM, Bittl JA, Kleiman NS et al. Comparison of bivalirudin versus heparin during percutaneous coronary intervention (the Randomized Evaluation of PCI Linking Angiomax to Reduced Clinical Events [REPLACE]–1 trial). Am J Cardiol 2004;93:1092–6.

28. Lincoff AM, Kleiman NS, Kottke-Marchant K et al. Bivalirudin with planned or provisional abciximab versus low-dose heparin and abciximab during percutaneous coronary revascularization: results of the Comparison of Abciximab Complications with Hirulog for Ischemic Events Trial (CACHET). Am Heart J 2002;143(5):847–53.

29. Lincoff AM, Bittl JA, Harrington RA et al. REPLACE–2 Investigators. Bivalirudin and provisional glycoprotein IIb/IIIa blockade compared with heparin and planned glycoprotein IIb/IIIa blockade during percutaneous coronary intervention: REPLACE–2 randomized trial. JAMA 2003;289(7):853–63.

4

Femoral vascular access and vascular bleeding complications

Jose A Silva and Christopher J White

Bleeding complications following common femoral arterial access • Hematoma • Pseudoaneurysm • Retroperitoneal bleeding • Conclusion

The common femoral artery (CFA) is the most frequently used vascular access for the performance of both coronary and peripheral vascular diagnostic angiography and interventional procedures. In a report from the 1990 Registry of the Society for Cardiac Angiography and Interventions, CFA access was used in 83% of diagnostic and 96% of interventional procedures.[1] Compared to upper extremity arterial access sites, the CFA vascular access has several advantages, including a larger diameter, allowing easier cannulation and the introduction of larger catheters, as well as the possibility of repeat vascular access in the same patient almost immediately. Its anatomic location over the femoral head allows for compression of the puncture site to achieve hemostasis after catheter removal.

The technique of CFA access is relatively simple and safe when properly performed and cardiologists, as well as other interventionalists, usually have a great deal of experience with it. However, bleeding complications do occur, which may vary in severity from self-limited hematomas to life-threatening retroperitoneal hemorrhages. In this chapter we will address the most common bleeding complications related to the femoral arterial vascular access.

Common femoral arterial access: practical tips

The technique for CFA vascular access has been described previously.[2] A few points are worth emphasizing. First, the operator must remember that the inguinal skin crease is highly variable in relation to the CFA and has been shown to be located caudal to the CFA bifurcation in up to 75% of patients (Figure 4.1).[3] Consequently, when access is attempted, after palpating the femoral pulse, identifying the femoral head under fluoroscopy is very helpful. It has been shown that puncturing the CFA at this level ensures access below the inguinal ligament and above the level of the CFA bifurcation.[4]

Antegrade CFA access is very useful for performing lower extremity vascular angiography and interventions of the mid to distal femoropopliteal or infrapopliteal arteries. However, it is more technically demanding and may carry a higher complication rate than retrograde CFA access. Complications such as retroperitoneal bleeding may occur if the access is 'too' proximal, or hematoma, pseudoaneurysm or

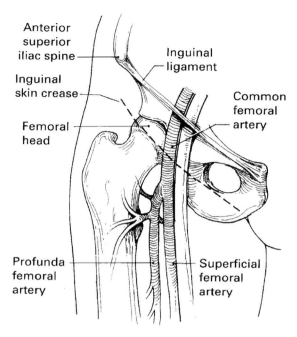

Figure 4.1   Right femoral area. Relation of the common femoral artery with the femoral head and inguinal ligament. Reproduced with permission from Silva JA, White CJ. Peripheral vascular intervention. In: Kern MJ, ed. The interventional cardiac catheterization handbook, 2nd edn. Philadelphia: Elsevier, 2004.

arteriovenous fistulas if the access is 'too' distal. When entering the CFA in an antegrade fashion, it is important to identify the femoral head under fluoroscopy.

Depending on the amount of subcutaneous tissue, a skin incision is made 1–2 cm superior or cranial to the femoral head. After the CFA pulse is located over the femoral head, the percutaneous needle is introduced through the skin incision and directed obliquely and caudally toward the center of the femoral head.[4] Once the CFA has been entered, a steerable guidewire is advanced under fluoroscopic guidance toward the superficial femoral artery (SFA) which is medial to the profunda femoris artery (PFA). It is important to emphasize that at their origin, there is overlapping of the SFA and PFA in the anteroposterior fluoroscopic view. Therefore, when performing antegrade access, the operator must use the ipsilateral oblique view (20–40°) in order to separate the origin of these two vessels. Relative contraindications to this approach include atherosclerotic disease of the CFA or proximal SFA and extreme obesity.

BLEEDING COMPLICATIONS FOLLOWING COMMON FEMORAL ARTERIAL ACCESS

Access site bleeding complications including hematomas, pseudoaneurysms, and retroperitoneal hemorrhage are the most frequent complications following vascular access from the CFA with a reported incidence of 2–6%.[5–7] In a series of surgically treated groin complications following percutaneous cardiac procedures, groin hematomas (11.2%), pseudoaneurysms (61.2%), and retroperitoneal bleeding (5.1%) accounted for nearly 80% of the cases.[8] In Table 4.1 we have summarized the most important risk factors for developing bleeding complications after CFA vascular access.[9,10] Although it seems intuitive to expect a lower bleeding rate when arterial access is obtained with a smaller vascular sheath,[11,12] some studies have found that a larger sheath size did not correlate with an increased risk for bleeding.[5,7] Other general measures, such as early sheath removal and discontinuation of heparin post procedure, are of utmost importance for decreasing bleeding complications.[13] In addition, numerous studies have now demonstrated that the dose of unfractionated heparin must be adjusted to no more than 70 iu/kg when platelet IIb/IIIa inhibitors are given.[14]

Table 4.1   Risk factors related to increase bleeding complications
Female gender
Hypertension
Older age
Obesity
Low body weight
Larger heparin dose
Use of fibrinolytics
Use of IIb/IIIa inhibitors
Prolonged in-dwelling sheath time
Larger sheath diameter

HEMATOMA

The incidence of hematoma, defined as a significant swelling in the femoral region requiring blood transfusion or a decrease ($\geq$15 points from baseline) in the hematocrit, has been reported to be in the range of 0.9–2.8%.[5,15] In the majority of patients, its occurrence is clinically obvious and if there is persistence of bleeding, hematoma enlargement can be managed with simple manual compression. In rare instances, particularly in morbidly obese patients, the development of this complication may be missed and patients may lose a significant amount of blood before the hemorrhage is detected and therapy instituted. The clinical signs are of an enlarging mass in the groin or in the thigh, with or without hypotension. In extreme cases hypovolemic shock may develop.

When significant bleeding is suspected, therapy must be commenced without delay, starting with manual compression of the groin and volume resuscitation with crystalloid solutions and blood replacement. In some cases, effective arterial compression may be difficult to achieve due to the patient's body habitus. An endovascular measure that we have found effective in achieving hemostasis for persistent bleeding is balloon occlusion of the CFA. This is accomplished by obtaining contralateral CFA access or brachial artery vascular access.

Patients with persistent bleeding after all conservative measures may be treated with covered stents or may be referred for surgical repair. It is important to remember that the use of stents in the CFA, although safe in selected patients,[16] may prevent future vascular access in this location. In addition, the use of covered stents may obstruct the origin of the PFA. Consequently, the interventionalist has to gauge whether covered stents are suitable in this particular location. Alternatively, the patient may be referred for surgical repair and hematoma evacuation since vascular laceration may be the underlying cause of bleeding.

PSEUDOANEURYSM

The reported incidence of femoral pseudoaneurysms ranges from 0.1% to 1.5% after diagnostic angiography and 2.1–6% following interventional procedures.[5,17,18] However, the incidence has been found to be higher (7.7%) when routine Doppler ultrasound is performed after noninterventional or interventional percutaneous procedures,[19] as well as with the use of IIb/IIIa inhibitors or with a higher procedural complexity.[7,20] This complication occurs as a result of blood accumulation around an unsealed arterial puncture, that creates a false lumen.

The clinical presentation of pseudoaneurysms is usually a painful pulsatile mass in the groin area. Often, a bruit is audible on auscultation of this area and, rarely, the pseudoanueyrsm will compress the femoral vein and/or nerve or cause deep vein thrombosis and/or neuropathic symptoms. The clinical findings of femoral pseudoaneurysms may be difficult to differentiate from those of hematomas; therefore the diagnosis is usually made by color flow Doppler which shows a characteristic echolucent, extraluminal cavity in communication with the adjacent common femoral artery.[21]

The treatment of this complication depends on the size of the pseudoaneursym and the presence of symptoms. As a general rule, pseudoaneursyms of ≤2 cm in diameter may be treated conservatively, with observation, since most of them resolve spontaneously. On the other hand, symptomatic pseudoaneurysms >2 cm in diameter usually need to be treated, since most of them do not resolve spontaneously.[10] The treatment may be surgical repair or nonsurgical therapy.

Ultrasound-guided compression

This nonsurgical treatment uses the ultrasound probe to compress the psuedoaneurysm neck. This compression causes sealing of the arterial neck (original puncture site), ultimately leading to stasis, thrombosis, and resolution of the false aneurysm. The technique was first described by Fellmeth et al in 1991[22] and has enjoyed mixed success and acceptance in the interventional community, with a reported success rate ranging from 55% to 90%.[17,22–25] There are several drawbacks with this therapy. It may be time consuming, as the average compression time has been reported to be approximately 30 minutes, with a range of 10–300 minutes.[18] The probe compression may cause a great deal of discomfort for which analgesia and sedation may be required. If long-term anticoagulation is necessary, close surveillance is crucial following compression, since the likelihood of recurrence and/or rupture of the pseudoaneurysm is enhanced.[25] Patients with significant obesity, large pseudoaneurysm size or severe groin discomfort during compression are at increased risk for failure with ultrasound compression.[17,18,25] Finally, ultrasound-guided compression therapy should be avoided in patients with a groin infection or with limb-threatening ischemia.

Ultrasound-guided thrombin injection

Thrombin injection into the pseudoaneurysm lumen under ultrasound guidance, although not FDA approved for this purpose, has been shown to be highly effective for treating pseudoaneurysms, with a reported success rate of 86–96%.[26–30] Under ultrasound guidance, the tip of the needle is positioned within the pseudoaneurysm. The operator then aspirates blood to confirm the position and then injects thrombin (500–1000 units) directly into the pseudoaneurysm. This causes immediate blood coagulation, with dramatic alleviation of the patient's symptoms. A potential complication of this form of therapy is that the injected thrombin may pass into the arterial lumen through the pseudoaneursym neck, leading to distal embolization. In a series of 70 pseudoaneurysms treated with this technique, no events of arterial thromboses were reported.[29] In another report of 23 pseudoaneurysms, two patients developed this complication.[30] The operator should try to minimize this complication by directing the needle away from the neck of the pseudoaneurysm.

In order to prevent thrombin from entering the arterial lumen, a balloon catheter may be inflated on the arterial side of the pseudoaneurysm neck. This is accomplished by obtaining vascular access from the contralateral CFA or brachial artery. Once the balloon catheter is inflated (sized 1:1 with the reference vessel diameter), the flow between the pseudoaneurysm and arterial lumen is impaired and thrombin can be injected safely into the pseudoaneurysm lumen. In a report from our institution, four patients were successfully treated using this technique.[31] The stasis induced by balloon occlusion facilitates thrombosis of the pseudoaneurysm, using a minimal amount of thrombin (Figure 4.2).

Another significant problem with the use of bovine thrombin is immunologic cross-reactivity and anaphylactic reactions. The former may manifest as bradycardia, hypotension, and by the formation of coagulation factor inhibitors.[32,33] The latter is a serious manifestation which usually occurs after repeated exposures to bovine thrombin, and it is recommended that all patients with previous exposures to bovine thrombin should undergo skin testing.[34]

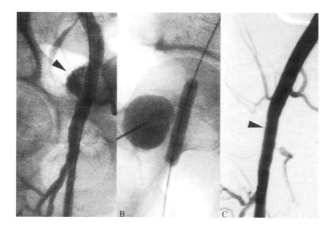

Figure 4.2 Pseudoaneurysm treated with thrombin after angiography and balloon occlusion of the CFA. Reproduced with permission.[10]

Biodegradable collagen injection

With this technique, biodegradable adhesive bovine collagen is injected percutaneously through an 11 F sheath, into the pseudoaneurysm, guided by angiography from the contralateral femoral access. In a report from The Netherlands, 107 of 110 (98%) pseudoaneurysms were successfully closed with this percutaneous therapy.[35] The major advantage of this technique is that the collagen plug has minimal chance of embolization to the arterial circulation through the pseudoaneurysm neck. The major disadvantage of this technique is the need for angiography from contralateral access and the large sheath for the collagen plug injection.

Covered stents

Covered stents are effective for excluding aneurysms and pseudoaneurysms in vascular territories with the increased risk of stent thrombosis.[36-38] More recently, it has been shown that covered stents may also be used for the treatment of femoral artery pseudoaneurysms in selected patients.[39,40] In one report, 26 of 29 postcatheterization femoral pseudoaneurysms (n=16) or arteriovenous fistulas (n=10), located in the superficial femoral (n=16), profunda (n=6) and common femoral (n=4) arteries, were successfully treated with covered stents.[40] In three patients, the procedure failed due to aneurysm location at the bifurcation of the CFA (n=2) or significant tortuosity of the iliac artery (n=1). At one-year follow-up, four patients (17%) had developed stent thrombosis.

The use of stents in the CFA is controversial and is only indicated in selected patients, when other treatment measures have failed.[16] Stents in the CFA may render further vascular access difficult or impossible, and may increase the likelihood of stent fracture, compression, thrombosis, and late restenosis since this vessel is located at a joint and subject to significant bending. Furthermore, the use of covered stents for the treatment of pseudoaneurysms in the bifurcation of the CFA may occlude the PFA. Consequently, the interventionalist must keep in mind all these pitfalls and potential complications before considering the use of covered stents as a treatment for pseudoaneurysms in the femoral artery.

Coil embolization

Pseudoaneurysms may be successfully closed with coil embolization.[39,41,42] The coils can be delivered by direct puncture of the pseudoaneurysm or in the aneurysm neck, through a guiding catheter advanced from the contralateral CFA access.[39,41] The major drawback of this technique is that it may be time consuming, and the coils may cause local discomfort and skin pressure necrosis if they are deployed superficially.

Surgical therapy

Until the advent of percutaneous interventional techniques, surgery was the treatment of choice for these patients. However, surgery is a relatively unattractive therapeutic option due to the surgical morbidity and mortality.[43,44] In addition, surgery is associated with a small incidence of local complications such as wound infection and postoperative discomfort, which may lead to a prolonged hospital stay. Surgical treatment of postcatheterization femoral artery pseudoaneurysms should be reserved for patients in whom percutaneous therapeutic modalities have failed or are not available.

RETROPERITONEAL BLEEDING

Retroperitoneal bleeding is a relatively unusual, but potentially fatal, complication after endovascular diagnostic or interventional procedures performed from CFA vascular access. The true incidence of retroperitoneal bleeding is difficult to determine; however, it has been reported to be in the range of 0.12–0.44% after percutaneous interventional procedures.[5,20,45–49] In a recent study of almost 11,000 unselected patients who underwent PCI, retroperitoneal bleeding occurred in 0.27%.[50]

The risk of bleeding into the retroperitoneal space increases with a high femoral puncture (above the inguinal ligament). In addition, several studies have found that older age (>80 years), female gender, peripheral vascular disease, postprocedural anticoagulation, low platelet count, use of fibrinolytic agents,[5,13,20,47] and more recently an activated clotting time during PCI with the use of IIb/IIIa platelet receptor inhibitors are all independent predictors for postprocedural development of retroperitoneal bleeding.[51–53]

The signs and symptoms of retroperitoneal bleeding usually consist of hypotension, nausea, vomiting, abdominal distension, fullness or abdominal pain. The ipsilateral lower quadrant or flank may appear mildly distended on simple inspection and this area may be tender to palpation. However, every patient who becomes hypotensive after a femoral vascular access procedure should raise the suspicion of retroperitoneal hemorrhage. If hemodynamically significant bleeding is suspected, therapy should be instituted without delay while the diagnosis is confirmed. The diagnosis of retroperitoneal bleeding may be confirmed with computed tomography, ultrasound of the abdomen and pelvis or selective angiography.

When the diagnosis of retroperitoneal blood loss is suspected, anticoagulation must be reversed or discontinued. These patients need close surveillance, preferably in the intensive care unit. Hypotension usually responds to volume resuscitation with crystaloid solutions and blood replacement. If necessary, pressors may be administered. Most patients respond well to these measures and in the majority of cases, this form of bleeding subsides spontaneously. In patients who fail conservative therapy, a severe form of bleeding should be suspected and more aggressive treatment must be started promptly, since death may occur in this group of patients.[49] The traditional treatment for patients with persistent retroperitoneal bleeding has been surgical repair.[43,44,46,54] However, since many of these individuals have significant coronary artery disease and other co-morbidities, surgical intervention in this group of patients may pose further risk, with some studies showing a surgical morbidity rate of 21%, including myocardial infarction and wound complications, and a mortality rate of 2–5%.[43,44]

Catheter-based approaches have recently been shown to offer an alternative treatment of this complication. Percutaneous therapy leads to rapid restoration of hemodynamic stability without exposing patients to the morbidity and mortality risk associated with surgery. At our institution, patients who remain hypotensive or have recurrence of hemodynamic instability after fluid resuscitation and blood transfusion are taken to the catheterization suite for angiographic confirmation of the bleeding site and, if possible, balloon tamponade of the bleeding site.[55,56] If bleeding persists after prolonged balloon inflation and the anatomy is favorable, the interventionalist may choose to place a covered stent (Figure 4.3).[10] If the anatomy is not favorable for deployment of a covered stent, the patient may be referred for surgical repair. It is important to keep the balloon inflated while awaiting surgery, and to proceed with balloon deflation in the operation room only when the surgeon has gained vascular access and is ready to proceed with repair.

Occasionally, laceration of a small branch arising from the CFA or the external iliac artery (such as the inferior epigastric artery) may be the culprit causing retroperitoneal bleeding. Successful hemostasis can be obtained by selectively engaging the vessel from contralateral access with a 6 F guiding catheter (JR-4, IMA) and proceeding with delivery of coils or balloon catheter delivery of thrombin (Figures 4.4, 4.5).[10,57]

Vascular closure devices and bleeding complications

Vascular access closure devices have gained popularity among invasive cardiologists, because they provide prompt hemostasis and early ambulation.[58–63] However, these

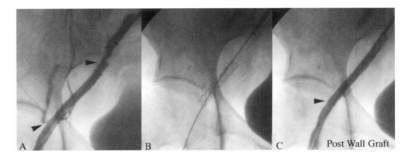

Figure 4.3   Retroperitoneal bleeding, treated with a covered stent. Reproduced with permission.[10]

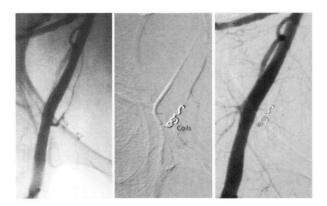

Figure 4.4   Retroperitoneal bleeding caused by laceration of the inferior epigastric artery, successfully treated with coil embolization. Reproduced with permission.[10]

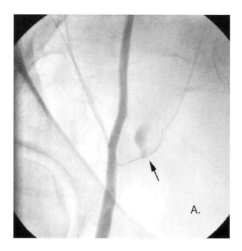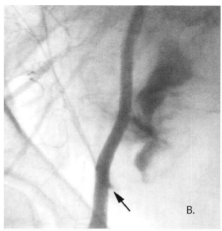

Figure 4.5   A. Retroperitoneal bleeding caused by laceration of the inferior epigastric artery. B. Successfully treated with catheter delivery of thrombin. Reproduced with permission.[16]

devices have not yet demonstrated a reduction in the bleeding complication rate when compared with manual compression. Furthermore, the use of these devices has introduced other complications which are specific to this technology, such as local infections which, although rare, may lead to significant morbidity.

In a retrospective report of 425 patients treated with a collagen plug closure device (Angioseal, Daig, St. Paul, MN), device failure occurred in 8%, bleeding complications in 0.2%, pseudoaneurysms in 0.5%, femoral artery stenoses in 1.4%, infections in 0.2%, and need for surgical repair in 1.6%.[58] In another prospective nonrandomized study, two collagen plug devices, the Vasoseal (Datascope, Montvale, NJ) (n=937) and the Angioseal (n=732), and a suture mediated device (Techstar, Perclose, Redwood City, CA) (n=1001) were compared with manual compression (n=1019) to achieve hemostasis.[59] The two collagen plug devices had a significantly higher complication rate (surgical repair, acute occlusion, transfusions, readmissions, and infections), and the suture-mediated device had a similar complication rate as the patients treated with manual compression (Figure 4.6).

In a retrospective series of 1200 patients using the Techstar suture-mediated device for vascular hemostasis, bleeding complications were reported in a significant number of patients (Table 4.2).[60] Another study comparing the Vasoseal and the Perclose with assisted manual compression (Femostop) after percutaneous coronary interventions requiring abciximab found a significantly higher success rate for the Femostop compression device (100%), compared to the Vasoseal (78.8%) and the Perclose (85.7%; $P <0.001$).[63]

CONCLUSION

The CFA is the most commonly used vascular access site for diagnostic and therapeutic invasive vascular procedures. Hematoma formation, pseudoaneurysm, and retroperitoneal hemorrhage are the most frequent complications following

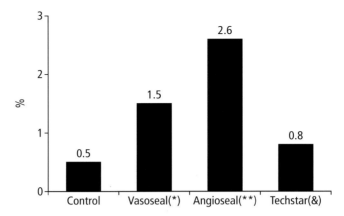

Figure 4.6 Complications of different vascular closure devices versus manual compression (control) to achieve hemostasis. (*) $P=0.02$ versus control; (**) $P=0.0002$ versus control; (&) $P=$NS versus control.[59]

Table 4.2 Complications related to vascular closure devices

Closure device	Hematoma	Retroperitoneal hemorrhage	Pseudoaneurysm	Infection
Angioseal[58]	–	0.2%	0.5%	0.2%
Techstar[60]	2.1%	0.3%	0.1%	0.5%
Duett[61]	4.7%	–	–	–

vascular access from the CFA, with a reported incidence of 2–6%. Although in the majority of the cases these complications are self-limited, some may carry significant risk of morbidity or may even be life-threatening, particularly retroperitoneal bleeding. Physicians must be vigilant for bleeding complications and have a low threshold to initiate therapy. Surgery, the traditional treatment of these complications, has been largely replaced with percutaneous catheter-based techniques.

REFERENCES

1. Noto TJ, Johnson LW, Krone R et al. Cardiac catheterization 1990: a report of the Registry of the Society for Cardiac Angiography and Interventions (SCA&I). Cathet Cardiovasc Diagn 1991;24:75–83.
2. Seldinger SI. Catheter placement of the needle in percutaneous arteriography. A new technique. Acta Radiol 1953;39:368–76.
3. Lechner G, Jantsch H, Waneck R, Kretschmer G. The relationship between the common femoral artery, the inguinal crease, and the inguinal ligament: a guide to accurate angiographic puncture. Cardiovasc Intervent Radiol 1988;11:165–9.
4. Spijkerboer AM, Scholten FG, Mali WPT, van Schaik JP. Antegrade puncture of the femoral artery: morphologic study. Cardiovasc Radiol 1990;176:50–60.
5. Popma JJ, Satler LF, Pichard AD et al. Vascular complications after balloon and new device complications. Circulation 1993;88:1568–78.

6. Johnson LW, Esente P, Giambartolomei A et al. Peripheral vascular complications of coronary angioplasty by the femoral and brachial techniques. Cathet Cardiovasc Diagn 1994;31:165–72.

7. Waksman R, King SB III, Douglas JS et al. Predictors of groin complications after balloon and new-device coronary intervention. Am J Cardiol 1995;75:886–9.

8. Lumsden AB, Miller JM, Kosinski AS et al. A prospective evaluation of surgically treated groin complications following percutaneous cardiac procedures. Am Surg 1994;60:132–7.

9. Wiley JM, White CJ, Uretsky BF. Noncoronary complications of coronary intervention. Cathet Cardiovasc Intervent 2002;57:257–65.

10. Samal AK, White CJ. Percutaneous management of access site complications. Cathet Cardiovasc Intervent 2002;57:12–23.

11. Metz D, Meyer P, Touati C et al. Comparison of 6F with 7F and 8F guiding catheters for elective coronary angioplasty: results of a prospective, multicenter, randomized trial. Am Heart J 1997;134:131–7.

12. Aguirre FV, Topol EJ, Ferguson JJ et al. Bleeding complications with the chimeric antibody to platelet glycoprotein IIb/IIIa integrin in patients undergoing percutaneous coronary intervention. Circulation 1995;91:2882–90.

13. Piper WD, Malenka DJ, Ryan TJ et al. Predicting vascular complications in percutaneous coronary interventions. Am Heart J 2003;145:1022–9.

14. EPILOG Investigators. Effects of platelet glycoprotein IIb/IIIa receptor inhibitor abciximab with lower heparin dosages on ischemic complications of percutaneous coronary revascularization. N Engl J Med 1997;336:1689–96.

15. Ricci MA, Trevisani TG, Pilcher DB. Vascular complications of cardiac catheterization. Am J Surg 1994;167:375–8.

16. Silva JA, White CJ, Quintana H et al. Percutaneous revascularization of the common femoral artery for limb ischemia. Cathet Cardiovasc Intervent 2004;62:230–3.

17. Chatterjee T, Do DD, Kaufmann U et al. Ultrasound-guided compression repair for treatment of femoral artery pseudoaneurysm: acute and follow-up results. Cathet Cardiovasc Diagn 1996;38:335–40.

18. Schaub F, Theiss W, Busch R et al. Management of 219 consecutive cases of postcatheterization pseudoaneurysm. J Am Coll Cardiol 1997;30:670–5.

19. Katzenschalager R, Ugurluoglu A, Ahmadi A et al. Incidence of pseudoaneurysm after diagnostic and therapeutic angiography. Radiology 1995;195:463–6.

20. Omoigui NA, Califf RM, Pieper K et al. Peripheral vascular complications in the Coronary Angioplasty Versus Excisional Atherectomy Trial (CAVEAT-I). J Am Coll Cardiol 1995;26:922–30.

21. Sheikh KM, Adams DB, McCann R et al. Utility of Doppler color flow imaging for identification of femoral arterial complications of cardiac catheterization. Am Heart J 1989;117:623–8.

22. Fellmeth BD, Baron SB, Brown PR et al. Repair of postcatheterization femoral pseudo-aneurysms by color flow ultrasound guided compression. Am Heart J 1992;123:547–51.

23. Feld R, Patton GM, Carabasi RA et al. Treatment of iatrogenic femoral artery injuries with ultrasound-guided compression. J Vasc Surg 1992;16:382–4.

24. Hajarizadeh H, LaRosa CR, Cardullo P et al. Ultrasound-guided compression of iatrogenic femoral pseudoaneurysm: failure, recurrence and long-term results. J Vasc Surg 1995;22:425–33.

25. Dean SM, Olin JW, Piedmonte M et al. Ultrasound-guided compression closure of postcatheterization pseudoaneurysm during concurrent anticoagulation: a review of seventy-seven patients. J Vasc Surg 1996;23:28–35.

26. Liau C, Ho F, Chen M et al. Treatment of iatrogenic femoral artery aneurysm with percutaneous thrombin injection. J Vasc Surg 1997;26:18–23.

27. Kang SS, Labropoulos N, Mansour MA et al. Percutaneous ultrasound guided thrombin injection: a new method for treating postcatheterization femoral pseudoaneurysm. J Vasc Surg 1998;27:1032–8.

28. Brophy DP, Sheiman RG, Amatulle P et al. Iatrogenic femoral pseudoaneurysm: thrombin injection after failed US-guided compression. Radiology 2000;214:278–82.
29. La Perna L, Olin JW, Goines D et al. Ultrasound-guided thrombin injection for the treatment of postcatheterization pseudoaneurysms. Circulation 2000;102:2391–5.
30. Pezzullo JA, Dupuy DE, Cronan JJ et al. Percutaneous injection of thrombin for the treatment of pseudoaneurysms after catheterization: an alternative to sonographic guided compression. Am J Roentgenol 2000;175:1035–40.
31. Samal AK, White CJ, Collins TJ et al. Treatment of femoral artery pseudoaneurysm with percutaneous thrombin injection. Cathet Cardiovasc Intervent 2001;53:259–63.
32. AHFS drug information. Hemostatics 1997;20:12–16.
33. Dorion RP, Hamati HF, Landis B et al. Risk and clinical significance of developing antibodies induced by topical thrombin preparations. Arch Pathol Lab Med 1998;12:887–94.
34. Pope M, Johnston KW. Anaphylaxis after thrombin injection of femoral pseudoaneurysm: recommendations for prevention. Vasc Surg 2000;32:190–1.
35. Hamraoui K, Ernst SM, van Dessel PF et al. Efficacy and safety of percutaneous treatment of iatrogenic femoral artery pseudoaneurysm by biodegradable collagen injection. J Am Coll Cardiol 2002;39:1297–304.
36. Marcade JP. Stent graft for popliteal aneurysms: six cases with Cragg Endopro System 1 Mintec. J Cardiovasc Surg 1996;37(Suppl 1):41–4.
37. Gasparini D, Lovaria A, Saccheri S et al. Percutaneous treatment of iliac aneurysms and pseudoaneurysms with Cragg Endopro System 1 stent grafts. Cardiovasc Intervent Radiol 1997;20:348–52.
38. Christensen L, Justensen P, Larsen KE. Percutaneous transluminal treatment of an iliac pseudoaneurysm with endovascular implantation: a case report. Acta Radiol 1996;37:542–4.
39. Waigand J, Uhlich F, Gross CM et al. Percutaneous treatment of pseudoaneurysms and arteriovenous fistulas after invasive vascular procedures. Cathet Cardiovasc Intervent 1999;47:157–64.
40. Thalhammer C, Kirchherr AS, Uhlich F et al. Postcatheterization pseudoaneurysms and arteriovenous fistulas: repair with percutaneous implantation of endovascular covered stents. Radiology 2000;214:127–31.
41. Murray A, Buckenham TM, Belli AM et al. Direct puncture coil embolization of iatrogenic pseudoaneurysms. J Intervent Radiol 1994;9:183–6.
42. Lemair JM, Dondelinger RF. Percutaneous coil embolization of iatrogenic femoral arteriovenous fistula or pseudoaneurysm. Eur J Radiol 1994;18:96–100.
43. Franco CD, Goldsmith J, Veith FJ, Calligaro KD, Gupta SK, Wengerter KR. Management of arterial injuries produced by percutaneous femoral procedures. Surgery 1993;113:419–25.
44. Lumsden AB, Miller JM, Kosinski AS et al. A prospective evaluation of surgically treated groin complications following percutaneous cardiac procedures. Am Surg 1994;60:132–7.
45. Babu SC, Piccorelli GO, Shah PM, Stein JH, Clauss RH. Incidence and results of arterial complications among 16,530 patients undergoing cardiac catheterization. J Vasc Surg 1989;10:113–16.
46. Kent KC, Moscucci M, Mansour KA et al. Retroperitoneal hematoma after cardiac catheterization: prevalence, risk factors, and optimal management. J Vasc Surg 1994;20:905–13.
47. Johnson LW, Esente P, Giambartolomei A et al. Peripheral vascular complications of coronary angioplasty by femoral and brachial techniques. Cathet Cardiovasc Diagn 1994;31:165–72.
48. Muller DM, Shamir KJ, Ellis SG, Topol EJ. Peripheral vascular complications after conventional and complex percutaneous coronary interventional procedures. Am J Cardiol 1992;69:63–8.
49. Sreeram S, Lumsden AB, Miller JS, Salam AA, Dodson TF, Smith RB. Retroperitoneal hematomas following femoral arterial catheterization: a serious and often fatal complication. Am Surg 1993;59:94–8.

50. Kinnaird TD, Stabile E, Mintz GS et al. Incidence, predictors, and prognostic implications of bleeding and blood transfusion, following percutaneous coronary interventions. Am J Cardiol 2003;92:930–5.

51. Hillegas WB, Brott BC, Chapman GD et al. Relationship between activated clotting time during percutaneous intervention and subsequent bleeding complications. Am Heart J 2002;144:501–7.

52. Choussat R, Black A, Bossi I, Fajadet J, Marco J. Vascular complications and clinical outcome after coronary angioplasty with platelet IIb/IIIa receptor blockade. Comparison of transradial vs transfemoral arterial access. Eur Heart J 2000;21:662–7.

53. Cote AV, Berger PB, Holmes DR et al. Hemorrhagic and vascular complications after percutaneous coronary intervention with adjunctive abciximab. Mayo Clin Proc 2001;76:890–6.

54. Ricci MA, Trevisani GT, Pilcher DB. Vascular complications of cardiac catheterization. Am J Surg 1994;167:375–8.

55. Davison AT. Direct intralumen balloon tamponade. A technic for the control of massive retroperitoneal hemorrhage. Am J Surg 1978;136:393–4.

56. Mak GY, Daly B, Chan W, Tse KK, Chung HK, Woo KS. Percutaneous treatment of post catheterization massive retroperitoneal hemorrhage. Cathet Cardiovasc Diagn 1993;29:40–3.

57. Silva JA, Stant J, Ramee SR. Endovascular treatment of a massive retroperitoneal bleeding: successful balloon-catheter delivery of intra-arterial thrombin. Cathet Cardiovasc Intervent 2005;64:218–22.

58. Eidt JF, Habibipour S, Saucedo JF et al. Surgical complications from hemostatic puncture closure devices. Am J Surg 1999;178:511–16.

59. Carey D, Martin JR, Moore CA et al. Complications of femoral artery closure devices. Cathet Cardiovasc Intervent 2001;52:3–8.

60. Fram DB, Giri S, Jamil G et al. Suture closure of the femoral arteriotomy following invasive cardiac procedures: a detailed analysis of efficacy, complications, and the impact of early ambulation in 1,200 consecutive unselected patients. Cathet Cardiovasc Intervent 2001;53:163–73.

61. Mooney MR, Ellis SG, Gershoney G et al. Immediate sealing of arterial puncture sites after cardiac catheterization and coronary interventions: initial U.S. feasibility trial using the Duett vascular closure device. Cathet Cardiovasc Intervent 2000;50:96–102.

62. Lehman KG, Heath-Lange SJ, Ferris ST. Randomized comparison of hemostasis techniques after invasive cardiovascular procedures. Am Heart J 1999;138:1118–25.

63. Chamberlain JR, Lardi AB, McKeever LS et al. Use of vascular sealing devices (VasoSeal and Perclose) versus assisted manual compression (Femostop) in transcatheter coronary interventions requiring abciximab (ReoPro). Cathet Cardiovasc Intervent 1999;343:180–4.

5

Specific complications of the radial approach: how to avoid them

Yves Louvard, Thierry Lefèvre and Marie-Claude Morice

Specifics of the transradial approach • Complications of the transradial approach. How to treat them? • Complications associated with postprocedure compression • Conclusion

Transradial diagnostic or interventional cardiac catheterization is associated with a reduction in the incidence and severity of bleeding and vascular complications.[1] It improves patient comfort and decreases procedural costs[2-5] without impeding the implementation of technical strategies currently in use in the field of interventional cardiology.[6] Only a slight increase in procedure time and x-ray exposure has been observed in transradial angiography.[5] The advantages of this approach are even greater in settings or subgroups considered high risk for the femoral approach,[7] such as patients requiring thrombolytics,[8] anticoagulation,[9] and antiplatelet treatment,[8,10] patients with hemostasis disorders, hypertension, female patients, elderly patients,[11-13] patients with low BMI, severe obesity, and chronic respiratory deficit.

The radial approach, however, does have its own inherent complications.[14] Some of these, such as external bleeding or hematomas, false aneurysms, arteriovenous fistulae and neurologic complications, are also associated with the femoral and brachial approaches, though with different causes in some instances. Others, such as the acute compartment syndrome of the forearm and artery rupture or avulsion, are specific to the radial approach.

As with any approach, the occurrence of such complications is directly related to the degree of operator experience.

SPECIFICS OF THE TRANSRADIAL APPROACH

In theory, the presence of a dual vascularization of the hand through the two palmar arcades precludes the risk of hand ischemia in cases of radial artery occlusion.

The radial artery is muscular and its vasomotor activity is mainly determined by alpha-1 adrenoreceptors and, to a lesser extent, by alpha-2 adrenoreceptors, the stimulation of which by circulating catecholamines induces vasoconstriction.[15] Patient anxiety as well as repeated local or distant stimulation are factors of radial spasm. The radial artery has a relatively small diameter[16] (2.9±0.6 mm in a series of 120 consecutive French patients) and diameter distribution in the general population allows the use of 8 F introducers in 25–65% of patients, 7 F in 57–77%, and 6 F in 82–92%. In 8–18% of patients, the radial artery is smaller than a 6 F introducer.

However, use of nitrates may result in a 16% enlargement of the radial artery diameter.[17] In most patients, the radial artery can be stretched except in the presence of substantial wall calcifications; nevertheless, catheter or introducer oversizing may generate friction, pain, spasm, and sometimes radial dissection.

In the current era where stents and 6 F guiding catheters are widely used, at least in Europe, the technical limitations of transradial PCI are scarce since all balloons and coronary stents are compatible with this approach as well as rotating atherectomy, cutting balloons, distal protection devices, thrombectomy catheters, and the kissing balloon inflation technique. Following radial catheterization, the radial artery presents functional modifications, reduction of endothelium-derived vasodilatation and nitroglycerin-derived vasodilatation which are reversible within 3–4 weeks.[17–19] Histologic modifications, such as neo-intimal hypertrophy reducing the inner artery diameter, may also occur in the wake of radial catheterization, which accounts for the reduced success rate of repeated transradial procedures and additional punctures[20,21] and may also preclude the use of this artery as a surgical bypass conduit.[22]

The right transradial approach may be complicated by anatomic variations which, though rarely observed, may assume a variety of forms, generate a number of technical difficulties, and result in complications. These variations may be congenital,[23] such as brachioradial arteries originating high in the vascular tree (11% of the radial arteries), brachial or axillary arteries associated or not with anastomosis with the brachio-ulnar vasculature (Figure 5.1). The upper brachial segment of these brachioradial arteries is often thin (remnant), especially in the presence of a large-diameter radio-ulnar anastomosis, which may cause friction and spasm (Figure 5.2). Radio-ulnar anastomoses, associated with brachioradial arteries in 25% of cases, often form loops (Figure 5.3). Sinuous segments and loops at the antebrachial, brachial or subclavian levels may also be observed in elderly patients (forearm) and

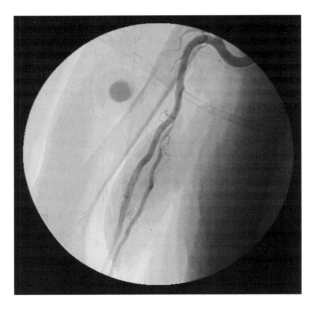

Figure 5.1   High take-off of a radial artery from the brachial artery (brachioradial artery).

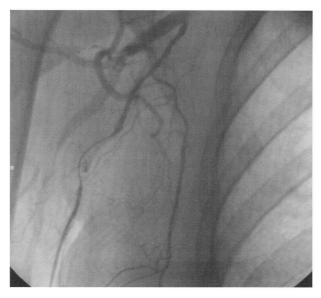

Figure 5.2   High take-off of a radial artery from the axillary artery (spasm).

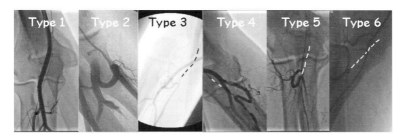

Figure 5.3   Different types of radio-ulnar anastomosis from the most simple to the most difficult (impossible) to cross.

patients with hypertension or increased BMI (subclavian loops).[24,25] Such loops may hinder guiding catheter and catheter advancement and account for a higher risk of dissection or perforation. Subclavian loops are rare on the left side.

Though the incidence of atherosclerosis is lower in the upper limbs, it is not an uncommon occurrence, especially at the subclavian level. Crossing of a stenosed segment may be associated with embolic events.

COMPLICATIONS OF THE TRANSRADIAL APPROACH. HOW TO TREAT THEM?

Discomfort and brachial pain

These are the most frequently reported complications and the most benign.[26]

Pain is caused by catheter friction during antero-, retrograde, and rotation maneuvers. Such friction may be related to spasm or to an excessively large introducer or catheter diameter, and occurs in the course of the procedure or during introducer ablation. In some instances, friction may be generated by loops, especially subclavian ones. Spasm can be brought about by patient anxiety, multiple puncture attempts, and lengthy catheter maneuvers and is, therefore, significantly related to operator inexperience.

Prevention

The catheter and introducer selected by the operator must be proportionate to the size of the patient's artery. Optimal selection can be made after palpation and according to patient stature and gender or with echography guidance.

Coronary angiograms can be performed with 4 F catheters and a high percentage of coronary angioplasties with 5 F guiding catheters.

The occurrence of spasm can be efficiently prevented by careful explanation of the procedure to the patient, ensuring a quiet environment, administration of premedication and local anesthesia using subcutaneous or percutaneous lidocaine (which should be applied at least 90 minutes prior to the procedure), intra-arterial antispasmodic treatment, and careful and restricted catheter maneuver.

It has been clearly demonstrated that spasm can be very efficiently prevented by the use of an intra-arterial medication cocktail which can be injected into the introducer before its insertion, or into the venous catheter used for puncture.[27,28] This cocktail is composed of nitrates or verapamil[29] or a combination of both and must be diluted before injection in order to reduce the burning sensation. Diltiazem[30] is equally efficient, but intra-arterial lidocaine has a vasoconstricting effect.[31] Administration of neuroleptanalgesia by an anesthetist during diagnostic or interventional catheterization prevents the occurrence of spasm. Hydrophilic coatings on introducers greatly facilitate insertion and withdrawal maneuvers.[32–34] Hydrophilic-coated catheters are also very useful in tortuous anatomies.[35] In order to limit the occurrence of spasm, the use of a single 'multipurpose' catheter has been recommended for cannulation of both arteries. This catheter can be a left Amplatz, Sones, Judkins or the recently developed Tiger (Terumo).

Treatment

Spasm is easier to prevent than to treat. Local administration of nitrates is usually efficient in eliminating spasm, but removal of the catheter and/or sheath can be painful. Once again, the most efficient option is to resort to the anesthetist who can administer general anesthesia of very short duration when sheath removal is painful.

In exceptional cases, axillary block or general anesthesia may be required for catheter ablation. Refractory spasm or, more probably, discrepancies between introducer and artery diameters have been reported to result in partial or total avulsion of the radial artery[36] (Figure 5.4). In instances of painful friction caused by subclavian loops, requesting the patient to take a deep breath may facilitate advancement or withdrawal of the catheter.

Severe bleeding complications

The incidence of severe bleeding complications is significantly lower compared with the femoral and brachial approaches.

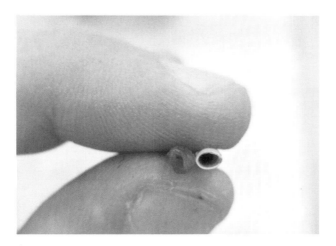

Figure 5.4   Surgical ablation of the radial artery to remove a 7 F sheath.

External bleeding may occur at the puncture site due to inadequate compression or after compression release. This can be easily remedied by reapplying compression. Maximal pressure must be exerted proximally to the cutaneous puncture site (arterial entry point). The radial artery is generally very easy to compress, at least when the puncture has been performed distally opposite the bone. More proximal compression is usually less efficient.

Small hematomas are relatively frequent and more easily visualized in the postprocedure phase than with the femoral approach. Though a rare occurrence, large hematomas may have severe consequences. They may be caused by inadequate compression of the radial artery distal to the arterial puncture site, excessively high puncture site, perforation of the main radial artery segment (Figure 5.5) or, in most instances, perforation of an antebrachial, brachial, thoracic parietal (especially with hydrophilic-coated wires) or even intrathoracic collateral branch.[37] The cause may also be the occurrence of radial arterial rupture in the forearm or rupture of a brachioradial artery in the arm as a consequence of diameter discrepancy between the vessel and the catheter. A sudden voluminous injection into the introducer may also cause microvascular rupture and result in hematoma (Figure 5.6).

In order to prevent the occurrence of such complications, the first puncture should be performed slightly proximal to the radial styloid. If the first attempt is unsuccessful, increasingly proximal punctures should be avoided.

Primary use of a hydrophilic wire is not recommended. When used, these wires should be advanced under x-ray guidance. In cases where wire advancement meets with some resistance, force should not be applied. A cautious injection of diluted contrast medium through the small catheter of the puncture kit, through the introducer or more proximally through a pressure-connected catheter, allows the identification of the obstacle. Sometimes x-ray visualization alone is enough to identify a problem (side branch wire penetration). Certain anatomic variations may call for guidewire insertion into a mammary (Figure 5.7) or, in most instances, a vertebral artery. Even if no resistance is felt, the x-ray tube should be positioned at patient shoulder level.

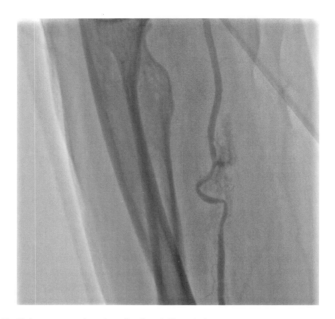

Figure 5.5   Radial artery perforation (hydrophilic wire).

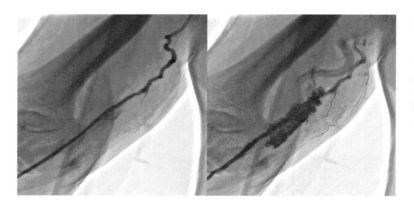

Figure 5.6   High take-off of a radial artery, resistance to catheter advancement, result of a brutal contrast injection.

Force should not be applied to a catheter which is incompatible with the arterial segment diameter (remnant, brachioradial artery), in the presence of spasm, loops and even at the ostium of a collateral branch. Identification of the problem by angiography may help the operator find a solution such as cross-over to the contralateral radial artery (congenital abnormalities are not bilateral) or to the femoral artery, simple catheter rotation to avoid the ostium, selection of a smaller catheter, identification of the main vessel, or attempt at crossing a radio-ulnar

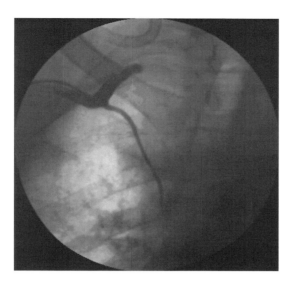

Figure 5.7 Distal subclavian take-off of the right internal mammary artery (risk of wire/catheter penetration).

anastomosis at elbow level. In the latter case, the anastomosis often forms a loop and the chances of success are commensurate with the anastomotic vessel size and inversely proportional to the loop diameter (Figure 5.8).

Treatment

When extravasation is identified during the procedure, compression using a large elastic adhesive arm band or a cuff, whilst carrying on with the procedure, may be useful as the introducer or catheter may limit the extent of extravasation. In cases of rupture, insertion of a long introducer[38] has proved efficient in several instances.

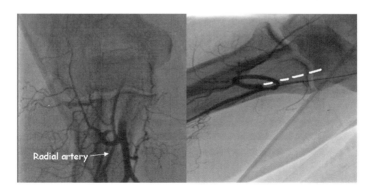

Radial artery →

Figure 5.8 Left: large vessel small diameter anastomotic radio-ulnar loop (easy to straighten). Right: large vessel large diameter anastomotic radio-ulnar loop (painful straightening).

When diagnosed after completion of the procedure, any hematoma should be measured immediately in order to monitor its evolution. An efficient means of stopping extravasation consists in inflating a cuff at arm or forearm level up to the degree of the patient's arterial pressure. In addition, previously injected heparin can be totally or partially antagonized (protamine).

The forearm should be carefully monitored for potential symptoms of hand ischemia (pain, late pallor, pulselessness, paralysis, paresthesia) and prompt diagnosis of the dangerous acute compartment syndrome,[39] which is a rare occurrence directly related to operator inexperience. If this occurs, a fasciotomy with delayed cutaneous closure should be performed by a surgeon (Figure 5.9). The use of leeches for decompressing hematomas has been recommended (Figure 5.10).

Globular transfusion is only exceptionally required in the case of bleeding complications associated with the transradial approach.

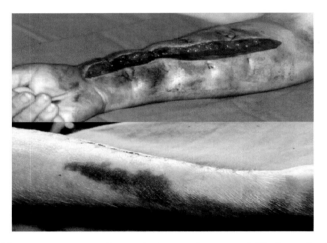

Figure 5.9   Volar compartment syndrome, fasciotomy (courtesy of G Barbeau, Quebec, Canada).

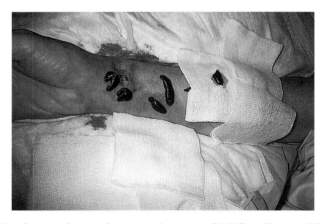

Figure 5.10   Leeches on a forearm hematoma (courtesy of D Hilton, Victoria, BC, Canada).

Radial artery occlusion and hand ischemia

Thrombosis is the most common cause of radial artery occlusion (Figure 5.11). However, dissection may occur (though sometimes impressive, this does not cause clinical complications as it is retrograde in most cases) (Figure 5.12) and even spasm. Several predictive factors of occlusion have been reported: absence of or inadequate anticoagulation, a too small internal artery diameter/catheter diameter ratio, procedure duration, and probably compression mode and duration. In the absence of anticoagulation with heparin, the rate of radial occlusion following angiography may be in excess of 70%. It is 24% with a heparin dosage of 2000–3000 iu and lower than 7% with a dosage ≥ 5000 iu.[40] It seems that this rate has been decreasing over time and

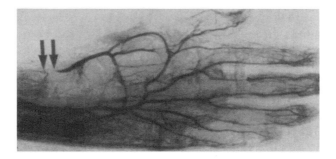

Figure 5.11   Radial artery occlusion.

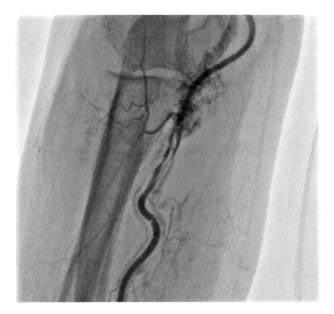

Figure 5.12   Dissection of a small brachioradial artery without any clinical consequence.

is currently estimated to be 1.3% with a similar dosage of 5000 iu, maybe due to improved puncture technique, catheter handling, and compression methods (reduced duration).[41] When the internal artery diameter/catheter diameter ratio is <1, the risk of severe reduction of radial artery flow is 13% vs 4% when it is higher.[42] Between 47% and 75% of occluded radial arteries resume normal perfusion spontaneously over the mid-term.[43]

The risk of hand ischemia is not only related to the risk of radial artery occlusion but also to the absence of alternative hand vascularization (risk of hand ischemia = percentage of radial artery occlusion × percentage of absence of collateral flow from the cubital artery). In our experience, we have never encountered a case of acute hand ischemia and such an occurrence has not been reported in patients undergoing diagnostic or interventional coronary transradial catheterization.

Hand ischemia has been observed following prolonged catheterization for anesthetic or intensive care purposes.[44]

Prevention of radial artery occlusion and its consequences

The use of heparin during transradial catheterization is indispensable. Heparin is frequently injected locally, simultaneously with antispasmodic medication, which may cause a burning sensation and possible spasm induced by the acidity of the product. It seems that the minimal dose is 5000 iu even for diagnostic procedures. This dose may be adjusted according to patient weight. There are no available data on radial artery patency following use of fractioned heparin. Selection of patients with double hand vascularization by the radial and cubital arteries is an alleged means of avoiding the occurrence of hand ischemia in cases of radial artery occlusion. The classic Allen's test is not predictive of the risk of hand ischemia.[45] This test induces ischemia in 13–14% of radial arteries. Barbeau proposed a more accurate assessment of collateral flow by means of pulse oximetry and plethysmography (thumb).[46]

Modification of the plethysmography curve during radial artery compression has been classified into four types: A, no damping; B, slight damping of pulse tracing; C, loss followed by recovery; or D, no recovery of pulse tracing within two minutes.[46] By allowing the radial approach in types A–C, this method leads to the exclusion of only 6.3% of radial arteries and 1.5% of patients. Some operators have not performed collateral flow evaluation tests for a long time in a large number of patients in whom no events have been reported. These two strategies are impossible to compare in a randomized study. However, the fact that both the radial and cubital approaches may be used in a single center warrants extreme caution at least in cases where collateral tests have not been performed.[47]

Treatment

Treatment of hand ischemia occurring after prolonged radial catheterization for monitoring purposes requires emergency surgery and can be complex.

False aneurysm

This is a relatively frequent complication of the transradial approach (<1%)[48] (Figure 5.13) The risk factors have not been identified but, as with the femoral approach, they are probably related to inadequate compression resulting in the formation of

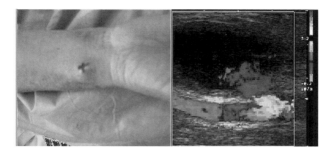

Figure 5.13   Radial artery false aneurysm.

hematoma. Though this may not always be efficient and is sometimes associated with cutaneous complications, prolonged compression may be attempted if performed less than 48 hours after the procedure. Local injection of thrombin resulting in the occlusion of the false aneurysm and of the radial artery has been attempted. Surgical treatment is sometimes required.

Arteriovenous fistulas

These are rarely observed given the absence of significant veins next to the radial artery (2/10,000). Predictive factors have not been identified. However, multiple injections of anesthetic agents and punctures may increase the risk. The rare cases of arteriovenous fistulas that we observed were resolved by spontaneous closure. Prolonged compression seems a logical option if performed early.

Neurologic complications

A recent registry comparing the radial and femoral approaches reported a higher neurologic risk with the radial approach (not confirmed in the last update).[49] Another small nonrandomized study reached the same conclusion after analyzing cerebral emboli of solid debris by means of intracranial Doppler.[50] An inverse trend was observed in a randomized study conducted in octogenarians by teams very experienced in the radial approach.[13] Comparison of clinical events by means of large randomized studies in high-risk populations or smaller studies conducted with intracranial Doppler control by operators very experienced in both approaches should allow the investigators to reach reliable conclusions.

The prevention of complications related to the transradial approach lies in the gradual introduction of complex cases according to the operator's experience and in the limitation of catheter maneuvers.

COMPLICATIONS ASSOCIATED WITH POSTPROCEDURE COMPRESSION

Circular compression of the wrist usually results in swelling of the hand which becomes cyanosed and painful. This type of compression may cause deep vein thrombosis.[51] The very rare instances of regional pain syndrome reported following transradial procedures were apparently related to compression.[52,53] Compression must be of short duration and performed on the radial edge of the hand with a thick pad and elastic bands or other types of dedicated pads (Figure 5.14). Certain types of adhesive elastic bands should be avoided, especially in elderly patients with fragile skin.

Catheter kinking

Catheter rotation during a transradial procedure is much more difficult to perform than via the femoral approach because of the friction generated by the size of the vessel. Catheter advancement around loops and in calcified segments must be monitored (the tip must rotate with the rest of the catheter!) by x-ray and pressure measurement.

Indeed, catheter kinking, which can also occur via the transfemoral approach, may have worse consequences. The catheter must not be withdrawn before being straightened up by rotating it in the opposite direction and by inserting a hydrophilic wire which should be advanced in a larger artery.

Nonhealing wounds

Nonhealing wounds combined with inflammatory reaction and sterile abscess resulting from a foreign body reaction to a hydrophilic arterial sheath have been described. This phenomenon appearing within two to three weeks of the transradial catheterization procedure is associated with the presence of subcutaneous silicone debris.[54,55] In order to minimize this risk, skin incision should be performed before placement or at least removal of the arterial sheath in order to avoid shedding of the silicone coating. In some instances, abscess drainage was required.

Coronary complications

There are no specific coronary complications inherent in the radial approach. However, the use of catheters originally designed for the femoral approach, in order to achieve coronary stability during catheterization in angioplasty procedures and sucessful catheterization of both arteries in coronary angiography, has been shown rarely to cause dissection of the right coronary artery and of the left main trunk (especially left Amplatz catheters).[56]

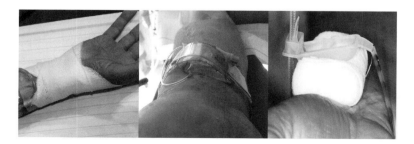

Figure 5.14   Different types of puncture site selective compression.

The current use of 'dedicated' catheters specifically designed for the radial approach, both for diagnostic and interventional procedures, has been associated with a reduction in the risk of dissection.

CONCLUSION

Transradial catheterization in percutaneous coronary interventions reduces the incidence and the severity of noncoronary complications related to the procedure.

Though rarely severe, the complications of the transradial approach are mainly associated with operator inexperience and lack of familiarity with the difficulties involved. These include small spastic muscular arteries, acquired or congenital anatomic variations which, though infrequent, may assume multiple forms (loops more than atheroma) and are associated with hypertension and advanced age. In order to ensure optimal safety, the operator should use small-caliber needles, wires, and catheters. Handling should be smooth and force should never be applied. Anatomic difficulties should be identified by x-ray or angiography before deciding on the approach and in order to select specific strategies according to the operator's experience. Like the femoral approach, the radial approach requires practice although the learning curve is longer. It is particularly adapted to high-volume operators who use it routinely.

Severe bleeding complications are rare because bleeding can be easily controlled provided that effective measures are immediately taken in order to prevent the occurrence of the most severe complication, namely the volar compartment syndrome. Cases of hand ischemia have never been reported.

Further randomized studies in high-risk patient subsets are warranted in order to quantify the respective neurologic risk of the radial and femoral approaches.

REFERENCES

1. Agostoni P, Biondi-Zoccai GG, de Benedictis ML et al. Radial versus femoral approach for percutaneous coronary diagnostic and interventional procedures; Systematic overview and meta-analysis of randomized trials. J Am Coll Cardiol 2004;44(2):349–56.
2. Kiemeneij F, Hofland J, Laarman GJ, Hupkens van der Elst D, Van der Lubbe H. Cost comparison between two modes of Palmaz Schatz coronary stent implantation: transradial bare stent technique vs. transfemoral sheath-protected stent technique. Cathet Cardiovasc Diagn 1995;35:301–8.
3. Tift Mann J III, Cubeddu G, Schneider JE, Arrowood M. Right radial access for PTCA: a prospective study demonstrates reduced complications and hospital charges. J Invasive Cardiol 1996;8(Suppl D):40D–44D.
4. Cooper CJ, El-Shiekh RA, Cohen DJ et al. Effect of transradial access on quality of life and cost of cardiac catheterization: a randomized comparison. Am Heart J 1999;138:430–6.
5. Louvard Y, Lefevre T, Allain A, Morice MC. Coronary angiography through the radial or the femoral approach: the Carafe Study. Cathet Cardiovasc Intervent 2001;52:181–7.
6. Kiemeneij F, Laarman GJ, Odekerken D, Slagboom T, van der Wieken R. A randomized comparison of percutaneous transluminal coronary angioplasty by the radial, brachial and femoral appproaches: the Access study. J Am Coll Cardiol 1997;29:1269–75.
7. Piper WD, Malenka DJ, Ryan TJ Jr et al, for the Northern New England Cardiovascular Disease Study Group. Predicting vascular complications in percutaneous coronary interventions. Am Heart J 2003;145(6):1022–9.

8. Charlat ML. Rescue percutaneous coronary intervention using transradial arterial access with glycoprotein IIb/IIIa inhibitor eptifibatide therapy initiated post-fibrinolysis. J Invasive Cardiol 2000;12(Suppl D):13D–15D.
9. Hildick-Smith DJ, Walsh JT, Lowe MD, Petch MC. Coronary angiography in the fully anticoagulated patient: the transradial route is successful and safe. Cathet Cardiovasc Intervent 2003;58(1):8–10.
10. Choussat R, Black A, Bossi I, Fajadet J, Marco J. Vascular complications and clinical outcome after coronary angioplasty with platelet IIb/IIIa receptor blockade. Comparison of transradial vs transfemoral arterial access. Eur Heart J 2000;21(8):662–7.
11. Caputo RP, Simons A, Giambartolomei A et al. Transradial cardiac catheterization in elderly patients. Cathet Cardiovasc Intervent 2000;51:287–90.
12. Klinke WP, Hilton JD, Warburton RN, Warburton WP, Tan RP. Comparison of treatment outcomes in patients >/=80 years undergoing transradial versus transfemoral coronary intervention. Am J Cardiol 2004;93(10):1282–5.
13. Louvard Y, Benamer H, Garot P et al. Comparison of transradial and transfemoral approaches for coronary angiography and angioplasty in octogenarians (the OCTOPLUS Study). Am J Cardiol 2004;94:1177–80.
14. Cox N, Resnic FS, Popma JJ, Simon DI, Eisenhauer AC, Rogers C. Comparison of the risk of vascular complications associated with femoral and radial access coronary catheterization procedures in obese versus nonobese patients. Am J Cardiol 2004;94:1174–7.
15. He GW, Yang CQ. Characteristics of adrenoreceptors in the human radial artery: clinical implications. J Thorac Cardiovasc Surg 1998;115:1136–41.
16. Saito S, Ikei H, Hosokawa G, Tanaka S. Influence of the ratio between radial artery inner diameter and sheath outer diameter on radial artery flow after transradial coronary intervention. Cathet Cardiovasc Intervent 1999;46(2):173–8.
17. Sanmartin M, Goicolea J, Ocaranza R, Cuevas D, Calvo F. Vasoreactivity of the radial artery after transradial catheterization. J Invasive Cardiol 2004;16(11):635–8.
18. Ko JY, Yoon J, Yoo BS et al. Effect of transradial coronary procedure on the vasodilatory function of the radial artery. Am J Cardiol 2001;88(Suppl 5A):112G.
19. Del Core MG, Price C, LaMadrid L, Ryshon K, Mohiuddin SM. Endothelial dysfunction following radial artery cannulization. J Am Coll Cardiol 2002;39:Suppl. A.
20. Wakeyama T, Ogawa H, Iida H et al. Intima-media thickening of the radial artery after transradial intervention: an intravascular ultrasound study. J Am Coll Cardiol 2003;41:1109–14.
21. Sakai H, Ohe H, Harada T et al. Incidence and reasons for drop out in successive transradial procedures in one arm. J Am Coll Cardiol 2001;37(2):1158.
22. Kamiya H, Ushijima T, Kanamori T et al. Use of the radial artery graft after transradial catheterization: is it suitable as a bypass conduit? Ann Thorac Surg 2003;76(5):1505–9.
23. Rodriguez-Niedenfuhr M, Vazquez T, Nearn L, Ferreira B, Parkin I, Sanudo JR. Variations of the arterial pattern in the upper limb revisited: a morphological and statistical study, with a review of the literature. J Anat 2001;199:547–66.
24. Cha KS, Park EH, Yang DK et al. Clinical predictors of severely tortuous right subclavian-innominate arteries in patients undergoing transradial coronary procedures and a reliable and safe technique for completing the procedures. Am J Cardiol 2002;90(Suppl 6A):68H.
25. Yoo BS, Ko JY, Kim JY et al. Anatomic consideration of the radial artery for transradial coronary procedures: arterial diameter, branching anomaly, and vessel tortuosity. Am J Cardiol 2002;90(Suppl 6A): 167H.
26. Ludman PF, Stephens NG, Harcombe A, Lowe MD, Schofield PM, Petch MC. Radial versus femoral approach for diagnostic coronary angiography in stable angina pectoris. Am J Cardiol 1997;79:1239–41.
27. Kiemeneij F, Vajifdar BU, Eccleshall SC et al. Measurement of radial artery spasm using an automatic pullback device. Cathet Cardiovasc Intervent 2001;54:437–41.
28. Kiemeneij F, Vajifdar BU, Eccleshall SC, Laarman G, Slagboom T, van der Wieken R. Evaluation of a spasmolytic cocktail to prevent radial artery spasm during coronary procedures. Cathet Cardiovasc Intervent 2003;58:281–4.

29. He GW. Verapamil plus nitroglycerin solution maximally preserves endothelial function of the radial artery: comparison with papaverine solution. J Thorac Cardiovasc Surg 1998;115:1321–7.

30. Mont'Alverne Filho JR, Assad JA, Zago A et al. Comparative study of the use of diltiazem as an antispasmodic drug in coronary angiography via the transradial approach. Arq Bras Cardiol 2003;81:59–63.

31. Abe S, Meguro T, Endoh N et al. Response of the radial artery to three vasodilatory agents. Cathet Cardiovasc Intervent 2000;49(3):253–6.

32. Dery JP, Simard S, Barbeau GR et al. Reduction of discomfort at sheath removal during transradial coronary procedures with the use of a hydrophilic-coated sheath. Cathet Cardiovasc Intervent 2001;54:289–94.

33. Kiemeneij F, Fraser D, Slagboom T, Laarman G, van der Wieken R. Hydrophilic coating aids radial sheath withdrawal and reduces patient discomfort following transradial coronary intervention: a randomized double-blind comparison of coated and uncoated sheaths. Cathet Cardiovasc Intervent 2003;59(2):161–4.

34. Koga S, Ikeda S, Futagawa K et al. The use of a hydrophilic-coated catheter during transradial cardiac catheterization is associated with a low incidence of radial artery spasm. Int J Cardiol 2004;96(2):255–8.

35. Barbeau G. Radial loop and extreme vessel tortuosity in the transradial approach: advantage of hydrophilic-coated guidewires and catheters. Cathet Cardiovasc Intervent 2003;59:442–50.

36. Dieter RS, Akef A, Wolff M. Eversion endarterectomy complicating radial artery access for left heart catheterization. Cathet Cardiovasc Intervent 2003;58:478–80.

37. Jao YT, Chen Y, Fang CC, Wang SP. Mediastinal and neck hematoma after cardiac catheterization. Cathet Cardiovasc Intervent 2003;58(4):467–72.

38. Calviño-Santos RA, Vázquez-Rodríguez JM, Salgado-Fernández J et al. Management of iatrogenic radial artery perforation. Cathet Cardiovasc Intervent 2004;61:74–8.

39. Lin YJ, Chu CC, Tsai CW. Acute compartment syndrome after transradial coronary angioplasty. Int J Cardiol 2004;97(2):311.

40. Spaulding C, Lefevre T, Funck F et al. Left radial approach for coronary angiography: results of a prospective study. Cathet Cardiovasc Diagn 1996;39:365–70.

41. Bertrand B, Sene Y, Huygue O, Monsegu J. Doppler ultrasound imaging of the radial artery after catheterization. Ann Cardiol Angiol 2003;52(3):135–8.

42. Saito S, Ikei H, Hosokawa G, Tanaka S. Influence of the ratio between radial artery inner diameter and sheath outer diameter on radial artery flow after transradial coronary intervention. Cathet Cardiovasc Intervent 1999;46:173–8.

43. Stella PR, Odekerken D, Kiemeneij F, Laarman GJ, Slagboom T, van der Wieken R. Incidence and outcome of radial artery occlusion following transradial coronary angioplasty. Cathet Cardiovasc Diagn 1997;40:156–8.

44. Ozbek S. Ischemia of the hand following radial artery catheterization. Ulus Travma Derg 2002;8(4):256–8.

45. Starnes SL, Wolk SW, Lampman RM et al. Noninvasive evaluation of hand circulation before radial artery harvest for coronary artery bypass grafting. Thorac Cardiovasc Surg 1999;117(2):261–6.

46. Barbeau GR, Arsenault F, Dugas L, Simard S, Lariviere MM. Evaluation of the ulnopalmar arterial arches with pulse oximetry and plethysmography: comparison with the Allen's test in 1010 patients. Am Heart J 2004;147(3):489–93.

47. Lanspa TJ, Reyes AP, Oldemeyer JB, Williams MA. Ulnar artery catheterization with occlusion of corresponding radial artery. Cathet Cardiovasc Intervent 2004;61:211–13.

48. Fagih B, Beaudry Y. Pseudoaneurysm: a late complication of the transradial approach after coronary angiography. J Invasive Cardiol 2000;12(4):216–17.

49. Lagerqvist B, Albertsson P, James S, Nilsson T. Increased risk of complications with a transradial approach in coronary procedures – a report from the Swedish coronary angiography and angioplasty registry. Paper presented at AHA meeting, November 2004.

50. Lund C, Bang Nes R, Pynten Ugelstad T et al. Cerebral emboli during left heart catheterization may cause acute brain injury. Eur Heart J 2005;26(13):1269–75.
51. Hall IR, Lo TS, Nolan J. Deep vein thrombosis in the arm following transradial cardiac catheterization: an unusual complication related to hemostatic technique. Cathet Cardiovasc Intervent 2004;62:346–8.
52. Papadimos TJ, Hofmann JP. Radial artery thrombosis, palmar arch systolic blood velocities, and chronic regional pain syndrome 1 following transradial cardiac catheterization. Cathet Cardiovasc Intervent 2002;57:537–40.
53. Sasano N, Tsuda T, Sasano H, Ito S, Sobue K, Katsuya H. A case of complex regional pain syndrome type II after transradial coronary intervention. J Anesth 2004;18(4):310–12.
54. Subramanian R, White CJ, Sternbergh III W et al. Nonhealing wound resulting from a foreign-body reaction to a radial arterial sheath. Cathet Cardiovasc Intervent 2003;59:205–6.
55. Kozak M, Adams DR, Ioffreda MD et al. Sterile inflammation associated with transradial catheterization and hydrophilic sheaths. Cathet Cardiovasc Intervent 2003;59(2):207–13.
56. Louvard Y. The Amplatz catheter as sole catheter for transradial coronary angiography. In: Hamon M, McFadden E, eds. Transradial approach for cardiovascular interventions. Carpiquet, France: ESM Editions 2003.

Section C
During the procedure

6

Abrupt vessel closure and no-reflow

Alexandre Berger, Morton Kern and Amir Lerman

• **Abrupt vessel closure** • **The no-reflow phenomenon** • **Conclusion**

Abrupt impairment of coronary blood flow during percutaneous coronary intervention (PCI) is a catastrophic complication. Two major causes, namely abrupt vessel closure and no-reflow phenomenon, are responsible for most cases. Since no-reflow might be diagnosed only after excluding abrupt epicardial closure, this chapter will briefly discuss the practical approach of this topic before focusing on the no-reflow phenomenon, its pathophysiology, recognition, prevention, and management.

ABRUPT VESSEL CLOSURE

Abrupt vessel closure is still the most common cause of major procedure-related complications despite increasing operator experience, technologic advancements, and wide-ranging use of adjunctive medications. Up to 11% of vessel closure was noted in the pre-stent area which is now lowered to less than 2% due to the widespread use of intracoronary stents.[1–4] Even if most of the cases occur during the intervention, late closure within hours or days may occur. The present discussion will focus on acute vessel closure in the catheterization laboratory.

Definition and pathophysiology

Most acute abrupt vessel closures are due to mechanically induced coronary dissections. Up to 40% of cases of routine coronary angioplasty are complicated with some degree of vessel dissection, generally due to injuries provoked by vigorous attempts to pass the guidewire or balloon inflation.[5] Deep injury of the media with hemorrhages such as intraplaque hematoma and tissue flaps (dissection type C to F) may compromise coronary blood flow.[6] Table 6.1 shows the relationship between the severity of coronary dissection and the risk of abrupt vessel closure.[7] Furthermore, the length of the dissection, the residual diameter stenosis (>30%), and the presence of unstable angina or chronic total occlusion are additional risk factors for major ischemic events in the presence of coronary dissection.[7,8] Other well-recognized causes for sudden impairment of coronary flow are macrothrombi, spasm, and air embolism. They all should be taken into account when considering prevention and management.

Table 6.1   Relationship between dissection type and risk of abrupt vessel closure (from reference 99)

Type A (0–2%)	Minor radiolucencies within lumen during angiography without dye persistence
Type B (2–4%)	Parallel tracks or double lumen separated by radiolucent area during angiography without dye persistence
Type C (10%)	Extraluminal cap with dye persistence
Type D (30%)	Spiral luminal filling defects
Type E (9%)	New persistent filling defects
Type F (69%)	Non A–E types that lead to impaired flow or total occlusion

Prevention

Anticipation is the key component in the prevention of complications. Therefore, interventional cardiologists should assess the global complication risk of each procedure. Even if no accurate prediction can be drawn, several well-recognized risk factors should be taken into account (Table 6.2). Those high-risk circumstances should be identified through a checklist in order to apply adequate precautions.

High-quality patient preparation and premedication are critical in preventing abrupt vessel closure. Preprocedural aspirin administration reduces its incidence by 50–75% and addition of clopidogrel or ticlopidine is mandatory to further prevent stent thrombosis.[9] Boluses of weight-adjusted heparin, with adjustment during the procedure based on activated clotting time (ACT) levels, have also been shown to decrease the risk of thrombotic events and are now part of the standard care.[10,11] GP IIb/IIIa platelet receptor inhibitors have also been demonstrated to be useful in preventing major complications and should be strongly considered in complex procedures.[12,13]

Management (Figure 6.1)

Development of abrupt vessel closure is usually associated with clinical signs of ischemia and acute chest pain, ST segment changes and, in some situations, arrhythmia and systemic hypotension. Therefore, the first concern should be the patient's clinical stabilization. Use of intravenous saline, inotropic drugs, a temporary pacemaker, and/or intra-aortic balloon pump may be needed to restore normal hemodynamic status. In some cases, re-establishing coronary blood flow may be sufficient. In such situations, it is recommended to wait another 10–20 minutes in the catheterization laboratory to confirm vessel patency. If coronary blood flow remains impaired despite clinical stabilization, a stepwise approach is mandatory.

Table 6.2   Risk factors for abrupt vessel closure (from reference 99)

Clinical
Cardiogenic shock, advanced age, congestive heart failure, renal dysfunction, female gender, diabetes, unstable angina, acute myocardial infarction

Angiographic
Multivessel disease, thrombus-containing lesion, older vein graft, bifurcation lesion, angulated lesion, lesion after tortuous segments, long lesion

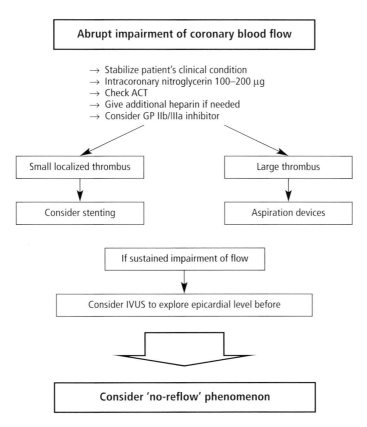

Figure 6.1 Algorithm for abrupt vessel closure.

1. Coronary spasm should be first ruled out through intracoronary nitroglycerin (100–200 µg) administration. Increasing doses of nitroglycerin or calcium channel blockers could be used for refractory spasm, taking the hemodynamic and rhythm status into account. In rare cases, when coronary spasm cannot be relieved by pharmacologic approaches, general anesthesia with muscle relaxants should be considered. It is important to remember that the presence of coronary spasm is usually associated with thrombus as a primary or secondary event.
2. Intracoronary thrombus should be considered if coronary blood flow does not return despite administration of coronary vasodilators. Therefore, the anticoagulation level should be checked and adjusted as soon as possible, even in the absence of visible thrombus at angiography. In the presence of visible thrombus and an adequate level of anticoagulation, GP IIb/IIIa platelet receptor inhibitors and aspiration devices should be considered.
3. The benefit of intravenous GP IIb/IIIa inhibitors has been well investigated, suggesting clinical benefit in large clinical trials. In particular, these drugs have been shown to decrease the incidence of abrupt vessel closure. Intracoronary rather than intravenous administration has been suggested in preliminary reports

but cannot be recommended systematically because of lack of randomized clinical trials.

4. If the thrombus is small and localized (ovoid filling defect), stent implantation may be undertaken. In the presence of large burden of thrombus, aspiration devices are recommended before stenting, because of the risk of fragmentation, distal microembolization, and development of angiographic no-reflow. The Angiojet coronary thrombectomy device (Possis Medical, Minneapolis, USA) removes clots and thrombus. A pump set delivers a high-pressure saline solution through a catheter and out the saline jets into the artery. This creates a strong vacuum in the artery, which breaks up the blood clot and pulls it out of the body through the catheter and into the pump set. The GuardWire® Temporary Occlusion and Aspiration System (GuardWire, Medtronic Inc., Santa Rosa, CA, USA) combines a distal balloon occlusion and an aspiration catheter. After distal occlusion, aspiration could be done before and after stenting, without any risk of distal microembolizations. The TriActiv® System (Kensey Nash Corporation, Exton, USA) is an embolic protection device that actively flushes and uniformly extracts a broad spectrum of debris sizes. This is accomplished with three integrated system features: a protection balloon, active flushing, and an automated extraction system to remove problematic debris from the treated vessel. The X-sizer (ev3 Europe SAS, Paris, France) system consists of a catheter with dual-lumen shaft connected permanently to a control module which houses a small motor and various safety switches. This system combines vacuum technology with a helical cutter housed in the tip of a small catheter. The outer lumen within the catheter body provides the path for excised debris to be aspirated with the use of vacuum. Finally, the Diver® catheter (Invatec Srl, Roncadelle, Italy) is a user-friendly, 6 F compatible catheter with a central lumen and side holes allowing aspiration of organized and fresh thrombus. Figure 6.2 depicts the different devices.

Coronary dissection, as mentioned above, is the most frequent cause of abrupt vessel closure. Multiple angiographic projections are sometimes needed to expose the dissection. The use of intravascular ultrasound (IVUS) is highly recommended and should serve as a gold standard diagnostic tool. Several specific findings should be considered and assessed. Special attention should be paid to the relationship between the lesion and stent lengths since the edges of the stent are more prone to spasm and thrombus formation. Struts stent should be fully opposed and special attention should be paid to the presence of intraplaque or intravascular hematoma. It is also crucial to image the proximal segments of the vessel (left main and the ostium of the right coronary artery) to exclude guiding catheter-induced dissection. Often, additional stent implantation should be considered.

THE NO-REFLOW PHENOMENON

In 1967, the concept of no-reflow was originally described in ischemic rabbit brains. Additional experimental studies in dogs extended the concept to the heart. No-reflow and persistent subendocardial perfusion defects were identified after 90 minutes of coronary vessel ligation.[14,15] In 1985, first clinical evidence of no-reflow in humans was described.[16] Sixteen patients undergoing thrombolysis for acute anterior myocardial infarction were assessed by scintigraphy. Absence of new thallium-201 uptake

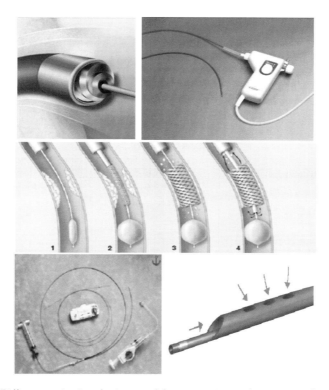

Figure 6.2 Different aspiration devices used for prevention and treatment of coronary blood flow impairment.

nonconcordant to technetium-99m scintigrams reflected lack of capillary reperfusion. In 1986 Bates and colleagues described the now classic angiographic appearance of no-reflow with the impairment of anterograde coronary blood flow.[17] No-reflow following angioplasty of native coronary vessels and during percutaneous coronary revascularization of acute myocardial infarction was then described.[18]

Definitions and physiopathology

No-reflow phenomenon refers to inadequate myocardial perfusion despite a patent epicardial coronary artery.[19,20] Two subsets of no-reflow should be defined.

- *Myocardial no-reflow phenomenon* refers to inadequate myocardial perfusion in the setting of pharmacologic or mechanical revascularization for acute myocardial infarction.[19] Its incidence varies from 4% to 25% depending on the definition used and the presence of high-risk features (age >70 years, diabetes, long time to reperfusion, initial low thrombolysis in myocardial infarction (TIMI) flow grade, depressed left ventricular function).[21] Electronic microscopy in animal models revealed severe capillary injuries inducing alterations of regional myocardial blood flow: endothelial cells with large intraluminal protrusions and decreased pinocytic vesicles, intraluminal fibrin thrombi, and swollen myocardial cells.[14,15] Furthermore, the reperfusion injuries expressed by myocyte contraction, fibrin, platelet and leukocytes plug, and oxygen-free radical production amplify the no-reflow phenomenon.[22-29]

- *Angiographic no-reflow phenomenon* refers to inadequate myocardial perfusion complicating percutaneous coronary intervention (PCI).[19] The pathophysiology of this entity is probably due to the release of thrombus, plaque debris, and potent vasoconstrictors such as endothelin-1 as well as inflammatory mediators distally into the coronary bed, closely related to the use of the percutaneous devices.[30] The incidence of angiographic no-reflow varies depending on the clinical setting: 0.3% for native coronary artery angioplasty, 0.3% for excimer laser, 7.7% for rotational atherectomy.[30,31] Furthermore, high-risk features like thrombus-containing lesions or degenerated saphenous vein grafts are associated with higher occurrence of no-reflow phenomenon.

Detection

Several techniques are available to identify inadequate myocardial perfusion characterizing the no-reflow phenomenon. Electrocardiographic ST segment alterations during coronary angioplasty and absence of complete ST segment resolution despite patent epicardial artery in the setting of acute myocardial infarction are important markers of impaired reperfusion.[32] Characteristically, no-reflow phenomenon is suspected when chest pain and ST segment modifications are associated with inadequate anterograde contrast progression at angiography.

TIMI flow and TIMI frame count grades were used to score the contrast progression.[33,34] Initially, TIMI 0–1 were associated with impaired reperfusion and TIMI 2–3 with successful reperfusion, but subsequent investigations have proven that this interpretation was misleading.[35] Even if the accepted angiographic definition of no-reflow is whenever TIMI flow is 0–2, grade 3 does not prove complete myocardial perfusion.[35,36] The TIMI perfusion grade, based on the assessment of the ground-glass appearance of the filling of the microcirculation (blush) distal to the culprit coronary artery was developed, allows additional risk stratification among patients with TIMI grade 3 flow.[37,38] If interpreted with caution and experience, coronary angiography is a fundamental tool for detecting and diagnosing coronary no-reflow phenomenon in any clinical setting.[39]

Additional devices, available in the catheterization laboratory, can be used to further investigate the integrity of the coronary microcirculation. Intracoronary Doppler guidewires are able to detect changes in coronary blood flow and its pattern. Appearance of systolic retrograde flow, diminished systolic anterograde flow, and rapid deceleration of diastolic flow characterize no-reflow.[40-42] Reduction in coronary flow reserve (CFR) following PCI is also highly correlated with evidence of myocardial ischemia.[43]

Intravascular ultrasound (IVUS) and intracoronary pressure measurements (fractional flow reserve: FFR) are very useful to exclude potential causes of inadequate contrast progression in the coronary bed, such as residual stenosis, macrothrombi or superimposed spasm, but no data demonstrate their utility in characterizing no-reflow.

Additional noninvasive techniques can help to identify the no-reflow phenomenon. Schofer and colleagues demonstrated the usefulness of myocardial scintigraphy to identify no-reflow, but it is now seldom used in clinical practice.[16,44] Myocardial contrast echocardiography played a pivotal role in demonstrating that angiography TIMI 3 flow was not always associated with complete reperfusion.[45] Indeed, intracoronary and intravenous contrast echocardiography have the ability to investigate the microvascular function and integrity via a real-time assessment of coronary blood flow.[46,47] Ito and colleagues identified advanced microvascular damage assessed by myocardial contrast echocardiography in patients with TIMI 2 flow following reperfusion of acute myocardial infarction. Their data confirmed that up to 30% of patients undergoing primary angioplasty lack complete myocardial reperfusion despite successful coronary revascularization.[48–50] Contrast-enhanced magnetic resonance was also tested in patients after successful primary PCI for acute myocardial infarction.[51–53] Left ventricular function, myocardial perfusion, and viability are achievable with this approach. Detection of impaired microvascular reperfusion is efficient and, when severe, associated with lack of recovery of left ventricular wall motion. Positron emission tomography can also be used in the investigation of reperfusion and no-reflow phenomenon.[54]

Prevention of no-reflow

Several strategies to prevent no-reflow have been tested: distal embolic protection devices, intracoronary and intravenous medications, and direct stenting.

Distal protection devices

Thrombotic distal embolizations are common during degenerated saphenous vein graft angioplasty due to the soft and friable nature of the lipid-rich plaque. Webb and colleagues were the first to demonstrate the potential benefit of distal protection devices (PercuSurge GuardWire, Medtronic Inc., Santa Rosa, USA).[55] In 93% of their cases, atheromatous and thrombotic debris were collected with the system.

Several investigations confirmed the benefit of using a protection device in the strategy of vein graft angioplasty, among them the SAFER study using the PercuSurge GuardWire system.[56] Of the 801 eligible patients, 406 were randomized to stent placement over the shaft of the protection system and 395 patients to stent placement over a conventional guidewire. A 42% reduction of combined end-point of death, myocardial infarction, emergency bypass surgery, and target vessel revascularization was noted in the protected group compared to the control group. Therefore, its use is now part of the standard care of saphenous vein graft angioplasty. The FIRE trial, including 651 patients, was able to compare the FilterWire EX (Boston Scientific Corp., Santa Clara, USA) to the PercuSurge system in the treatment of diseased saphenous aortocoronary bypass grafts.[57] Similar efficacy was demonstrated for both. Nevertheless, up to 10% of major cardiac events are still noted despite the use of these devices and therefore research continues. The TriActiv system (Kensey Nash Corporation, Exton, USA) was investigated in comparison to the PercuSurge and FilterWire EX systems for saphenous vein graft treatment in the PRIDE study.[58] The TriActiv system met the criteria of noninferiority to a control cohort using the Medtronic GuardWire Plus or the Boston Scientific FilterWire EX for the prevention of major adverse cardiac events within 30 days.

Even though these devices are effective and definitely indicated in the treatment of degenerated saphenous vein graft (angiographic no-reflow), their value is yet to be established in primary PCI for acute myocardial infarction. A first feasibility trial showed encouraging results with improved ST segment resolution, reduction in peak CK release, and increased left ventricular ejection fraction.[59] Several pilot studies further confirmed that embolic debris retrieved with the distal protection device (70%) resulted in greater TIMI flow and blush, ST segment resolution, and improved left ventricular function.[60,61] However, the only published multicenter randomized trial comparing primary PCI with a protection device (PercuSurge) versus PCI alone in the setting of acute myocardial infarction (EMERALD trial) failed to confirm these previous encouraging results.[62] Five hundred and five patients were included within six hours of chest pain onset and primary or rescue PCI. In 83% of cases, GP IIb/IIIa inhibitors were given through the procedure. Despite an effective retrieval of embolic debris (70% of cases in the protected group), no significant difference was noted on ST segment resolution at 30 minutes, left ventricular ejection fraction or major cardiac events at six months. Numerous explanations were raised in order to understand the lack of benefit in the setting of acute myocardial infarction.[63] The currently unpublished, smaller PROMISE trial also failed to demonstrate any beneficial effect of distal protection on markers of myocardial ischemia as well as on the coronary microcirculation.[64]

There are currently no data supporting the systematic use of distal protection devices during PCI in native coronary arteries. Their use should remain reserved for cases where important thrombus burden is suspected. The issue of distal protection will be further discussed in the following chapters.

Medications

The role of GP IIb/IIIa antagonists in preventing angiographic no-reflow remains unclear. A large randomized trial did not show any benefit of GP IIb/IIIa antagonist pretreatment in diseased saphenous vein graft angioplasty.[65] In contrast, several investigations have shown their positive impact on coronary blood flow and occurrence of no-reflow in the setting of acute myocardial infarction.[66,67] Neumann and colleagues investigated prospectively the effect of abciximab in 200 patients treated by primary PCI. Improvements in coronary flow velocity and wall motion score were noted.[66] A recent study of 300 patients randomized to abciximab versus placebo before primary PCI confirmed this benefit with a significantly better TIMI flow grade at the end of the procedure in patients pretreated by the GP IIb/IIIa receptor inhibitor.[68] Therefore, even if GP IIb/IIIa inhibitors are not useful in saphenous vein graft angioplasty, their efficacy in the setting of acute myocardial infarction is proven due to improved epicardial and microvascular perfusion. Several other drugs (adenosine, verapamil, nicorandil) have been tested in the prevention of no-reflow.[69–71] Despite encouraging results, no specific recommendation can be given in the routine prevention of no-reflow. Larger randomized trials based on clinical end-point should be planned.

Others

Loubeyre and colleagues investigated 206 patients with acute myocardial infarction randomized to direct stenting versus predilatation before stenting. An improved myocardial reperfusion was noted in patients treated with direct stenting.[72] These data were confirmed by other investigators emphasizing that direct stenting is feasible and associated with lower microvascular damages and no-reflow.[73,74]

Finally, intra-aortic balloon counterpulsation has been recommended for drug-resistant no-reflow.[75,76]

Treatment of no-reflow (Figure 6.3)

Any drug should be given as distal as possible into the coronary bed in order to specifically act on the microcirculation (Figure 6.4). Different perfusion microcatheters are available for this purpose.

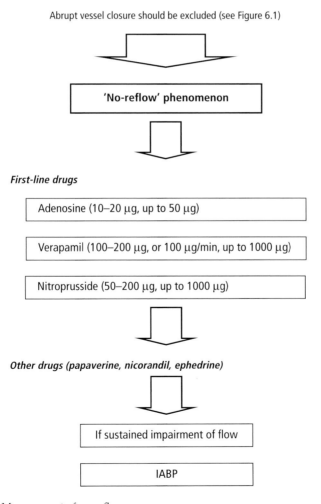

Figure 6.3   Management of no-reflow.

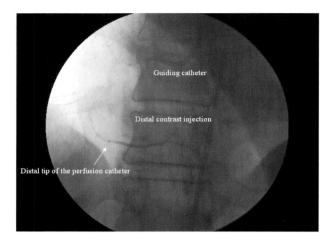

Figure 6.4   Perfusion catheter allowing distal injection of contrast or medications into the coronary bed.

Adenosine

Natural endogenous nucleoside which, first, slows the conduction through the AV and sinus pacemaker cells and, second, mediates local metabolic control of coronary blood flow (vasodilatation) through interaction with the adenosine receptors on coronary arteriolar smooth muscle cells.

The first evidence of the potential benefit of adenosine as adjunctive treatment for acute myocardial infarction came out of the AMISTAD study.[77] Two hundred and thirty-six patients with acute myocardial infarction treated by thrombolysis were randomized to adenosine versus placebo. The active drug resulted in a significant reduction of infarct size compared to placebo. Although some small studies also suggested the benefit of adenosine, the AMISTAD II study did not confirm its usefulness in the management of acute myocardial infarction.[77-80] A population of 2118 patients with evolving anterior myocardial infarction treated by thrombolysis or primary angioplasty was randomized to adenosine versus placebo. No differences in terms of clinical outcome were noted between the two groups, but infarct size was reduced in the group of patients receiving 70 µg/kg/min of adenosine. Adenosine was also tested in the setting of saphenous vein graft angioplasty and rotational atherectomy, with positive results.[81-83]

Nicorandil

Adenosine triphosphate (ATP)-sensitive K+ channel opener with nitrate effects which acts as arterial and venous dilator with coronary blood flow improvement.

Nicorandil was tested in acute myocardial infarction with encouraging results in small studies including 354 patients.[84,85] Ito and colleagues published the single randomized study, including 81 acute myocardial infarction patients. Nicorandil (intravenous bolus of 4 mg followed by 6 mg/24 h) or placebo was given before primary angioplasty.[86] The group treated with nicorandil had a better functional and clinical outcome compared to patients managed only with angioplasty.

Nicorandil has been compared to several other drugs. Adenosine-nicorandil association was shown to be superior to adenosine alone on occurrence of no-reflow and short-term clinical outcome.[87] Nicorandil was also compared to verapamil in 61 patients who had undergone rotational atherectomy. No GP IIb/IIIa inhibitor was given to the studied population. No or slow flow was observed significantly less in the group of patients receiving nicorandil.[88]

Verapamil

Calcium ion influx inhibitor that modulates the influx of ionic calcium across the cell membrane of the arterial smooth muscle (vasodilator) as well as in conductible and contractile myocardial cells.

Based on trials including patients with acute myocardial infarction, verapamil seems to be beneficial in the treatment of no-reflow.[89] One report of 40 patients showed benefit of 500 µg intracoronary verapamil compared to placebo. Improved coronary flow measured by myocardial contrast echocardiography was noted.[90] One trial tested the effect of verapamil compared to nitroglycerin in the treatment of no-reflow during saphenous vein graft angioplasty. Intragraft verapamil was superior in restoring flow with 88% success.[91] Other calcium channel blockers (diltiazem, nicardipine) were also tested, with positive effects on no-reflow.[92,93] Papaverine, which is structurally close to verapamil and relaxes the smooth muscle cells directly, has also been shown to be beneficial.[94]

Nitroprusside

Chemical nitric oxide (NO) donor that vasodilates the coronary muscle cells.

A retrospective study suggested that nitroprusside was effective in the treatment of acute myocardial no-reflow.[95] Two prospective studies, including 208 and 11 patients, confirmed that intracoronary injection of nitroprusside is feasible, safe, and effective.[96,97] In a study by Pasceri and colleagues, TIMI flow grade and TIMI frame count were significantly improved in almost all treated patients. One study compared adenosine and nitroprusside in angiographic no-reflow: 21 patients received adenosine alone and 20 patients a combination of adenosine and nitroprusside.[98] The latter association was safe and provided better improvement in coronary flow. Despite its nitric oxide-mediated pathway, nitroglycerin is ineffective in the treatment of no-reflow since it has few physiologic effects on the arterial microcirculation.

Thus many drugs have shown a positive impact in the treatment of no-reflow. However, as for the prevention of no-reflow, data from large randomized studies with clinical end-points are currently unavailable. Therefore, none of these drugs has become the gold standard for the treatment of no-reflow. Adenosine (10–20 µg IC bolus), verapamil (100–200 µg IC bolus or 100 µg/min, up to 1000 µg) and nitroprusside (50–200 µg IC bolus, up to 1000 µg) have shown the most convincing results and should therefore be used alone or potentially in combination through a super-selective injection.

CONCLUSION

In spite of advances in interventional cardiology, the incidence of slow coronary blood flow following percutaneous procedures and during acute myocardial infarction continues to cause adverse cardiac events following PCI. Identifying those patients at risk and paying particular attention to the coronary flow and not only to the anatomic results should minimize adverse events. Moreover, the appropriate diagnostic tools and pharmacologic agents should be readily available in every cardiac catheterization laboratory.

REFERENCES

1. Lincoff AM, Popma JJ, Ellis SG et al. Abrupt vessel closure complicating coronary angioplasty: clinical, angiographic and therapeutic profile. J Am Coll Cardiol 1992;20:926–35.
2. Simpfendorfer C, Belardi J, Bellamy G et al. Frequency, management, and follow-up of patients with acute coronary occlusions after percutaneous transluminal coronary angioplasty. Am J Cardiol 1987;59:267–9.
3. De Feyter PJ, van den Brand M, Laarman GH et al. Acute coronary artery occlusion during and after percutaneous transluminal angioplasty: frequency, prediction, clinical course, management and follow up. Circulation 1991;83:927–36.
4. Anderson HV, Shaw RE, Brindis RG et al. A contemporary overview of percutaneous coronary interventions. The American College of Cardiology-National Cardiovascular Data Registry (ACC-NCDR). J Am Coll Cardiol 2002;39:1096–103.
5. Sharma SK, Israel DH, Kamean JL et al. Clinical, angiographic, and procedural determinants of major and minor coronary dissection during angioplasty. Am Heart J 1993;126:39–47.
6. Ferguson JJ, Barash E, Wilson JM et al. The relation of clinical outcome to dissection and thrombus formation during coronary angioplasty. J Invasive Cardiol 1995;7:2–10.
7. Huber MS, Mooney JF, Madison J et al. Use of a morphologic classification to predict clinical outcome after dissection from coronary angioplasty. Am J Cardiol 1991;68:467–71.
8. Bell M, Berger PB, Reeder GS et al. Coronary dissection following PTCA: predictors of major ischemic complications. Circulation 1991;84:II–130.
9. Mishkel GJ, Aguirre FV, Ligon RW et al. Clopidogrel as adjunctive antiplatelet therapy during coronary stenting. J Am Coll Cardiol 1999;34:1884–90.
10. Smith SC Jr, Dove JT, Jacobs AK et al. ACC/AHA guidelines for percutaneous coronary intervention: a report of the American College of Cardiology/American Heart Association Task Force on Practice Guidelines (Committee to Revise the 1993 Guidelines for Percutaneous Transluminal Coronary Angioplasty). J Am Coll Cardiol 2001;37:2215–39.
11. Boccara A, Benamer H, Juliard JM et al. A randomized trial of a fixed high dose versus a weight-adjusted low dose of intravenous heparin during coronary angioplasty. Eur Heart J 1997;18:631–5.
12. Topol EJ, Ferguson JJ, Weisman HF et al. Long-term protection from myocardial ischemic events in a randomized trial of brief integrin beta3 blockade with percutaneous coronary intervention. EPIC Investigator Group. Evaluation of Platelet IIb/IIIa Inhibition for Prevention of Ischemic Complication. JAMA 1997;278:479–84.
13. Topol EJ, Mark DB, Lincoff AM et al. Outcomes at 1 year and economic implications of platelet glycoprotein IIb/IIIa blockade in patients undergoing coronary stenting: results from a multicentre randomised trial. EPISTENT Investigators. Evaluation of Platelet IIb/IIIa Inhibitor for Stenting. Lancet 1999;354:2019–24.
14. Kloner RA, Ganote CE, Jennings RB. The 'no-reflow' phenomenon after temporary coronary occlusion in dogs. J Clin Invest 1974;54:1496–508.
15. Willerson JT, Watson JT, Hutton I et al. Reduced myocardial reflow and increased coronary vascular resistance following prolonged myocardial ischemia in the dog. Circ Res 1975;36:771–81.
16. Schopfer J, Montz R, Mathey D. Scintigraphic evidence of the 'no-reflow' phenomenon in human beings after coronary thrombolysis. J Am Coll Cardiol 1985;5:593–8.

17. Bates ER, Krell MJ, Dean EN et al. Demonstration of 'no reflow' phenomenon by digital coronary arteriography. Am J Cardiol 1986;57:177–8.
18. Feld H, Lichstein E, Schachter J et al. Early and late angiographic findings of the 'no-reflow' phenomenon following direct angioplasty as the primary treatment for acute myocardial infarction. Am Heart J 1992;123:782–4.
19. Eeckhout E, Kern MJ. The coronary no-reflow phenomenon: a review of mechanisms and therapies. Eur Heart J 2001;22:729–39.
20. Rezkalla SH, Kloner RA. No-reflow phenomenon. Circulation 2002;105:656–62.
21. Mehta RH, Harjai KJ, Cox D et al. Clinical and angiographic correlates and outcomes of suboptimal coronary flow in patients with acute myocardial infarction undergoing primary percutaneous coronary intervention. J Am Coll Cardiol 2003;42:1739–46.
22. Ambrosio G, Weisman HF, Mannisi JA et al. Progressive impairment of regional myocardial perfusion after initial restoration of postischemic blood flow. Circulation 1989;80:1846–61.
23. Gregorini L, Marco J, Kozakova M et al. Alpha-adrenergic blockade improves recovery of myocardial perfusion and function after coronary stenting in patients with acute myocardial infarction. Circulation 1999;99:482–90.
24. Murohara T, Buerke M, Lefer AM. Polymorphonuclear leukocyte induced vasocontraction and endothelial dysfunction. Role of selectins. Arterioscler Thromb 1994;14:1509–19.
25. Seydoux C, Goy J-J, Davies G. Platelet and neutrophil imaging techniques in the investigation of the response to thrombolytic therapy and the no-reflow phenomenon. Am Heart J 1993;125:1142–7.
26. Michaels AD, Gibson CM, Barron HV. Microvascular dysfunction in acute myocardial infarction: focus on the roles of platelet and inflammatory mediators in the no-reflow phenomenon. Am J Cardiol 2000;85:50b–60b.
27. Engler RL, Schmid-Schönbein GW, Pavelec RS. Leukocyte capillary plugging in myocardial ischemia and reperfusion in the dog. Am J Pathol 1983;111:98–111.
28. Sheridan FM, Cole PG, Ramage D. Leukocyte adhesion to the coronary microvasculature during ischemia and reperfusion in an in vivo canine model. Circulation 1996;93:1784–7.
29. Engler RL, Dahlgren MD, Morris DD et al. Role of leukocytes in response to acute myocardial ischemia and reflow in dogs. Am J Physiol 1986;251:H314–H322.
30. Abbo KM, Dooris M, Glazier S. Features and outcome of no-reflow after percutaneous coronary intervention. Am J Cardiol 1995;75:778–82.
31. Leopold JA, Berger CJ, Cupples LA et al. No-reflow during coronary intervention: observations and implications. Circulation 2000;102:II–604.
32. Santoro GM, Valenti R, Buonamici P et al. Relation between ST-segment changes and myocardial perfusion evaluated by myocardial contrast echocardiography in patients with acute myocardial infarction treated with direct angioplasty. Am J Cardiol 1998;82:932–7.
33. Gibson CM, Cannon CP, Daley WL et al. The TIMI frame count: a quantitative method of assessing coronary artery flow. Circulation 1996;93:879–88.
34. Gibson CM, Murphy SA, Rizzo MJ et al. The relationship between the TIMI frame count and clinical outcomes after thrombolytic administration. Circulation 1999;99:1945–50.
35. Lincoff AM, Topol EJ, Califf RM et al. Significance of a coronary artery with thrombolysis in myocardial infarction grade 2 flow 'patency' (outcome in the Thrombolysis and Angioplasty in Myocardial Infarction trials). Thrombolysis and Angioplasty in Myocardial Infarction Study Group. Am J Cardiol 1995;75:871–6.
36. Piana R, Paik GK, Moscucci M et al. Incidence and treatment of 'no-reflow' after percutaneous coronary intervention. Circulation 1994;89:2514.
37. Gibson CM, Cannon CP, Murphy SA et al. Relationship of the TIMI myocardial perfusion grades, flow grades, frame count, and percutaneous coronary intervention to long-term outcomes after thrombolytic administration in acute myocardial infarction. Circulation 2002;105:1909.
38. Van't Hof AW, Liem A, Suryapranata H et al. Angiographic assessment of myocardial reperfusion in patients treated with primary angioplasty for acute myocardial infarction: myocardial blush grade. Circulation 1998;97:2302–6.

39. Tan WA, Moliterno DJ. TIMI flow and surrogate end points: what you see is not always what you get. Am Heart J 1998;136:570–3.
40. Sherman JR, Anwar A, Bret JR et al. Distal vessel pullback angiography and pressure gradient measurements: an innovative diagnostic approach to evaluate the no-reflow phenomenon. Cathet Cardiovasc Diagn 1996;39:1–6.
41. Iwakura K, Ito H, Takiuchi S et al. Alteration in the coronary blood flow velocity pattern in patients with no reflow and reperfused acute myocardial infarction. Circulation 1996;94:1269–75.
42. Iwakura K, Ito H, Nishikawa N et al. Early temporal changes in coronary flow velocity patterns in patients with acute myocardial infarction demonstrating the 'no-reflow' phenomenon. Am J Cardiol 1999;84:415–19.
43. Herrmann J, Haude M, Lerman A et al. Abnormal coronary flow velocity reserve following coronary intervention is associated with cardiac marker elevation. Circulation 2001;103:2339–45.
44. Kondo M, Nakano A, Saito D et al. Assessment of 'microvascular no-reflow phenomenon' using technetium-99m macroaggregated albumin scintigraphy in patients with acute myocardial infarction. J Am Coll Cardiol 1998;32:898–903.
45. Santoro GM, Valenti R, Buonamici P et al. Relation between ST-segment changes and myocardial perfusion evaluated by myocardial contrast echocardiography in patients with acute myocardial infarction treated by direct angioplasty. Am J Cardiol 1998;82:932–7.
46. Porter TR, Li S, Kricsfeld D et al. Detection of myocardial perfusion in multiple echocardiographic windows with one intravenous injection of microbubbles using transient response second harmonic imaging. J Am Coll Cardiol 1997;29:791–9.
47. Villanueva FS, Glasheen WP, Sklenar J et al. Characterization of spatial patterns of flow within the reperfused myocardium by myocardial contrast echocardiography: implications in determining extent of myocardial salvage. Circulation 1993;88:2596–606.
48. Ito H, Tomooka T, Sakai N et al. Lack of myocardial perfusion immediately after successful thrombolysis: a predictor of poor recovery of left ventricular function in anterior myocardial infarction. Circulation 1992;85:1699–705.
49. Ito H, Maruyama A, Iwakura K et al. Clinical implications of the 'no reflow' phenomenon: a predictor of complications and left ventricular remodeling in reperfused anterior wall myocardial infarction. Circulation 1996;93:223–8.
50. Kenner MD, Zajac EJ, Kondos GT et al. Ability of the no-reflow phenomenon during an acute myocardial infarction to predict left ventricular dysfunction at one-month follow-up. Am J Cardiol 1995;76:861–8.
51. Taylor AJ, Al-Saadi N, Abdel-Aty H et al. Detection of acutely impaired microvascular reperfusion after infarct angioplasty with magnetic resonance imaging. Circulation 2004;109:2080–5.
52. Wu KC, Zerhouni EA, Judd RM et al. Prognostic significance of microvascular obstruction by magnetic resonance imaging in patients with acute myocardial infarction. Circulation 1998;97:765–72.
53. Bremerich J, Wendland MF, Arheden H et al. Microvascular injury in reperfused infarcted myocardium: non-invasive assessment with contrast-enhanced echoplanar magnetic resonance imaging. J Am Coll Cardiol 1998;32:787–93.
54. Jeremy RW, Links JM, Becker CC. Progressive failure of coronary flow during reperfusion of myocardial infarction: documentation of the no-reflow phenomenon with positron emission tomography. J Am Coll Cardiol 1990;16:695–704.
55. Webb JG, Carere RG, Virmani R et al. Retrieval and analysis of particulate debris after saphenous vein graft intervention. J Am Coll Cardiol 1999;34:468–75.
56. Baim DS, Wahr D, George B et al. Randomized trial of a distal embolic protection device during percutaneous intervention of saphenous vein aorto-coronary bypass grafts. Circulation 2002;105:1285–90.
57. Stone GW, Rogers C, Hermiller J et al. Randomized comparison of distal protection with a filter-based catheter and a balloon occlusion and aspiration system during percutaneous

intervention of diseased saphenous vein aorto-coronary bypass grafts. Circulation 2003;108:548–53.

58. Carrozza JP, Caussin C, Braden G et al. Embolic protection during saphenous vein graft intervention using a second-generation balloon protection device: results from the combined US and European pilot study of the TriActiv Balloon Protected Flush Extraction System. Am Heart J 2005;149:1136–7.
59. Limbruno U, Micheli A, de Carlo M et al. Mechanical prevention of distal embolisation during primary angioplasty: safety, feasibility, and impact on myocardial reperfusion. Circulation 2003;108:171.
60. Nakamura T, Kubo N, Seki Y et al. Effects of a distal protection device during primary stenting in patients with acute anterior myocardial infarction. Circ J 2004;68:763–8.
61. Yip HK, Wu CJ, Chang HW et al. Effect of the PercuSurge GuardWire device on the integrity of microvasculature and clinical outcomes during primary transradial coronary intervention in acute myocardial infarction. Am J Cardiol 2003;92:1331–5.
62. Stone GW, Webb J, Cox DA et al. Distal microcirculatory protection during percutaneous coronary intervention in acute ST-segment elevation myocardial infarction: a randomised controlled trial. JAMA 2005;293:1063.
63. Schömig A, Kastrati A. Distal embolic protection in patients with acute myocardial infarction: attractive concept but no evidence of benefit. JAMA 2005;293:1116–17.
64. Gick M, Jander N, Bestehorn HP et al. Randomized study on the effectiveness of a filter device for distal protection during direct percutaneous catheter intervention for acute myocardial infarction: results of the PROMISE (Protection Devices in PCI-Treatment of Myocardial Infarction for Salvage of Endangered Myocardium) Study. Presented at Late Breaking Clinical Trials, 54th Annual Scientific Session of the American College of Cardiology, March 6–9, 2005, Orlando, FL.
65. Roffi M, Mukherjee D, Chew DP et al. Lack of benefit from intravenous platelet glycoprotein IIb/IIIa receptor inhibition as adjunctive treatment for percutaneous interventions of aortocoronary bypass grafts. Circulation 2002;106:3063–7.
66. Neumann F-J, Blasini R, Schmitt C et al. Effect of glycoprotein IIb/IIIa receptor blockade on recovery of coronary flow and left ventricular function after the placement of coronary-artery stents in acute myocardial infarction. Circulation 1998;98:2695–701.
67. De Lemos JA, Antman EM, Gibson M et al. Abciximab improves both epicardial flow and myocardial reperfusion in ST-elevation myocardial infarction: observations from the TIMI 14 trial. Circulation 2000;101:239–43.
68. Montalescot G, Barragan P, Wittenberg O et al. Platelet glycoprotein IIb/IIIa inhibition with coronary stenting for acute myocardial infarction. N Engl J Med 2001;344:1895–903.
69. Michaels AD, Appleby M, Otten MH et al. Pretreatment with intragraft verapamil prior to percutaneous coronary intervention of saphenous vein graft lesions: results of the randomized, controlled vasodilator prevention on no-reflow (VAPOR) trial. J Invasive Cardiol 2002;14:299–302.
70. Marzilli M, Orsini E, Marraccini P et al. Beneficial effects of intracoronary adenosine as an adjunct to primary angioplasty in acute myocardial infarction. Circulation 2000;101:2154–9.
71. Taniyama Y, Ito H, Iwakura K et al. Beneficial effect of intracoronary verapamil on microvascular and myocardial salvage in patients with acute myocardial infarction. J Am Coll Cardiol 1997;30:1193–9.
72. Loubeyre C, Morice MC, Lefevre T et al. A randomized comparison of direct stenting with conventional stent implantation in selected patients with acute myocardial infarction. J Am Coll Cardiol 2002;39:15–21.
73. Antoniucci D, Valenti R, Migliorini A et al. Direct infarct artery stenting without predilation and no-reflow in patients with acute myocardial infarction. Am Heart J 2001;142:684–90.
74. Timurkaynak T, Ozdemir M, Cengel A et al. Conventional versus direct stenting in AMI: effect on immediate coronary blood flow. J Invasive Cardiol 2002;14:372–7.
75. Port SC, Patel S, Schmidt DH. Effects of intracoronary balloon counterpulsation on

myocardial blood flow in patients with severe coronary artery disease. J Am Coll Cardiol 1984;3:1367–74.

76. Kern MJ, Aguirre F, Bach R et al. Augmentation of coronary blood flow by intra-aortic balloon pumping in patients after coronary angioplasty. Circulation 1993;87:500–11.

77. Mahaffey KW, Puma JA, Barbagelata A et al. Adenosine as an adjunct to thrombolytic therapy for acute myocardial infarction. J Am Coll Cardiol 1999;34:1711–20.

78. Assali AR, Sdringola S, Ghani M et al. Intracoronary adenosine administered during percutaneous intervention in acute myocardial infarction and reduction in the incidence of 'no reflow' phenomenon. Cathet Cardiovasc Intervent 2000;51:27–31.

79. Ross AM, Gibbons RJ, Stone GW et al. A randomized, double-blind, placebo-controlled multicenter trial of adenosine as an adjunct to reperfusion in the treatment of acute myocardial infarction (AMISTAD-II). J Am Coll Cardiol 2005;45:1775–80.

80. Marzilli M, Orsini E, Marraccini P et al. Beneficial effects of intracoronary adenosine as an adjunct to primary angioplasty in acute myocardial infarction. Circulation 2000;101:2154–9.

81. Fischell TA, Carter AJ, Foster MT et al. Reversal of 'no-reflow' during vein graft stenting using high velocity boluses of intracoronary adenosine. Cathet Cardiovasc Diagn 1998;45:366–7.

82. Sdringola S, Assali A, Ghani M et al. Adenosine use during aortocoronary vein graft interventions reverses but does not prevent the slow no-reflow phenomenon. Cathet Cardiovasc Intervent 2000;51:394–9.

83. Hanna GP, Yhip P, Fujise K et al. Intracoronary adenosine administration during rotational atherectomy of complex lesions in native coronary arteries reduces the incidence of no-reflow phenomenon. Cathet Cardiovasc Intervent 1999;48:275–8.

84. Sakata Y, Kodama K, Ishikura F et al. Disappearance of the 'no-reflow' phenomenon after adjunctive intracoronary administration of nicorandil in a patient with acute myocardial infarction. Jpn Circ J 1997;61:455–8.

85. Sugimoto K, Ito H, Iwakura K et al. Intravenous nicorandil in conjunction with coronary reperfusion therapy is associated with better clinical and functional outcomes in patients with acute myocardial infarction. Circ J 2003;67:295–300.

86. Ito H, Taniyama Y, Iwakura K et al. Intravenous nicorandil can preserve microvascular integrity and myocardial viability in patients with reperfused anterior wall myocardial infarction. J Am Coll Cardiol 1999;33:654–60.

87. Lim SY, Bae EH, Jeong MH et al. Effect of combined intracoronary adenosine and nicorandil on no-reflow phenomenon during percutaneous coronary intervention. Circ J 2004;68:928–32.

88. Tsubokawa A, Ueda K, Sakamoto H et al. Effect of intracoronary nicorandil administration on preventing no-reflow/slow flow phenomenon during rotational atherectomy. Circ J 2002;66:1119–23.

89. Demir I, Yilmaz H, Ermis C et al. Treatment of no-reflow phenomenon with verapamil after primary stent deployment during myocardial infarction. Jpn Heart J 2002;43:573–80.

90. Taniyama Y, Ito H, Iwakura K et al. Beneficial effect of intracoronary verapamil on microvascular and myocardial salvage in patients with acute myocardial infarction. J Am Coll Cardiol 1997;30:1193–9.

91. Kaplan BM, Benzuly KH, Kinn JW et al. Treatment of no-reflow in degenerated saphenous vein graft intervention: comparison of intracoronary verapamil and nitroglycerin. Cathet Cardiovasc Diagn 1996;39:113–18.

92. McIvor ME, Undemir C, Lawson J et al. Clinical effects and utility of intracoronary diltiazem. Cathet Cardiovasc Diagn 1995;35:287–91.

93. Fugit MD, Rubal BJ, Donovan DJ. Effects of intracoronary nicardipine, diltiazem and verapamil on coronary blood flow. J Invasive Cardiol 2000;12:80–5.

94. Ishihara M, Sato H, Tateishi H et al. Attenuation of the no-reflow phenomenon after coronary angioplasty for acute myocardial infarction with intracoronary papaverine. Am Heart J 1996;132:959–63.

95. Hillegass WB, Dean NA, Liao L et al. Treatment of no-reflow and impaired flow with the

nitric oxide donor nitroprusside following percutaneous coronary interventions: initial human clinical experience. J Am Coll Cardiol 2001;37:1335–43.

96. Wang HJ, Lo PH, Lin JJ et al. Treatment of slow/no-reflow phenomenon with intracoronary nitroprusside injection in primary coronary intervention for acute myocardial infarction. Cathet Cardiovasc Intervent 2004;63:171–6.

97. Pasceri V, Pristipino C, Pelliccia F et al. Effects of the nitric oxide donor nitroprusside on no-reflow phenomenon during coronary interventions for acute myocardial infarction. Am J Cardiol 2005;95:1358–61.

98. Barcin C, Denktas AE, Lennon RJ et al. Comparison of combination therapy of adenosine and nitroprusside with adenosine alone in the treatment of angiographic no-reflow phenomenon. Cathet Cardiovasc Intervent 2004;61:484–91.

99. Klein LW. Coronary complications of percutaneous coronary intervention: a practical approach to the management of abrupt closure. Cathet Cardiovasc Intervent 2005;64:395–401.

7

Management of stent loss and foreign body retrieval

Bruno Farah, Jean Fajadet and Jean Marco

• **Removal of embolized material from the coronary system** • **Removal of embolized material from the iliac vessel** • **Conclusion**

In the year 2000, the incidence of stent embolization was estimated at 1.2%.[1] It is significantly lower with the premounted stent system compared to hand-crimped stents.[2] Dislodgement of a stent may result in systemic or intracoronary embolization. While systemic embolization may cause severe cerebrovascular events, intracoronary embolization is associated with a high risk of coronary thrombosis and subsequent myocardial infarction. Moreover, interventional cardiologists are sometimes approached to remove various materials, accidentally embolized into the vascular system (for example, central venous line embolized in the right heart chambers). Percutaneous management of this rare complication can avoid bail-out cardiac surgery.

The first goal is to safely bring the embolized material to the iliac artery. At that level, further manipulations can be attempted without any major risk as peripheral embolization usually is not associated with apparent clinical side effects.[3] The embolized material may be removed from the introducer, or by a simple surgical access.

All of the techniques discussed below are used as references for interventional cardiologists. They include standard methods with commercial snares and some exotic techniques, which may be necessary due to lack of appropriate equipment. The selection of a particular method or piece of equipment depends on the patient's clinical condition, the operator's experience of retrieval equipment, and availability of equipment in the cardiac catheterization laboratory. Different options in the management of embolized materials are listed in Table 7.1.

Table 7.1 Therapeutic options in the management of embolized materials
1. No treatment for peripherally embolized small stents
2. Deployment of the embolized stent in a nonconsequential location (wire inside the stent)
3. Compression of the unexpanded stent by another stent
4. Removal of the stent by inflating a small balloon distally (wire inside the stent)
5. Removal of the stent by a snare
6. Removal of the stent by a myocardial biopsy forceps
7. Removal of the stent with two twisted wires (wires inside the stent)

REMOVAL OF EMBOLIZED MATERIAL FROM THE CORONARY SYSTEM

When a problem with defective equipment arises inside the coronary system or the ascending aorta, it is best to remove the entire system to the iliac artery in order to avoid any risk of cerebral embolization. In the case of a stent that slips off the delivery balloon, it cannot be brought to the iliac artery by simply withdrawing the whole system. Pulling the wire will leave a free stent behind.

Different techniques have been used for percutaneous retrieval of embolized materials, using conventional and nonconventional equipment. The conventional equipment includes Amplatz gooseneck snares and myocardial biopsy forceps, designed to grasp embolized material. The unconventional equipment is not designed for the purpose of grasping an object, and includes small size angioplasty balloon catheter, angioplasty wires, and guiding catheters.

Position of the wire

The position of the wire inside the stent will be very helpful in managing the retrieval techniques. Moreover, some easy techniques (low-profile balloon technique, two twisted wires) are not possible in case of inadvertent retraction of the guidewire.

So the first goal is to keep the wire inside the stent and across the lesion for prompt access of rescue hardware.

Removal of the stent with a low-profile angioplasty balloon[4–6]

This is often the primary approach because this technique does not require specific material. A small size balloon (1.5–2.0 mm) is advanced on the guidewire and then passed through beyond the stent. The stent is attached to the retrieval balloon by inflation to 1–2 atmospheres and is gently withdrawn out of the coronary system toward the guiding catheter. Once the stent is well secured between the balloon and the guiding catheter, it can be brought to the iliac artery and removed through the arterial sheath. The balloon catheter technique can also be used to advance the embolized stent directly and deploy it at the target lesion site or in a nonconsequential location. A limitation of balloon-assisted stent retrieval is the inadvertent retraction of the guidewire. In such cases, a gooseneck snare may be preferred or the stent loss can be managed by compressing the unexpanded stent against the vessel wall by another stent, without compromising coronary blood flow.

Removal of the stent or embolized fragment by a snare

This approach is often preferred in cases of inadvertent loss of the guidewire position. The Amplatz gooseneck snare (Microvena Corporation, White Bear Lake, MN, USA) is a nitinol retrieval device that includes a 4 F transport end-hole catheter and a snare loop 2 mm in diameter angulated at 90° to the shaft axis. This right angle of the loop facilitates the grasping of the target object. The 4 F catheter tapers to a 2.3 F tip and can easily fit inside a 6 F guiding catheter.[7]

Technique with the wire still inside the embolized stent

The position of the wire inside the stent will help the retrieval technique by giving prompt access to the defective stent and limiting the free movement of the stent to the longitudinal axis of the wire.

The loop of the gooseneck snare is passed over the angioplasty wire, encircles it and advances up to the coronary ostium. The snare is manipulated under fluoroscopic guidance to pass over the distal end of the embolized stent. Once the loop is in the right position, the transport catheter is advanced to tighten the loop around the stent.

If there is difficulty in positioning the snare, a second wire can be placed beside the original wire to provide a rail on which the snare device can be moved without shifting the position of the stent.[8]

When the stent is secured by the snare, it can be withdrawn as a whole to the iliac artery. Sometimes, it may be difficult or impossible to retrieve the stent through the 6 F or 7 F femoral sheath; at this point, the sheath can be changed to a larger one (9 F) through which the embolized stent can be removed.

Technique with a free stent or embolized material

In cases of a free stent (not on angioplasty wire) or embolized material, their capture depends on correct alignment of the loop to the free end of these fragments.

The following technical tips are important for success.

- Careful evaluation under fluoroscopy for locating the free end of the embolized material, which usually pulsates.
- Identifying the position of the snare. The plane of the snare is held at right angles to the estimated plane of the embolized material. To do this, the embolized fragment should be seen in its full length under fluoroscopy. Then the snare is held in such a way that it is shown as a straight line or a closed loop, confirming its vertical plane in relation to the embolized fragment. This position allows the capture of the embolized fragment. If the snare loop is parallel to the plane of the embolized material, ensnarement is impossible (Figure 7.1).

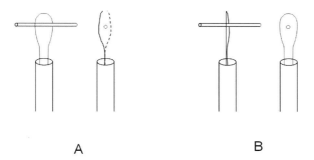

A   B

Figure 7.1   Importance of the plane of the snare loop in relation to the embolized material or stent. The snare is shown under fluoroscopy as a straight line or a closed loop, confirming its vertical plane in relation to the fragment or stent.[9]

- Securing the embolized fragment. The next important step is to be sure that the snare has encircled the embolized material. The transport catheter is advanced, causing the embolized fragment to bend when the snare is engaged. Withdrawing the ends of the wire to capture the embolized fragment is not recommended because it can cause disengagement[9] (Figure 7.2).
- Removal of protruding material with a pigtail or left Amplatz catheter. These catheters can be used to help the removal of embolized material protruding into the aorta or the right heart chambers. The catheter is twisted to wind the embolized fragment, then the fragment can be pulled down by the catheter to the iliac artery or vein (Figure 7.3). Once brought to the iliac vessel, the embolized material could be removed easily by a snare or a myocardial forceps or could be extracted with a mini-invasive surgical vascular access.

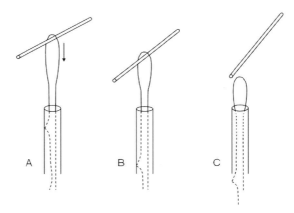

Figure 7.2 Incorrect technique of ensnarement. Withdrawing the ends of the wire to capture the embolized material or stent can cause disengagement.[9]

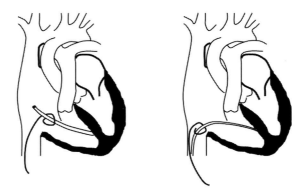

Figure 7.3 Technique of ensnarement with a pigtail catheter. The pigtail catheter is twisted to wind the embolized fragment (venous line embolized into the right heart chambers), then the pigtail and the entwined fragment are pulled down to the iliac vessel.

Stent removal with two twisted wires

When a snare is not available to retrieve the embolized stent, it may be possible to withdraw the stent with a second wire twisting around the stent to immobilize it against the first wire.[10,11]

A second wire is advanced and carefully manipulated through the struts of the free stent. The two wires outside the guiding catheter are bound together by a torquing device which is rotated clockwise about 15–20 times, until the wires are observed twisting together near the proximal end of the stent. Then both wires are pulled together and the guiding catheter advanced forward. The stent twisted between the two wires and the guiding catheter are pulled out gently as a single unit (Figure 7.4). Once the stent is brought to the level of the common iliac artery, it can be removed by conventional methods after the wires are untwisted.[10] The key point for snaring the stent is the second wire placement through the struts of the unexpanded stent and not through the central lumen. When the two wires are removed slowly, the guiding catheter should engage deeper into the ostium. This is the sign that the stent is properly snared. If the second wire goes through the central lumen, both wires can easily be pulled out, leaving the free stent behind.

REMOVAL OF EMBOLIZED MATERIAL FROM THE ILIAC VESSEL

Once the embolized material is brought to the iliac artery or vein, the main problem is to remove it through the vascular sheath without the need for vascular cut-down. If the 6 F or 7 F sheath is too small, it should be changed for a 9 F sheath.

Alligator forceps or a cardiac bioptome are suitable for retrieving the stent through a 'biting jaws' action.[5,12,13] The limitations of these instruments are the need to directly grasp small material and the possibility of endovascular trauma during manipulation. Hence other techniques are more commonly used for stent retrieval.

Retraction of the stent into the guiding catheter

This is a crucial moment in the retrieval technique as the stent can be dislodged if it impacts on the tip of the guiding catheter. This phase should be done at the level of the iliac vessel as further manipulations would not cause any cerebrovascular complication.

Retraction of the stent into the guiding catheter is feasible if there is a favorable alignment between the stent and the guiding catheter. Without an excellent co-axial

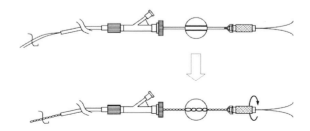

Figure 7.4   The double-wire technique.[14]

relationship, the stent can be dislodged. Sometimes, the retraction of the guiding catheter into the arterial sheath will straighten the tip of the guiding catheter and facilitate the stent retrieval[15] (Figure 7.5).

Removal of material from the iliac vessel with a gooseneck snare

Once the embolized stent has been brought to the iliac vessel, it can be removed with a gooseneck snare system. The snare should be placed above the embolized stent and tightened at its distal end under fluoroscopic guidance. By pulling the distal end, the operator can manipulate this end to enter the tip of the femoral sheath. If the stent is snared at its proximal part, it is more difficult to manipulate it to enter the sheath. If the stent is crushed at the proximal part, the whole stent will collapse and its large mass will pass with difficulty through the femoral sheath. If the stent is crushed at the distal end, the area of damage is smaller and it could be still manipulated to enter into the sheath. Upsizing the sheath (9 F) could be helpful in case of difficulty.

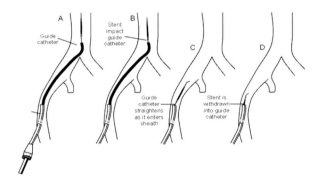

Figure 7.5   Attempts to remove a stent into a guiding catheter require excellent co-axial alignment between the stent and the tip of the guiding catheter. Sometimes, the guiding catheter needs to be retracted into the arterial sheath so the angulation of the tip can be straightened out.[15]

CONCLUSION

Embolization of coronary stents or various materials is a rare but technically challenging complication with hazardous potential for the patient. Different methods for percutaneous retrieval of these embolized fragments have been described. The selection of a particular method or piece of equipment depends on the patient's clinical condition, the operator's experience of retrieval equipment, and availability of the equipment in the cardiac catheterization laboratory.

Acknowledgments

The authors thank Stéphanie Gilliume for technical assistance and excellent secretarial support.

REFERENCES

1. Chevalier B, Glatt B, Guyon P et al. Current indications of stent retrieval techniques. J Am Coll Cardiol 2000;35 (Suppl 2):64A.
2. Sick P, Zindler G, Zotz R. Randomized comparison of 4 different stent designs in 966 stenoses. J Am Coll Cardiol 2000;35 (Suppl 2):55A.
3. Cantor WJ, Lazzam C, Cohen EA et al. Failed coronary stent deployment. Am Heart J 1998;136:1088–95.
4. Cishek MB, Laslett L, Gershony G. Balloon catheter retrieval of dislodged coronary stents: a novel technique. Cathet Cardiovasc Diagn 1995;34:350–2.
5. Berder V, Bedossa M, Gras D et al. Retrieval of a lost coronary stent from the descending aorta using a PTCA balloon and a biopsy forceps. Cathet Cardiovasc Diagn 1993;28:351–3.
6. Eggebrecht H, Haude M, von Birgelen C et al. Nonsurgical retrieval of embolized coronary stents. Cathet Cardiovasc Intervent 2000;51:432–40.
7. Elsner M, Pfeifer A, Kasper W. Intracoronary loss of balloon-mounted stents: successful retrieval with a 2 mm 'Microsnare' device. Cathet Cardiovasc Diagn 1996;39:271–6.
8. Bogart DB, Jung SC. Dislodged stent: a simple retrieval technique. Cathet Cardiovasc Intervent 1999;47:323–4.
9. Gerlock AJ, Mirfakhraee M. Foreign body retrieval. In: Gerlock AJ, Mirfakhraee M, eds. Essentials of Diagnostic and Interventional Angiographic Techniques. Philadelphia PA: WB Saunders, 1985.
10. Veldhuijzen FLMJ, Bonnier HJRM, Michels HR et al. Retrieval of undeployed stents from the right coronary artery. Report of two cases. Cathet Cardiovasc Diagn 1993;30:245–8.
11. Wong PHC. Retrieval of undeployed intracoronary Palmaz-Schatz stents. Cathet Cardiovasc Diagn 1995;35:218–23.
12. Foster-Smith KW, Garrath KN, Higano ST et al. Retrieval techniques for managing flexible intracoronary stent misplacement. Cathet Cardiovasc Diagn 1993;30:63–8.
13. Eeckhout E, Stauffer JC, Goy JJ. Retrieval of a migrated coronary stent by means of an alligator forceps. Cathet Cardiovasc Diagn 1993;30:166–8.
14. Grines C, Safian R. PTCA exotica: unusual problems in the invasive laboratory. In: Freed M, Grines C, Safian R, eds. The New Manual of Interventional Cardiology. Physician Press, 1996.
15. Garratt K, Bachrach M. Stent retrieval: devices and technique. In: Heuser R, ed. Peripheral Vascular Stenting for Cardiologists. London: Martin Dunitz, 1999.

8

Coronary perforation: incidence, predictive factors, management, and prevention

François Schiele and Nicolas Meneveau

- **Physiopathology, classification, consequences, and incidence** • **Management strategy** • **Prevention**

Coronary perforation is a rare but potentially life-threatening complication of percutaneous cardiovascular intervention (PCI). It includes a wide variety of pathologic situations, ranging from mere vessel puncture to large vessel rupture with brisk blood extravasation, tamponade, and hemodynamic compromise.

Over the past two decades, many changes in angioplasty techniques, driven by the quest for an easier immediate success and the fight against restenosis, have modified the incidence, risk factors, and management of coronary perforation. Indeed, different types of perforation result from different mechanisms, of which a proper understanding may serve to avoid this complication.

PHYSIOPATHOLOGY, CLASSIFICATION, CONSEQUENCES, AND INCIDENCE

Physiopathology and classification

Except in exceptional cases, coronary atherosclerosis does not spontaneously develop towards perforation,[1] and cases of traumatic perforation[2,3] or after diagnostic angiography[4,5] are rare. In the majority of cases, perforation occurs as a complication of coronary angioplasty and is related to several possible mechanisms:

- perforation of the arterial wall by a sharp object, such as the end of a guidewire
- excessive ablation of parietal tissue by an atherectomy device
- perforation caused by excessive stretching of the vessel wall by an oversized balloon or stent.

Ellis et al[6] proposed an angiographic classification of perforations into four types (Table 8.1), and this classification has since been adopted by the majority of other studies in this area.

- *Type 1*: extraluminal crater without extravasation. Type 1 perforations are generally without consequence and can be treated conservatively, although type 1 perforation has been reported to result in pericardial effusion.[7]

Table 8.1	Classification of perforations
Type 1	Extraluminal crater without extravasation
Type 2	Pericardial or myocardial blush without contrast jet extravasation
Type 3	Extravasation through frank (>1 mm) perforation
Cavity spilling	Perforation into an anatomic cavity chamber, coronary sinus, etc.
Subtype A	Directed toward the pericardium
Subtype B	Directed toward the myocardium

Adapted from Ellis et al[6] with permission

- *Type 2*: pericardial (subtype A; Figure 8.1) or myocardial[8,9] (subtype B) (Figure 8.2) blush without contrast jet extravasation. Can be observed at the site of angioplasty or may be distant, when resulting from arterial perforation with the end of a guidewire (Figure 8.3).
- *Type 3*: extravasation through frank (>1 mm) perforation (Figures 8.4 and 8.5). Generally accompanied by pericardial effusion that forms very rapidly, and complicated by tamponade, with unfavorable short-term prognosis.[6,9–13]

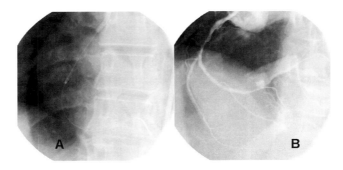

Figure 8.1   Type 2 perforation after use of thrombectomy system (X-Sizer) in a bifurcation (primary angioplasty and occluded right coronary artery). A. The X-Sizer catheter advanced in the right coronary artery. B. Type 2 perforation located at the ostium of the posterior descending artery.

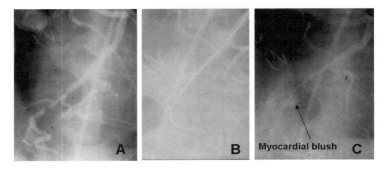

Figure 8.2   Type 2, subtype B perforation: intramyocardial blush after balloon rupture in distal left circumflex artery. A. Lesion before angioplasty. B. Balloon rupture. C. Myocardial blush and intramyocardial hematoma following perforation.

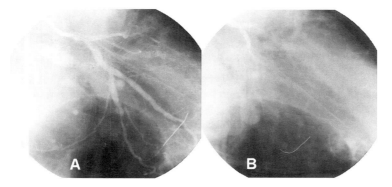

Figure 8.3   Type 2 perforation by the tip of a hydrophilic guidewire. A. Misplacement of the guidewire in a very small distal branch. B. Type 2 perforation after withdrawal of the wire.

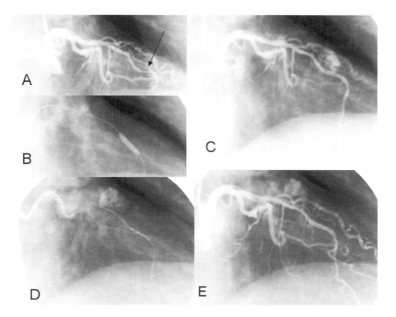

Figure 8.4   Type 3 perforation by balloon oversizing in the left anterior descending artery, treated by covered stent implantation. A. Lesion location in a tortuous mild left anterior descending artery in a woman. B. Oversized balloon inflated: balloon-to-artery ratio = 1.4. C. Type 3 perforation with frank extravasation. D. Polytetrafluoroethylene (PTFE)-covered stent placement. E. Final result.

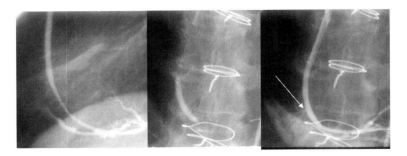

Figure 8.5   Perforation of a saphenous vein graft after stent implantation. Left: long lesion in a vein graft on right coronary artery. Middle: stent implantation (not oversized). Right: type 3 perforation (arrow).

- The fourth type corresponds to a perforation into an anatomic cavity chamber, such as the coronary sinus, and this phenomenon is termed 'cavity spilling'.

Diagnosis and consequences

In most cases, perforation is revealed immediately during PCI, although it can occur later, generally revealed by the presence of pericardial effusion.[6,7,14] Late pericardial effusion requires close monitoring for 24–48 hours. Furthermore, coronary perforation can also be accompanied by myocardial ischemia due to a coronary occlusion at the level of the perforation, or distant. The risk of death from perforation is related to the extent and tolerance of the pericardial effusion, and thus is correlated to the type of perforation, with a low risk of death for type 1 perforations and a high risk (45%) in types 2 and 3.[6,10]

Incidence and predictive factors

The incidence of coronary perforation is low, at about 0.5%, and several large-scale cohort studies were necessary to determine the predictive factors of perforation.[6,9–12,14–16] Among these risk factors, some are related to the patient anatomy, but the type of procedure is key in determining the risk.

Clinical features

Most reports show that the incidence of perforation is related to age and sex, with elderly patients and females being most at risk of this complication.[6,10,12,14] This increased risk could also be due to the coronary anatomy. Perforations are more frequent in tortuous or calcified arteries, and in vessels of small diameter[6,10–12] (Figure 8.4). Numerous cases of perforation during angioplasty on a saphenous vein graft have been reported, caused by the use of balloons and/or oversized stents, as well as atherectomy devices, reflecting the particular fragility of bypass grafts. When the perforation is of type 2 or 3, the effusion accumulates in the pericardium[17] (Figure 8.5).

Type of procedure

Pooled data from the various published series report a global incidence of perforation of 0.37%. Depending on the type of angioplasty procedure performed and the material used, the rate varies from 0.2% with an angioplasty balloon, to 0.88% after atherectomy, 0.08% with a stent and 0.29% for a guidewire alone (Table 8.2). Thus, it can be seen that the risk of perforation is ten times higher after atherectomy than with an angioplasty balloon (absolute difference of 0.68% [0.51–0.86]), and twice as high with a balloon as with a stent (absolute difference 0.12% [0.06–0.18]). Perforations caused by the guidewire alone occur with a similar frequency to those caused by the angioplasty balloon.

Atherectomy techniques

Many types of atherectomy procedures have been used in the past, but the advent of the stent has led to the disappearance of most of these strategies.

Among the atheroablative techniques used, the excimer laser (ELCA) was associated with the highest incidence of perforation, 1–2%,[18–21] generally of heat-related origin.[22] Similar frequency has been reported after procedures using directional atherectomy (DCA) and transluminal extraction catheter (TEC).[6,9,11,12,14,23,24] Perforations following directional atherectomy are generally of type 1, because the cut extends into the media of the artery in about half of all cases, and calcified and 'bend lesions' are at higher risk.[24]

Perforations related to rotational atherectomy (Rotablator) can be explained by the lateral pressure exerted by the burr in arterial bends (Figure 8.6), and special caution is warranted when using large-caliber burrs in tortuous arteries.

Lastly, the X-sizer thrombectomy catheter has a similar mode of action to mechanical atherectomy systems, and can also cause perforations[25] (Figure 8.1).

Guidewires

Many cases have been reported of perforation resulting from an injury caused by the guidewire, initially with stiff guidewires during attempts to recanalize the artery, and reported frequency was around 1%.[26] This risk can be minimized by exercising special care when advancing the guidewire.

Hydrophilic guidewires are particularly supple, but carry a risk of distal perforation by direct injury to the artery.[27,28] In the majority of cases, the resulting perforation

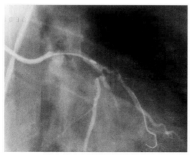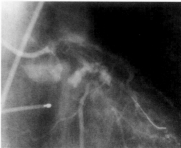

Figure 8.6 Type 3 perforation after rotational atherectomy. Right: approach of a 1.50 mm burr.

Table 8.2 Incidence of perforations according to the type of angioplasty (atherectomy devices, balloon, stent and guidewire)

Author	Year	Perforation	Atherectomy devices	Balloon	Stent	Guidewire
Gehl[45]	1982	27/6675 (0.4%)				
Ellis[6]	1994	62/12,900 (0.5%)	48/3084 (1.5%)	14/9080 (0.1%)		
Ajluni[23]	1994	35/8932 (0.4%)	12/1023 (1.17%)	11/7905 (0.14%)		
Gruberg[12]	2000	84/30,746 (0.29%)	16/4210 (0.38%)			
Dippel[10]	2001	36/6214 (0.58%)	13/489 (2.65%)	8/6160 (0.13%)	2/3852 (0.05%)	13/6214 (0.21%)
Gunning[14]	2002	52/6245 (0.8%)	3/254 (1.2%)	21/5991 (0.35%)		
Fukutomi[11]	2002	69/7443 (0.93%)	7/440 (1.59%)	20/4895 (0.41%)	4/810 (0.49%)	27/7443 (0.36%)
Fejka[9]	2002	31/25,697 (0.12%)	8/2691 (0.29%)	15/11,336 (0.13%)	8/11,653 (0.07%)	
Witzke[16]	2004	39/12,658 (0.3%)				
Total		435/117,510 (0.37%)	107/12,191 (0.88%)	89/45,367 (0.20%)	14/16,315 (0.09%)	40/13,657 (0.29%)

is of type 2 (Figure 8.3), sometimes complicated by cardiac tamponade. Recent reports suggest that guidewires could be responsible for up to 50% of all perforations.[16]

Balloons

Angioplasty balloons can cause coronary perforation by several mechanisms.

- Balloon oversizing as compared to the artery diameter is the classic mechanism (Figure 8.4). In this situation, the type of arterial remodeling plays an important role. The use of intravascular ultrasound to guide the procedure makes it possible to employ oversized balloons (adapted to the total diameter of the vessel) without an increased risk of perforation, and with similar results to those obtained with stenting.[29]
- In cases of angioplasty of an occlusive lesion, it is not only difficult to evaluate the size of the artery, but when there is no distal flow, the guidewire can end up in a branch with a small diameter (Figure 8.7).
- Finally, rupture of the balloon can cause dissection or perforation through a jet effect (Figure 8.2). However, this situation has become extremely rare thanks to the improved resistance of modern angioplasty balloons.

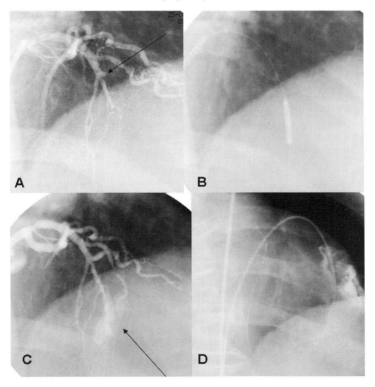

Figure 8.7 Perforation type 3 due to a misplaced balloon. A. Occlusion of the left anterior descending artery (arrow). B. A 3.0 × 20 mm balloon is misplaced (in a small septal branch instead of left anterior descending) and inflated at 12 atmospheres. C. Type 3 (subtype B) perforation. Patency of the left anterior descending artery, with significant lesion (arrow). D. Percutaneous pericardial drainage with a pigtail catheter.

Stents

The use of stents, apart from the obvious advantages of simplicity and efficacy, also seems to reduce the risk of perforation as compared to balloon alone. Nonetheless, cases of perforation caused by stenting have been reported, especially after excessive overdilatation[30,31] (Figure 8.8) or after implantation of an oversized stent compared to the caliber of the artery. This is a clinical situation that has the potential to occur frequently, especially in cases of direct stenting of an occlusive lesion (chronic occlusion and direct angioplasty).

To date, no cases of perforation after implantation of an active stent have been reported. It is likely that the efficacy of active stents in preventing restenosis will reduce the need for stent overexpansion.

Antithrombotic medication

The systematic use of an association of heparin, aspirin and clopidogrel, with the optional addition of GP IIb/IIIa inhibitors during angioplasty, does not appear to have had any effect on the incidence of coronary perforation. However, when perforation occurs, accompanied by tamponade, neutralizing the effect of these compounds can pose difficulties, although prognosis is related more to the type of perforation than to the medication used, such as GP IIb/IIIa inhibitors, for example.[10]

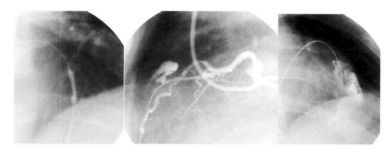

Figure 8.8 Type 3 perforation after overdilatation for maximal stent expansion. Left: incomplete stent expansion despite high balloon inflation pressure. Middle: type 3 perforation located at the distal edge of the stent. Right: percutaneous pericardial drainage using a pigtail catheter.

MANAGEMENT STRATEGY

Treatment of coronary perforation depends on the size of the perforation, the extent of contrast medium extravasation, and the hemodynamic status of the patient. The management strategy is dictated by the need to stop coronary extravasation and to relieve hemodynamic compromise. Hence, initial management of coronary perforation should focus on sealing the perforation as quickly as possible to prevent cardiac tamponade. Generally, this can be achieved by means of prolonged balloon inflation and, if necessary, a perfusion balloon catheter to reduce myocardial ischemia. Anticoagulation should be reversed and normal platelet function restored in cases of severe perforation. The cardiac surgeons should be notified immediately and the operative room prepared for possible emergency surgery. The advent of covered stents has been a significant advance and may avoid the need for surgical intervention. Foam or microcoil embolization may also be helpful in selected cases.

Prolonged balloon inflation

A balloon should immediately be positioned at the perforation site – even prior to pericardiocentesis, placement of an intra-aortic balloon pump or cardiopulmonary resuscitation – and inflated at the lowest possible pressure to promote hemostasis, generally less than 5 atm, for at least 10 minutes. Detection of residual extravasation should be evaluated by repeated injections of contrast medium at several time intervals. In cases of incomplete sealing, the use of a perfusion balloon catheter has been advocated to allow prolonged (15–45 minutes) inflation with reduced myocardial ischemia.[32]

Pericardiocentesis

Pericardial effusion is usually visible by angiography. Nonetheless, echocardiographic evaluation should be performed immediately at the bedside during and following balloon catheter inflation at the site of perforation. Even if pericardial hemorrhage is evident, pericardiocentesis should only be performed in the presence of hemodynamic or echocardiographic cardiac compromise. In the setting of hemodynamically significant cardiac tamponade, immediate pericardiocentesis and pericardial catheter drainage are life-saving maneuvers.[33] The need for percutaneous pericardiocentesis is a life-threatening situation that requires immediate intervention by a qualified operator. The pericardiocentesis needle should be exchanged for a multiple side hole catheter, allowing continuous aspiration and monitoring of pericardial blood (Figure 8.8). Continuous pericardial catheter aspiration should remain in place overnight and can be removed the next morning in the absence of echocardiographic evidence of fluid reaccumulation. Observation for an additional 24 hours with repeat echocardiography prior to discharge on the day following pericardial catheter removal is recommended.[10]

Reversal of antithrombotic treatment

Reversal of unfractionated heparin anticoagulation is rapidly achieved through the intravenous administration of protamine sulfate.[34] Protamine has been safely administered to facilitate hemostasis following coronary stent deployment without adverse ischemic sequelae.[35] If contrast extravasation persists despite prolonged balloon inflations, incremental doses of protamine should be administered with a target activated clotting time value of <150 seconds. Complete reversal of anticoagulation is not possible for patients treated with low molecular weight heparin, fondaparinux or bivalirudin.

Antiplatelet agents should not be discontinued in the absence of pericardial effusion. Conversely, after successful drainage of cardiac tamponade, oral antiplatelet therapy with aspirin, clopidogrel or ticlopidine should be reintroduced for stented patients prior to discharge.

Platelet IIb/IIIa receptor antagonists should be discontinued once perforation occurs. The strategy of platelet transfusion applies specifically to abciximab-treated patients. Indeed, the effect of abciximab can be reversed by platelet transfusion (6–10 units), although there is no antidote for eptifibatide or tirofiban.

Covered stent implantation

In the past few years, covered stent implantation has emerged as an alternative strategy to surgery when conservative approaches fail. Some case reports have shown promising results with autologous venous-covered stents[36,37] or radial artery graft-covered stents.[38] However, this strategy may be difficult to perform in emergency situations and requires a long time interval from vein harvest to stent deployment.

More recently, the efficacy of the polytetrafluoroethylene (PTFE)-covered stent was compared with that of noncovered stents to treat coronary perforations.[39] All vessel ruptures treated with PTFE-covered stent implantation were successfully sealed (Figure 8.4). The occurrence of cardiac tamponade and the necessity for emergency surgery were significantly lower in the PTFE group than in the non-PTFE group. None of the patients effectively treated with the PTFE-covered stent implantation had experienced any major adverse cardiac events at follow-up. However, the profile of this stent makes it unsuitable for use in tortuous and distal lesions. In addition, there is a lack of data concerning evolution of patency in the long term.

In rare cases, additional noncovered stents have been used to seal a coronary perforation.[40] Such a procedure may not be desirable, as balloon-expandable stents could potentially increase the size of the vessel rupture.

Microcoil embolization

Distal embolization using GelFoam,[41] a microcoil[42] or clotted autologous blood[43] is a reasonable therapeutic strategy in very selected cases of guidewire perforations. Trufill pushable coils (Cordis) are made from platinum alloy and synthetic fibers to promote maximum thrombogenicity and are designed for neuroradiology and peripheral vascular applications.[44] Coil embolization can be used safely in coronary perforation located in a distal segment or side branch of the vessel, because it results in occlusion of the artery. Indeed, the use of this technique in free coronary perforation or a perforation located in the proximal segment of the vessel is not recommended.

Surgical indications

The primary surgical indication in coronary perforation is a large perforation associated with severe ischemia, hemodynamic compromise, and arterial hemorrhage that persists despite nonoperative measures. Emergency surgery should be performed to control hemorrhage, repair the perforation or ligate the vessel, and bypass all vessels containing significant stenoses. A balloon catheter should be positioned and inflated at low pressure whenever possible while waiting for surgery. Operative management may be required in up to 30–40% of patients who develop perforation,[6] generally because of persisting myocardial ischemia.

PREVENTION

Any insertion of material into the coronary arteries can cause a perforation at any time during the procedure, from the first insertion of the guidewire until the end of the angioplasty procedure. The systematic use of stents has rarely been associated with perforations and has also contributed to the progressive disappearance of many atheroablative techniques, but the risk of perforation persists nonetheless.

The risk factors can be related to the patient, and to the medication and material or devices used (see Table 8.3).

Cardiac tamponade is a much-feared complication of perforation,[45] and its poor prognosis emphasizes the importance of taking steps to prevent this complication, such as careful guidewire advancement and positioning, avoidance of balloon or device oversizing, and meticulous attention to device selection and technique.

High-risk situations

Certain clinical situations carry a particularly high risk of perforation. Female gender, older age, tortuous and calcified arteries, bifurcations and angulated lesions, small vessels, acute or chronic occlusions, saphenous vein grafts or mammary anastomoses are often reported as being factors that contribute to a higher risk of coronary perforation.

Table 8.3   Risk factors

Patient related
- Female gender
- Coronary anatomy:
  - vessel tortuosity
  - calcifications
  - lesion located in a bend
  - occlusion (acute or chronic)

Medication related
The medication used is not directly related to the risk of perforation, but may increase the complexity of management in case of pericardial effusion or may promote late pericardial effusion
- Low molecular weight heparin, fondaparinux or bivalirudin: cannot be effectively neutralized by protamine sulfate
- Combination of antiplatelet agents (aspirin, clopidogrel, glycoprotein IIb/IIIa inhibitors): requires platelet transfusion to be reversed quickly

Device related
- Guidewire
  - Stiff guidewire used for total chronic occlusion
  - Stiff guidewire for dissection
  - Floppy hydrophilic wire in very distal branches
- **Balloon**
  - Balloon rupture (excessive inflation pressure, very calcified lesions)
  - Balloon oversizing: balloon-to-artery ratio >1.2 without intravascular ultrasound guidance
  - Balloon oversizing: balloon inflation without opacification of the distal bed (total occlusion)
- **Stent**
  - Stent oversizing (direct stenting in total occlusion)
  - Stent overdilatation or correction of focal incomplete stent expansion in calcified lesion
- **Atherectomy devices**
  - X-Sizer in small, angulated arteries or bifurcations
  - Directional atherectomy: excessive ablation or use in angulated or calcified lesions
  - Rotational atherectomy: burr oversizing in angulated lesions

Guidewire positioning

During all percutaneous coronary interventions, the tip of the guidewire should advance smoothly beyond the stenosis and retain torque response. The likelihood of perforation increases with stiffer guidewires. Maintaining guiding catheter back-up, step-by-step increase in guidewire stiffness, and changing the stiff wire as soon as possible may help to prevent perforation. If there is buckling of the guidewire, restricted tip movement or resistance to advancement, the wire may have entered a false lumen and should be withdrawn and repositioned. The balloon inflation should not be started until the guidewire is in place, since balloon inflation within a false lumen may result in coronary artery rupture and rapid clinical deterioration. When using hydrophilic guidewires, attention must be paid not to let the tip of the guidewire advance too far or into a very small branch.

Device oversizing

A device-to-artery ratio ≥ 1.2 for balloon and/or stent increases the risk of coronary perforation. Therefore, high-risk lesions (e.g. diffuse, bifurcated, angulated lesions or total occlusions) are best approached using a balloon-to-artery ratio of 1.0 for PCI, and device-to-artery ratios of 0.5–0.6 for devices that alter the integrity of the vascular wall (DCA, Rotablator). In such cases, it may be helpful to use gradually increasing device size, and achieve optimal lumen enlargement by adjunctive balloon angioplasty rather than upsizing to a larger device.

Other device considerations

Knowledge of balloon material and the specific rated and actual mean burst pressure is required to avoid balloon rupture and resulting jet effect. Perforations related to stent overexpansion may be avoided by paying particular attention to stent position or by using intravascular ultrasound guidance. Stents should not be used when the distal extent of a dissection cannot be identified angiographically.

REFERENCES

1. Semple T, Williams BO, Baxter RH. Spontaneous coronary artery perforation with tamponade. Demonstration by necropsy selective coronary arteriography. Br Heart J 1978;40:1423–5.
2. Gelsomino S, Romagnoli S, Stefano P. Right coronary perforation due to a toothpick ingested at a barbecue. N Engl J Med 2005;352:2249–50.
3. Steinwender C, Hofmann R, Leisch F. Pseudo-pericardial tamponade after perforation of the right coronary artery. Heart 2004;90:e36.
4. Escher DJ, Shapiro JH, Rubinstein BM, Hurwitt ES, Schwartz SP. Perforation of the heart during cardiac catheterization and selective angiocardiography. Circulation 1958;18:418–22.
5. Morettin LB, Wallace JM. Uneventful perforation of a coronary artery during selective arteriography. A case report. Am J Roentgenol Radium Ther Nucl Med 1970;110:184–8.
6. Ellis SG, Ajluni S, Arnold AZ et al. Increased coronary perforation in the new device era. Incidence, classification, management, and outcome. Circulation 1994;90:2725–30.
7. van Suylen RJ, Serruys PW, Simpson JB, de Feyter PJ, Strauss BH, Zondervan PE. Delayed rupture of right coronary artery after directional atherectomy for bail-out. Am Heart J 1991;121:914–16.

8. Sutton J, Russel E, Ellis SG. Textbook of Interventional Cardiology. Vol, 2nd ed. Philadelphia, PA: Saunders, 1993:576–99.
9. Fejka M, Dixon SR, Safian RD et al. Diagnosis, management, and clinical outcome of cardiac tamponade complicating percutaneous coronary intervention. Am J Cardiol 2002;90:1183–6.
10. Dippel EJ, Kereiakes DJ, Tramuta DA et al. Coronary perforation during percutaneous coronary intervention in the era of abciximab platelet glycoprotein IIb/IIIa blockade: an algorithm for percutaneous management. Cathet Cardiovasc Intervent 2001;52:279–86.
11. Fukutomi T, Suzuki T, Popma JJ et al. Early and late clinical outcomes following coronary perforation in patients undergoing percutaneous coronary intervention. Circ J 2002;66:349–56.
12. Gruberg L, Pinnow E, Flood R et al. Incidence, management, and outcome of coronary artery perforation during percutaneous coronary intervention. Am J Cardiol 2000;86:680–2, A8.
13. Seshadri N, Whitlow PL, Acharya N, Houghtaling P, Blackstone EH, Ellis SG. Emergency coronary artery bypass surgery in the contemporary percutaneous coronary intervention era. Circulation 2002;106:2346–50.
14. Gunning MG, Williams IL, Jewitt DE, Shah AM, Wainwright RJ, Thomas MR. Coronary artery perforation during percutaneous intervention: incidence and outcome. Heart 2002;88:495–8.
15. Von Sohsten R, Kopistansky C, Cohen M, Kussmaul WG 3rd. Cardiac tamponade in the 'new device' era: evaluation of 6999 consecutive percutaneous coronary interventions. Am Heart J 2000;140:279–83.
16. Witzke CF, Martin-Herrero F, Clarke SC, Pomerantzev E, Palacios IF. The changing pattern of coronary perforation during percutaneous coronary intervention in the new device era. J Invasive Cardiol 2004;16:257–301.
17. Lowe R, Hammond C, Perry RA. Prior CABG does not prevent pericardial tamponade following saphenous vein graft perforation associated with angioplasty. Heart 2005;91:1052.
18. Bittl JA, Ryan TJ Jr, Keaney JF Jr et al. Coronary artery perforation during excimer laser coronary angioplasty. The Percutaneous Excimer Laser Coronary Angioplasty Registry. J Am Coll Cardiol 1993;21:1158–65.
19. Baumbach A, Oswald H, Kvasnicka J et al. Clinical results of coronary excimer laser angioplasty: report from the European Coronary Excimer Laser Angioplasty Registry. Eur Heart J 1994;15:89–96.
20. Holmes DR Jr, Reeder GS, Ghazzal ZM et al. Coronary perforation after excimer laser coronary angioplasty: the Excimer Laser Coronary Angioplasty Registry experience. J Am Coll Cardiol 1994;23:330–5.
21. Litvack F, Eigler N, Margolis J et al. Percutaneous excimer laser coronary angioplasty: results in the first consecutive 3,000 patients. The ELCA Investigators. J Am Coll Cardiol 1994;23:323–9.
22. Isner JM, Donaldson RF, Funai JT et al. Factors contributing to perforations resulting from laser coronary angioplasty: observations in an intact human postmortem preparation of intraoperative laser coronary angioplasty. Circulation 1985;72:II191–9.
23. Ajluni SC, Glazier S, Blankenship L, O'Neill WW, Safian RD. Perforations after percutaneous coronary interventions: clinical, angiographic, and therapeutic observations. Cathet Cardiovasc Diagn 1994;32:206–12.
24. Ellis SG, De Cesare NB, Pinkerton CA et al. Relation of stenosis morphology and clinical presentation to the procedural results of directional coronary atherectomy. Circulation 1991;84:644–53.
25. Constantinides S, Lo TS, Been M, Shiu MF. Early experience with a helical coronary thrombectomy device in patients with acute coronary thrombosis. Heart 2002;87:455–60.
26. Melchior JP, Meier B, Urban P et al. Percutaneous transluminal coronary angioplasty for chronic total coronary arterial occlusion. Am J Cardiol 1987;59:535–8.
27. Tamura M, Oda H, Miida T, Sato H, Higuma N, Toeda T. Coronary perforation to the left ventricular cavity by a guide wire during coronary angioplasty. Jpn Heart J 1993;34:633–7.

28. Wong CM, Kwong Mak GY, Chung DT. Distal coronary artery perforation resulting from the use of hydrophilic coated guidewire in tortuous vessels. Cathet Cardiovasc Diagn 1998;44:93–6.
29. Schiele F, Meneveau N, Gilard M et al. Intravascular ultrasound-guided balloon angioplasty compared with stent: immediate and 6-month results of the multicenter, randomized Balloon Equivalent to Stent Study (BEST). Circulation 2003;107:545–51.
30. Goldberg SL, Di Mario C, Hall P, Colombo A. Comparison of aggressive versus nonaggressive balloon dilatation for stent deployment on late loss and restenosis in native coronary arteries. Am J Cardiol 1998;81:708–12.
31. Reimers B, von Birgelen C, van der Giessen WJ, Serruys PW. A word of caution on optimizing stent deployment in calcified lesions: acute coronary rupture with cardiac tamponade. Am Heart J 1996;131:192–4.
32. Stack RS, Quigley PJ, Collins G, Phillips HR 3rd. Perfusion balloon catheter. Am J Cardiol 1988;61:77G–80G.
33. Altman F, Yazdanfar S, Wertheimer J, Ghosh S, Kotler M. Cardiac tamponade following perforation of the left anterior descending coronary system during percutaneous transluminal coronary angioplasty: successful treatment by pericardial drainage. Am Heart J 1986;111:1196–7.
34. Stoelting RK. Allergic reactions during anesthesia. Anesth Analg 1983;62:341–56.
35. Briguori C, Di Mario C, De Gregorio J, Sheiban I, Vaghetti M, Colombo A. Administration of protamine after coronary stent deployment. Am Heart J 1999;138:64–8.
36. Caputo RP, Amin N, Marvasti M, Wagner S, Levy C, Giambartolomei A. Successful treatment of a saphenous vein graft perforation with an autologous vein-covered stent. Cathet Cardiovasc Intervent 1999;48:382–6.
37. Colombo A, Itoh A, Di Mario C et al. Successful closure of a coronary vessel rupture with a vein graft stent: case report. Cathet Cardiovasc Diagn 1996;38:172–4.
38. Stefanadis C, Toutouzas K, Tsiamis E et al. Implantation of stents covered by autologous arterial grafts in human coronary arteries: a new technique. J Invasive Cardiol 2000;12:7–12.
39. Briguori C, Nishida T, Anzuini A, Di Mario C, Grube E, Colombo A. Emergency polytetrafluoroethylene-covered stent implantation to treat coronary ruptures. Circulation 2000;102:3028–31.
40. Hammoud T, Tanguay JF, Rios F, Bilodeau L. Repair of left anterior descending coronary artery perforation by Magic Wallstent implantation. Cathet Cardiovasc Intervent 1999;48:304–7.
41. Dixon SR, Webster MW, Ormiston JA, Wattie WJ, Hammett CJ. Gelfoam embolization of a distal coronary artery guidewire perforation. Cathet Cardiovasc Intervent 2000;49:214–17.
42. Aslam MS, Messersmith RN, Gilbert J, Lakier JB. Successful management of coronary artery perforation with helical platinum microcoil embolization. Cathet Cardiovasc Intervent 2000;51:320–2.
43. Hadjimiltiades S, Paraskevaides S, Kazinakis G, Louridas G. Coronary vessel perforation during balloon angioplasty: a case report. Cathet Cardiovasc Diagn 1998;45:417–20.
44. Assali AR, Moustapha A, Sdringola S, Rihner M, Smalling RW. Successful treatment of coronary artery perforation in an abciximab-treated patient by microcoil embolization. Cathet Cardiovasc Intervent 2000;51:487–9.
45. Gehl L, Iskandrian AS, Goel I et al. Cardiac perforation with tamponade during cardiac catheterization. Cathet Cardiovasc Diagn 1982;8:293–8.

Section D
Device-related complications

9

How to perform optimal directional atherectomy

Antonio Colombo and Ioannis Iakovou

Historical notes and rationale for atherectomy • Directional coronary atherectomy equipment and technique • Clinical atherectomy studies • Optimal atherectomy • Avoiding procedural complications with directional coronary atherectomy • Is there a role for directional coronary atherectomy in today's clinical practice? • Associated pharmacologic treatment • Conclusion • What you should remember

HISTORICAL NOTES AND RATIONALE FOR ATHERECTOMY

John Simpson first introduced the concept of removing obstructive tissue by a catheter-based excision technique.[1,2] The idea was to overcome several caveats of the conventional balloon angioplasty (PTCA). The first directional atherectomy of human vessels was performed in a superficial femoral artery in 1985, and in human coronary arteries the next year.[1,2] The peripheral device was approved by the Food and Drug Administration (FDA) in 1987 and the coronary device in 1990.[1-4] Despite the initial enthusiasm for this first nonballoon percutaneous coronary interventional device, the early randomized clinical trials of directional coronary atherectomy (DCA) failed to demonstrate a clinically significant reduction in late angiographic or clinical restenosis after DCA versus PTCA.[5-9] These negative findings for DCA, combined with the approval of the Palmaz-Schatz coronary stent (Cordis Corporation, Miami Lakes, FL) in 1994, resulted in a rapid decrease in the usage of this unique technology.

Ironically, the most promising results with DCA were obtained using the combined strategy of DCA plus stenting.[10-15] Intuitively, DCA and stent implantation should be complementary in reducing restenosis. Both intravascular ultrasound (IVUS) and histopathologic studies[16,17] have shown that in-stent restenosis is mainly due to neo-intima formation, not chronic stent recoil. Pathologic specimens from stented arterial segments showed that the amount of neo-intima is greater when the medial layer of the vessel wall is damaged, the result of aggressive stent implantation to optimize final dimensions.[17] Conversely, studies using serial planar and volumetric IVUS indicated that late lumen loss following DCA is mainly due to negative arterial remodeling and, to a lesser extent, cellular proliferation.[18-23] Furthermore, IVUS studies showed that both preintervention and postintervention plaque burden are predictors of restenosis after stent implantation.[24-28] Plaque burden may also play an important role in the restenosis process by amplifying negative remodeling.[8]

One of the major limitations of IVUS-guided stenting is that optimal and symmetric stent expansion cannot be achieved in a large percentage of patients. For example, in the Multicenter Ultrasound Stenting In Coronaries (MUSIC) study, criteria for optimal stent deployment were achieved only in 80% of the lesions.[29] The amount of plaque behind the stent is the logical limitation.[21] The stretching force needed to expand the vessel is proportional to the vessel wall resistance, which depends on the amount and structure of the atherosclerotic plaque.[8,21,23] The presence of a large plaque burden may prevent optimal stent expansion even with the use of high inflation pressures or large balloons.[21] As stents reduce restenosis by opposing late negative remodeling, it was reasonable to assume that stent implantation following optimal lesion debulking (to minimize vessel wall trauma during optimal stenting) would be a promising approach to improve long-term clinical outcomes.[8,21,23]

DIRECTIONAL CORONARY ATHERECTOMY EQUIPMENT AND TECHNIQUE

The prototype of the DCA catheter was the Simpson Coronary AtheroCath (Devices for Vascular Interventions, Temecula, CA), which consists of a metal housing with a fixed support balloon, a nose cone collection chamber, and a hollow torque tube that accommodates a 0.014″ guidewire. A cup-shaped cutter inside the housing was attached to a flexible drive shaft and was activated by a hand-held battery-operated motor drive unit. A lever on the motor drive unit allowed the operator to slowly advance the cutter through the lesion as it rotated at 2000 revolutions per minute (rpm). Excised atheroma was stored in the distal nose cone collection chamber. The Simpson AtheroCath was the first device after balloon angioplasty to receive FDA approval for coronary intervention.

The second-generation AtheroCath (SCA-EX) was characterized by an improved nose cone design, and the third-generation device (SCA-GTO) had a redesigned shaft with better support and torque control than the EX. The Bantam catheter had a smaller shaft, allowing 9 F guiding catheter compatibility.

A more recent device is the Flexi-Cut. It has a cutter coated with titanium nitride (Figure 9.1) and a shaft diameter slightly smaller than 6 F (0.076″, 1.94 mm). The shaft

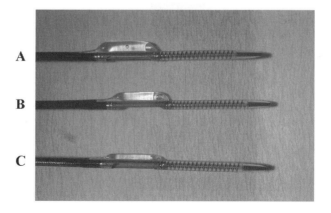

Figure 9.1   The Flexi-Cut catheter (Guidant, Temecula, CA). A. Large size: ≥3.5 mm. B. Medium size: 3.0–3.5 mm. C. Small size: 2.5–3.0 mm.

has not increased in size with larger devices. Rather, increasing diameter of the opposing balloon (2.5, 3.0, and 3.5 mm) adapted this device to larger vessels. As a result, the Flexi-Cut device was compatible with 8 F large-lumen (>0.87″ internal diameter) guiding catheters. The rigid part of the cutting chamber was also shorter than in the GTO catheter (13 mm vs 16 mm), improving tip flexibility while maintaining the length of the cutting window (9 mm).

The SilverHawk Plaque Excision System (Fox Hollow Technologies Inc., Redwood City, CA) is a new atherectomy device with a different concept (Figure 9.2). This device received CE mark approval for use in the coronary arteries in December 2002 and is currently available for coronary usage in Europe but not in the US where its use is still limited to peripheral interventions. A family of three different SilverHawk catheters (compatible with both 6 F and 8 F guiding catheters) is available for coronary use. The SilverHawk catheter does not need an external balloon to establish vessel wall contact, and can be advanced over a short PTCA wire as a monorail

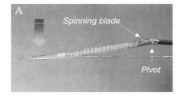

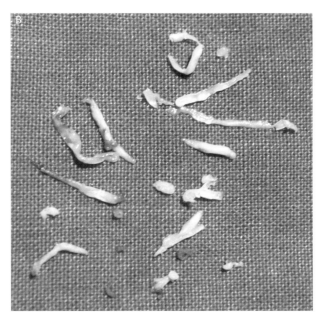

Figure 9.2 A. The SilverHawk catheter (FHT, Fox Hollow Technologies Inc., Redwood City, CA). B. 68 mg of tissue retrieved with the SilverHawk catheter from a single atherosclerotic lesion.

device. When the motor drive unit is activated and the positioning lever is retracted, the distal portion of the cutter deflects, bringing the device into apposition with the lesion and exposing the inner rotating cutter. While the blade is spinning, the entire catheter is slowly advanced across the lesion, 'shaving' the occlusive material from the artery and capturing the excised tissue in the tip of the catheter. Advancing the positioning lever, bringing the inner cutter back into the housing, and restoring the 'nondeflected' configuration completes the cutting process. Preliminary clinical experience with the SilverHawk catheter showed that plaque debulking can be performed safely and effectively in relatively small vessels and complex lesions located in mid-distal artery segments, with six-month clinical outcome similar to prior atherectomy devices.[30]

CLINICAL ATHERECTOMY STUDIES

The efficacy of DCA in removing noncalcified atherosclerotic plaque has been confirmed in several large-scale randomized trials comparing the results of this device with balloon angioplasty.[6,9,31,32] Angiographic restenosis and target lesion revascularization rates in the major atherectomy studies are shown in Figures 9.3 and 9.4.

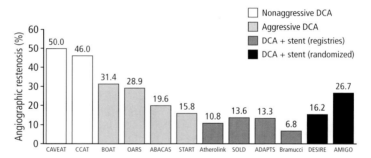

Figure 9.3   Angiographic restenosis rates in the major atherectomy studies.

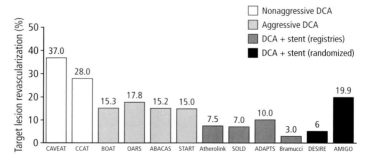

Figure 9.4   Target lesion revascularization rates in the major atherectomy studies.

In an early randomized trial comparing coronary angioplasty with directional atherectomy (the Coronary Angioplasty Versus Excisional Atherectomy Trial, CAVEAT-I), removing coronary plaque led to a larger acute gain in lumen diameter and a small but not significant reduction in angiographic restenosis at six-month follow-up, with no benefit in clinical outcomes.[9] Moreover, DCA was associated with a higher rate of in-hospital myocardial infarction, increased hospitalization costs, and an excess in mortality at one-year follow-up (2.2% vs 0.6%, $P=0.035$).[5] An increase in acute complications with DCA was not confirmed in the Canadian Coronary Atherectomy Trial (CCAT) which compared coronary angioplasty with DCA in nonostial left anterior descending coronary artery lesions.[31] One major limitation of these early studies was the use of a limited (or 'nonaggressive') debulking approach. In the CAVEAT-I study, the larger 7 F atherectomy device was used in only 47% of the lesions. Directional coronary atherectomy has, however, subsequently evolved toward a more 'optimal' technique (larger devices, more extensive tissue removal, and routine postdilatation to obtain final diameter stenosis <20%).

The Optimal Atherectomy Restenosis Study (OARS) was a registry that showed that use of an 'optimal' atherectomy technique (using IVUS guidance and adjunctive balloon postdilatation, if necessary) to produce larger acute lumen diameters translated into a lower restenosis rate at six months (28.9%) than previously seen with this device, without an increase in early or late major adverse events (2.5% and 23.6%, respectively).[33] Optimal DCA – defined as <15% residual stenosis (by the angiographic core laboratory), with adjunctive balloon dilatation if necessary – was achieved in 82% of lesions.

These favorable results led to the Balloon vs Optimal Atherectomy Trial (BOAT), which evaluated the short- and long-term outcomes of optimal DCA compared with balloon angioplasty. In this study, the encouraging results of the OARS study were confirmed in reduced angiographic restenosis rates with atherectomy compared to balloon angioplasty (31.4% vs 39.8% respectively, $P=0.01$), without an increase in early adverse events (death, Q-wave myocardial infarction or emergent coronary artery bypass graft surgery; 2.8% vs 3.3% respectively, $P=0.7$).[6] However, this study did not show a difference in six-month clinical outcomes (death, Q-wave myocardial infarction or target vessel revascularization): 21.1% vs 24.8% respectively, $P=0.1$.

In the OARS trial, despite 'optimal directional coronary atherectomy' by angiographic criteria, the residual plaque burden assessed by IVUS remained high (58%). This lead to the Adjunctive Balloon Angioplasty after Coronary Atherectomy Study (ABACAS), an IVUS-guided aggressive directional atherectomy comparing balloon postdilatation versus no adjunctive balloon postdilatation. ABACAS showed a further decrease in the six-month angiographic restenosis rate in both arms (23.6% vs 19.6%, respectively, $P=NS$), as well as in the target lesion revascularization rate (20.6% vs 15.2%, respectively, $P=NS$).[34]

Finally, the STent versus directional coronary Atherectomy Randomized Trial (START) was designed to compare stenting (62 lesions) with optimal IVUS-guided directional coronary atherectomy (60 lesions) in vessels suitable for both techniques.[35] Although the postprocedural lumen diameters were similar (2.79 mm vs 2.90 mm respectively), the follow-up minimal luminal diameter was significantly smaller in the stent arm (1.89 mm vs 2.18 mm, $P=0.02$). IVUS revealed that intimal proliferation was significantly larger in the stent arm than in the DCA arm (3.1 mm^2 vs 1.1 mm^2, $P<0.0001$), accounting for the significantly smaller follow-up lumen area in the stent arm (5.3 mm^2 vs 7.0 mm^2, $P=0.03$). Restenosis was significantly lower (32.8% vs 15.8%,

P=0.032), and target vessel failure at one year tended to be lower with directional atherectomy compared to stenting (33.9% vs 18.3%, *P*=0.056). The authors of this study concluded that aggressive DCA might provide superior angiographic and clinical outcomes compared to primary stenting.

Nevertheless, the most promising results with DCA were obtained using the combined strategy of DCA plus stenting.[10–15] Kiesz et al were among the pioneers to postulate that debulking before stenting would facilitate complete stent expansion and further decrease elastic recoil at the treated site without the necessity for aggressive stent postdilation.[10] In the Acute Directional coronary Atherectomy Prior To Stenting in complex coronary lesions study (ADAPTS), DCA plus stenting was performed in 60 consecutive patients with 89 lesions considered high risk for restenosis (aorto-ostial lesions, total chronic occlusions, long lesions, and lesions containing thrombus) and the restenosis rate was 13.3%.[10] Similar restenosis rates after DCA and stenting were reported by Bramucci et al (6.8%),[13] Hopp et al (Atherolink Registry, 8.4%) and Airoldi et al (13.8%).[36] In the Stenting after Optimal Lesion Debulking (SOLD) registry, 128 patients with 168 complex lesions were enrolled and restenosis rate was 13.6%.[12]

The encouraging results of DCA and stenting seen in registries led to the initiation of two large, prospective, randomized clinical trials comparing DCA before stenting with stenting alone: the Atherectomy Before MULTI-LINK Improves Lumen Gain and Clinical Outcomes (AMIGO) trial[37] and the Debulking and Stenting In Restenosis Elimination (DESIRE) trial.[3] The AMIGO trial randomized 753 patients to either DCA followed by stenting or stenting alone.[37] At eight-month follow-up, there was no difference in angiographic or clinical restenosis between the two groups (Figures 9.5 and 9.6). However, this study failed to support the original findings and hypothesis. Optimal debulking (defined as post-DCA diameter stenosis <25%) was achieved in only 26.5% of patients despite the fact that the study protocol required this end-point in all patients who were randomized to the DCA arm. Suboptimal debulking was associated with a significantly higher restenosis rate (32%) compared with optimal

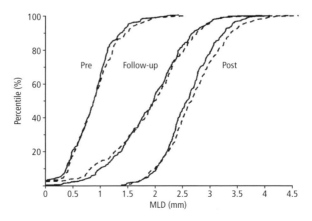

Figure 9.5 The AMIGO trial: cumulative distribution of minimal luminal diameter (MLD) before and after the procedure and at follow-up for the atherectomy-plus-stent group (dashed line) and the stent-alone group (solid line).

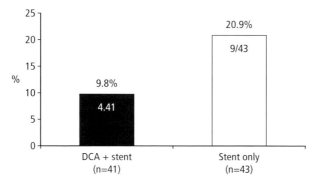

Figure 9.6   The AMIGO trial: angiographic restenosis rates in patients with bifurcation lesions treated with DCA plus stenting (black column) and stent alone (white column).

debulking (16%, *P*=0.01). Furthermore, cumulative major adverse cardiovascular events (death, myocardial infarction or urgent target vessel revascularization) to 30 days post procedure were slightly more frequent in the DCA-treated patients.

The DESIRE trial randomized 500 patients to IVUS-guided DCA followed by stenting or stenting alone. Despite the achievement of a lower loss index at quantitative coronary angiography follow-up in the DCA/stent group (0.34 vs 0.41, *P*=0.05), this did not translate into clinical benefit at six-month follow-up (Figure 9.7). The main problem of DCA which may also have affected the results of the AMIGO trial is that the technique is very operator dependent and the amount of tissue removal varies with the commitment of the operator to perform extensive debulking.

In summary, the available evidence indicates that DCA does not improve late angiographic outcome when performed before bare metal stent implantation unless optimal debulking is achieved and relatively higher risk lesions are treated. To support this second statement, we have only indirect data.

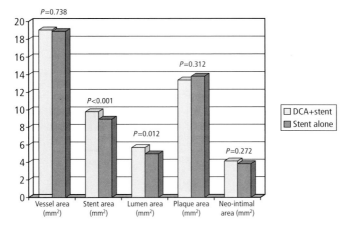

Figure 9.7   The DESIRE trial: six-month intravascular ultrasound data.

OPTIMAL ATHERECTOMY

Although adjunctive angioplasty after DCA was initially discouraged, angioplasty may actually improve DCA outcome and can often result in better immediate angiographic results. In addition, angioplasty has been shown to convert suboptimal DCA to optimal DCA and improve the clinical outcome. Furthermore, stenting (bare metal) following DCA resulted in superior lumen enlargement compared to angioplasty alone. In the era of drug-eluting stents (DES) we believe that DCA alone (without the use of subsequent DES implantation) has a minimal role. Nevertheless, we still occasionally combine atherectomy and DES when the anatomic setting is appropriate, such as a left main stenosis with a large plaque burden demonstrated by IVUS with the characteristics to be suitable for removal with current directional atherectomy devices. Intravascular ultrasound plays an important role in the correct sizing of the device according to the vessel size as well as in the characterization of the plaque. However, this finding has not been invariably demonstrated since other studies suggested that comparable lumen enlargement can be achieved using angiography alone. Despite some of these encouraging statements, we cannot deny that the use of coronary atherectomy is in a steady decline.

When the operator considers it appropriate to perform DCA, some general guidelines must be noted. First, initial cuts should be directed towards angiographically apparent plaque (as guided by multiple orthogonal views). The goal of optimal atherectomy is to create a large lumen diameter without complications. However, the operator should be careful in upsizing the device since there is always the possibility of complications such as perforations. In addition, it is worth noting that deep wall components (media and adventitia) can be identified in up to two-thirds of DCA specimens. Although immediate postprocedure lumen diameter is an important determinant of restenosis and is the central theme of the bigger-is-better hypothesis, there is a certain concern that achieving large lumen with partial excision of vessel wall tissue may increase the risk for procedural complications, aneurysm formation, and restenosis.

AVOIDING PROCEDURAL COMPLICATIONS WITH DIRECTIONAL CORONARY ATHERECTOMY

Dissection

With the early DCA devices, the rates of nonocclusive dissection and severe dissection leading to abrupt closure were 20% and 0–7% of cases respectively.[38] In CAVEAT-I, abrupt closure was more common with DCA compared to angioplasty (8% vs 3.8%, P=0.005) and occurred at a site other than the target lesion in 42%.[39] Dissections can be caused by the guiding catheter, the guidewire, and the atherectomy device itself (from the cutting mechanism, the nose cone or, more rarely, from the integrated balloon in the case of the Flexi-Cut device). Avoidance of deep seating and over-rotation of the guiding catheter can minimize the catheter-induced injury. It is always important not to overinflate the balloon. A maximum of three atmospheres is frequently all that is needed to establish appropriate plaque contact. Avoiding cuts at very angulated segments will also minimize the risk of dissections and vessel perforation.

Distal embolization and no-reflow phenomenon

This complication occurred in 0–13.4% of the DCA cases in the earlier studies,[38–43] usually due to dislodgment of thrombus or soft plaque from the target lesion, or incomplete capture of material from the cone of the device.[41] No-reflow is more frequent in vein grafts and thrombosis-containing lesions. There are numerous treatments proposed for this complication that invariably include the intracoronary administration of a vasodilator such as nitroprusside, verapamil or adenosine.

Non Q-wave myocardial infarction and side branch occlusion

Side branches were compromised at a rate of 0.7–7.7% after DCA.[32,33,38,39,41–43] Careful selection of cases, such as avoidance of DCA in the treatment of bifurcations with side branches with diseased origin, can help in reducing the rate of this complication unless the operator is able to perform initial cuts toward the origin of the side branch. This condition is a typical situation where experience plays a fundamental role: paradoxically, a condition where the side branch could become totally occluded can be converted into the ideal setting for atherectomy if handled appropriately.

DCA has been implicated in CAVEAT-I with a higher incidence of non Q-wave myocardial infarction compared to traditional angioplasty.[5] However, these results were not reproduced in CAVEAT-II and CCAT.[5,44] Risk factors for CK-MB release were complex lesion morphology and *de novo* lesions.

Perforation

A coronary artery perforation occurred in less than 1% of the cases in early DCA studies.[5,10,33,39,44,45] With the newer devices (i.e. SilverHawk) and with the use of standard workhorse wires, this complication is rare. Careful checking of the distal end of the wire is a prudent choice. Free mobility of the distal guidewire should be maintained at all times. Loss of free mobility may suggest that the collection chamber is full.

As previously suggested, it is important to avoid cutting in very angulated segments, especially when utilizing the Flexi-Cut device which has a longer straight housing compared to the SilverHawk.

Vasospasm

Severe vasospasm occurred in less than 2% with the use of the early DCA devices.[2,32,43,46] Spasm will respond readily to intracoronary nitroglycerin or other vasodilators or even gentle low pressure balloon inflations.

Thrombosis

Thrombosis occurred in approximately 2% and accounted for half of the abrupt closure cases in the early studies of DCA.[2,32,43,46] With the optimization of antiplatelet therapy and especially with the addition of clopidogrel or ticlopidine to aspirin, this problem seems to have been reduced dramatically. In the absence of other procedural complications, strict adherence to optimal double antiplatelet pretreatment will minimize the risk of intraprocedural thrombosis. The use of IIb/IIIa inhibitors is certainly a reasonable idea to lower the risk of this complication. In our experience we kept the use of IIb/IIIa inhibitors quite low and rarely on an elective base (less than 10%) due to the consequences if a perforation should occur.

IS THERE A ROLE FOR DIRECTIONAL CORONARY ATHERECTOMY IN TODAY'S CLINICAL PRACTICE?

Despite the lack of scientific evidence supporting the advantage of plaque debulking in today's clinical practice, our experience in this setting has been favorable and we still occasionally combine atherectomy and DES when the anatomic setting is appropriate, such as with specific ostial, bifurcation, and left main lesions. Despite this statement we should recognize that the use of atherectomy, even in suitable lesions, continues to decrease.

Ostial lesions

Percutaneous interventions on ostial, especially aorto-ostial, lesions is frequently limited by lesion rigidity and elastic recoil, leading to suboptimal results.[47–49] For noncalcified ostial lesions in vessels >3 mm, DCA is associated with procedural success in 87% and major complications in <1% of patients.[47,48] Although immediate angiographic results in highly selected lesions are excellent, DCA of ostial lesions is limited by a high incidence of restenosis. We have recently shown that this problem seems to be eliminated by the implantation of DES with or without prior DCA in the setting of aorto-ostial lesions.[50]

Bifurcation lesions

Angioplasty on bifurcation lesions is often complicated by the 'snow-plough' effect or plaque shifting which can be complicated with side branch occlusion, and suboptimal final angiographic results.[51,52] These problems continue, although to a lesser extent, with the treatment of bifurcations with DES. It is worth noting that we recently showed that bifurcation treatment with DES was an independent predictor of stent thrombosis at nine months.[53] The risk of side branch occlusion with DCA is greatest when the side branch originates from the target lesion or if it is itself significantly diseased (stenosis >50%). In our practice, we occasionally treat the main branch with DCA when there is a large plaque burden, to avoid plaque shifting.

Left main lesions

Stenosis in the left main coronary artery is well suited for DCA because of its proximal location and large vessel caliber. We still occasionally combine atherectomy and DES when treating a left main stenosis with a large plaque burden demonstrated by intravascular ultrasound with the characteristics to be suitable for removal with DCA.[54,55]

Case examples of ostial and bifurcation lesions treated with DCA followed by stenting are presented in Figures 9.8–10.

ASSOCIATED PHARMACOLOGIC TREATMENT

When performing DCA with stenting, we do not usually change our protocol of periprocedural heparin administration (100 U/kg without elective IIb/IIIa and

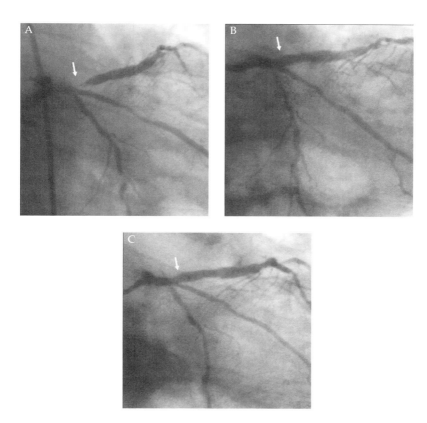

Figure 9.8   A. A lesion involving the ostium of the left anterior descending artery. B. Final angiographic result following atherectomy and stenting. C. Minimal late loss at eight-month follow-up angiogram.

70 U/kg with elective IIb/IIIa). Glycoprotein IIb/IIIa inhibitors are sometimes administered when the final result appears suboptimal and for various clinical or anatomic reasons the operator feels it unnecessary to implant another stent. In addition, the use of glycoprotein IIb/IIIa inhibitors prior to DCA has been shown to reduce the incidence of non Q-wave myocardial infarction.[56] As we pointed out above, the elective use of IIb/IIIa inhibitors is low in our experience due to the possible consequences of an occasional perforation.

We pay a lot of attention to periprocedural preparation with thienopyridines and if in doubt, we administer a 600 mg loading dose of clopidogrel in the catheterization laboratory. The duration of combined thienopyridine and aspirin treatment following stent implantation after DCA varies according to the length of the stent implanted, the type of stent used, and the clinical conditions of the patient (acute coronary syndrome at the time of stenting or diabetes mellitus).

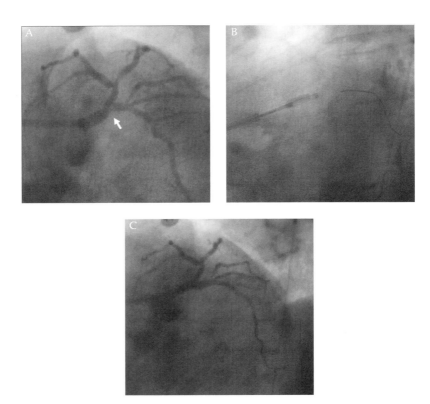

Figure 9.9 A. A lesion involving the ostium of the left circumflex coronary artery. B. The tip of the atherectomy catheter across the lesion during cutting. C. Final angiographic result following stenting.

CONCLUSION

Procedural complexity and long-term recurrence remain major concerns when stents are implanted in 'complex lesion subsets', such as long lesions, ostial lesions, bifurcations, and calcified or nondilatable lesions. Pretreatment of these complex lesions with high-pressure balloon inflation before stent implantation is certainly an option, but it is not always successful. Suboptimal dilatation, acute recoil, plaque shift, dissections, and vessel perforation are all potential shortcomings with this approach. To remedy this problem, directional atherectomy in noncalcified lesions and rotational atherectomy in calcified lesions have been developed to prepare complex plaques before stent implantation. However, the encouraging results of many single-center experiences[57] were not reproduced in the context of randomized studies.[3,13]

The technique is very operator dependent and the amount of tissue removal varies with the commitment of the operator to perform extensive debulking. In addition, except for the very recent introduction of the SilverHawk device, no further development in the devices available occurred for a long time. The introduction of DES has further challenged any additional complex approach.

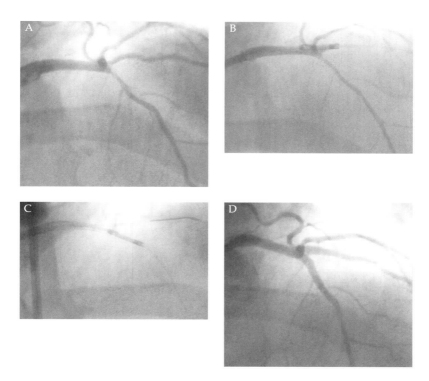

Figure 9.10 A typical bifurcation lesion involving the left anterior descending artery and diagonal branch (A), which is treated with atherectomy (B and C), followed by stenting on both branches (D).

Despite these concerns and the lack of scientific evidence supporting the advantage of plaque debulking in bifurcation lesions, our experience in this setting has been favorable and we still occasionally combine atherectomy and DES when the anatomic setting is appropriate, such as a left main stenosis with a large plaque burden demonstrated by IVUS with the characteristics to be suitable for removal with current directional atherectomy devices.

The rationale of plaque debulking with atherectomy is as appealing as ever. Whether technologic advances in this field will result in breakthrough in the treatment of coronary artery disease remains to be seen. For the moment, the role of DCA is only complementary to the 'Holy Grail' of PCI, which by any standard is the drug-eluting stent.

WHAT YOU SHOULD REMEMBER

General

1. Optimal DCA and stenting are associated with low restenosis rates despite the fact that we have been unable to demonstrate this statement in randomized trials. The main problem is that performing optimal DCA is complex and can be risky.

2. The need to perform DCA remains minimal due to the excellent results with DES (Cypher and Taxus). In very rare circumstances DES cannot or should not be implanted; the possibility of using DCA in these settings should be kept in mind.
3. There are selected lesions in which the use of DCA with or without stenting appears ideal. Despite this reasonable statement, most of these lesions are currently successfully treated with DES.

Technical

1. DCA requires a formal training with direct supervision. Incorrect usage of DCA can lead to major complications without easy solution.
2. Correct guiding catheter choice and manipulation are important. Major dissections can occur due to incorrect manipulation of the guide catheter.
3. Support wires such as the Iron Man (Guidant, Tamecula, CA) are essential for the Flexi-Cut device but not necessarily for the SilverHawk which can frequently be used with any type of guidewire.
4. In some situations DCA can be the only way to gain access to a side branch by removing the plaque in the main branch.
5. In any doubtful setting, consider evaluation of the artery size and results with intravascular ultrasound.
6. Even with contemporary DCA devices, calcium remains a major limitation and contraindication if extensive.
7. Do not force the device through the lesion; rotate, align, and accept that DCA cannot be performed in some lesions.
8. Do not perform DCA in very angulated lesions.
9. Make sure you have PTFE-covered stents available, know where they are located, and consider their deliverability at the site where you are planning to perform DCA. Remember also perfusion balloons (Guidant, Tamecula, CA).

REFERENCES

1. Simpson J, Johnson D, Thapliyal H. Transluminal atherectomy: a new approach in the treatment of atherosclerotic vascular disease (abstract). Circulation 1985;72:III111.
2. Honda Y, Fitzgerald PJ. The renaissance of directional coronary atherectomy: a second look from the inside. J Invasive Cardiol 2001;13:748–51.
3. Moses JW, Carlier S, Moussa I. Lesion preparation prior to stenting. Rev Cardiovasc Med 2004;5(Suppl 2):S16–21.
4. Moussa I, Di Mario C, Colombo A. Plaque removal prior to stent implantation in native coronary arteries: why? When? And how? Semin Interv Cardiol 1998;3:57–63.
5. Elliott JM, Berdan LG, Holmes DR et al. One-year follow-up in the Coronary Angioplasty Versus Excisional Atherectomy Trial (CAVEAT I). Circulation 1995;91:2158–66.
6. Baim DS, Cutlip DE, Sharma SK et al. Final results of the Balloon vs Optimal Atherectomy Trial (BOAT). Circulation 1998;97:322–31.
7. Colombo A, Iakovou I. Ten years of advancements in interventional cardiology. J Endovasc Ther 2004;11(Suppl 2):II10–18.
8. Mintz GS. Remodeling and restenosis: observations from serial intravascular ultrasound studies. Curr Interv Cardiol Rep 2000;2:316–25.

9. Topol EJ, Leya F, Pinkerton CA et al. A comparison of directional atherectomy with coronary angioplasty in patients with coronary artery disease. The CAVEAT Study Group. N Engl J Med 1993;329:221–7.

10. Kiesz RS, Rozek MM, Mego DM, Patel V, Ebersole DG, Chilton RJ. Acute directional coronary atherectomy prior to stenting in complex coronary lesions: ADAPTS Study. Cathet Cardiovasc Diagn 1998;45:105–12.

11. Kobayashi Y, Moussa I, Akiyama T et al. Low restenosis rate in lesions of the left anterior descending coronary artery with stenting following directional coronary atherectomy. Cathet Cardiovasc Diagn 1998;45:131–8.

12. Moussa I, Moses J, Di Mario C et al. Stenting after optimal lesion debulking (sold) registry. Angiographic and clinical outcome. Circulation 1998;98:1604–9.

13. Bramucci E, Angoli L, Merlini PA et al. Adjunctive stent implantation following directional coronary atherectomy in patients with coronary artery disease. J Am Coll Cardiol 1998;32:1855–60.

14. Hopp HW, Baer FM, Ozbek C, Kuck KH, Scheller B. A synergistic approach to optimal stenting: directional coronary atherectomy prior to coronary artery stent implantation–the AtheroLink Registry. AtheroLink Study Group. J Am Coll Cardiol 2000;36:1853–9.

15. Takeda Y, Tsuchikane E, Kobayashi T et al. Effect of plaque debulking before stent implantation on in-stent neointimal proliferation: a serial 3-dimensional intravascular ultrasound study. Am Heart J 2003;146:175–82.

16. Hoffmann R, Mintz GS, Dussaillant GR et al. Patterns and mechanisms of in-stent restenosis: a serial intravascular ultrasound study. Circulation 1996;94:1247–54.

17. Farb A, Sangiorgi G, Carter AJ et al. Pathology of acute and chronic coronary stenting in humans. Circulation 1999;99:44–52.

18. Kimura T, Kaburagi S, Tamura T et al. Remodeling of human coronary arteries undergoing coronary angioplasty or atherectomy. Circulation 1997;96:475–83.

19. de Vrey EA, Mintz GS, von Birgelen C et al. Serial volumetric (three-dimensional) intravascular ultrasound analysis of restenosis after directional coronary atherectomy. J Am Coll Cardiol 1998;32:1874–80.

20. Lansky AJ, Mintz GS, Popma JJ et al. Remodeling after directional coronary atherectomy (with and without adjunct percutaneous transluminal coronary angioplasty): a serial angiographic and intravascular ultrasound analysis from the Optimal Atherectomy Restenosis Study. J Am Coll Cardiol 1998;32:329–37.

21. Mintz GS, Kimura T, Nobuyoshi M, Leon MB. Intravascular ultrasound assessment of the relation between early and late changes in arterial area and neointimal hyperplasia after percutaneous transluminal coronary angioplasty and directional coronary atherectomy. Am J Cardiol 1999;83:1518–23.

22. von Birgelen C, Mintz GS, de Vrey EA et al. Preintervention lesion remodelling affects operative mechanisms of balloon optimised directional coronary atherectomy procedures: a volumetric study with three dimensional intravascular ultrasound. Heart 2000;83:192–7.

23. Mintz GS, Kimura T, Nobuyoshi M, Dangas G, Leon MB. Relation between preintervention remodeling and late arterial responses to coronary angioplasty or atherectomy. Am J Cardiol 2001;87:392–6.

24. Fitzgerald PJ, Yock PG. Mechanisms and outcomes of angioplasty and atherectomy assessed by intravascular ultrasound imaging. J Clin Ultrasound 1993;21:579–88.

25. Hoffmann R, Mintz GS, Mehran R et al. Intravascular ultrasound predictors of angiographic restenosis in lesions treated with Palmaz-Schatz stents. J Am Coll Cardiol 1998;31:43–9.

26. Prati F, Di Mario C, Moussa I et al. In-stent neointimal proliferation correlates with the amount of residual plaque burden outside the stent: an intravascular ultrasound study. Circulation 1999;99:1011–14.

27. Dangas G, Mintz GS, Mehran R et al. Preintervention arterial remodeling as an independent predictor of target-lesion revascularization after nonstent coronary intervention: an analysis of 777 lesions with intravascular ultrasound imaging. Circulation 1999;99:3149–54.

28. Shiran A, Weissman NJ, Leiboff B et al. Effect of preintervention plaque burden on subsequent intimal hyperplasia in stented coronary artery lesions. Am J Cardiol 2000;86:1318–21.

29. de Jaegere P, Mudra H, Figulla H et al. Intravascular ultrasound-guided optimized stent deployment. Immediate and 6 months clinical and angiographic results from the Multicenter Ultrasound Stenting in Coronaries Study (MUSIC Study). Eur Heart J 1998;19:1214–23.

30. Orlic D, Reimers B, Stankovic G et al. Initial experience with a new 8 French-compatible directional atherectomy catheter: immediate and mid-term results. Cathet Cardiovasc Intervent 2003;60:159–66.

31. Adelman AG, Cohen EA, Kimball BP et al. A comparison of directional atherectomy with balloon angioplasty for lesions of the left anterior descending coronary artery. N Engl J Med 1993;329:228–33.

32. Holmes DR Jr, Topol EJ, Califf RM et al. A multicenter, randomized trial of coronary angioplasty versus directional atherectomy for patients with saphenous vein bypass graft lesions. CAVEAT-II Investigators. Circulation 1995;91:1966–74.

33. Simonton CA, Leon MB, Baim DS et al. 'Optimal' directional coronary atherectomy: final results of the Optimal Atherectomy Restenosis Study (OARS). Circulation 1998;97:332–9.

34. Suzuki T, Hosokawa H, Katoh O et al. Effects of adjunctive balloon angioplasty after intravascular ultrasound-guided optimal directional coronary atherectomy: the result of Adjunctive Balloon Angioplasty After Coronary Atherectomy Study (ABACAS). J Am Coll Cardiol 1999;34:1028–35.

35. Tsuchikane E, Sumitsuji S, Awata N et al. Final results of the STent versus directional coronary Atherectomy Randomized Trial (START). J Am Coll Cardiol 1999;34:1050–7.

36. Airoldi F, Di Mario C, Stankovic G et al. Clinical and angiographic outcome of directional atherectomy followed by stent implantation in de novo lesions located at the ostium of the left anterior descending coronary artery. Heart 2003;89:1050–4.

37. Chung CM, Nakamura S, Tanaka K et al. Stenting alone versus debulking and debulking plus stent in branch ostial lesions of native coronary arteries. Heart Vessels 2004;19:213–20.

38. Rowe MH, Hinohara T, White NW, Robertson GC, Selmon MR, Simpson JB. Comparison of dissection rates and angiographic results following directional coronary atherectomy and coronary angioplasty. Am J Cardiol 1990;66:49–53.

39. Holmes DR Jr, Simpson JB, Berdan LG et al. Abrupt closure: the CAVEAT I experience. Coronary Angioplasty Versus Excisional Atherectomy Trial. J Am Coll Cardiol 1995;26:1494–500.

40. Ellis SG, De Cesare NB, Pinkerton CA et al. Relation of stenosis morphology and clinical presentation to the procedural results of directional coronary atherectomy. Circulation 1991;84:644–53.

41. Garratt KN, Holmes DR Jr, Bell MR et al. Results of directional atherectomy of primary atheromatous and restenosis lesions in coronary arteries and saphenous vein grafts. Am J Cardiol 1992;70:449–54.

42. Garratt KN, Kaufmann UP, Edwards WD, Vlietstra RE, Holmes DR Jr. Safety of percutaneous coronary atherectomy with deep arterial resection. Am J Cardiol 1989;64:538–40.

43. Kaufmann UP, Garratt KN, Vlietstra RE, Menke KK, Holmes DR Jr. Coronary atherectomy: first 50 patients at the Mayo Clinic. Mayo Clin Proc 1989;64:747–52.

44. Cohen EA, Sykora K, Kimball BP et al. Clinical outcomes of patients more than one year following randomization in the Canadian Coronary Atherectomy Trial (CCAT). Can J Cardiol 1997;13:825–30.

45. Meuwissen M, Piek JJ, van der Wal AC et al. Recurrent unstable angina after directional coronary atherectomy is related to the extent of initial coronary plaque inflammation. J Am Coll Cardiol 2001;37:1271–6.

46. Repetto A, Ferlini M, Ferrario M, Angoli L, Bramucci E. Directional coronary atherectomy in 2005. Ital Heart J 2005;6:494–7.

47. Stephan WJ, Bates ER, Garratt KN, Hinohara T, Muller DW. Directional atherectomy of coronary and saphenous vein graft ostial stenoses. Am J Cardiol 1995;75:1015–18.

48. Popma JJ, Dick RJ, Haudenschild CC, Topol EJ, Ellis SG. Atherectomy of right coronary ostial stenoses: initial and long-term results, technical features and histologic findings. Am J Cardiol 1991;67:431–3.

49. Zampieri P, Colombo A, Almagor Y, Maiello L, Finci L. Results of coronary stenting of ostial lesions. Am J Cardiol 1994;73:901–3.

50. Iakovou I, Ge L, Michev I et al. Clinical and angiographic outcome after sirolimus-eluting stent implantation in aorto-ostial lesions. J Am Coll Cardiol 2004;44:967–71.

51. Ge L, Tsagalou E, Iakovou I et al. In-hospital and nine-month outcome of treatment of coronary bifurcational lesions with sirolimus-eluting stent. Am J Cardiol 2005;95:757–60.

52. Yamashita T, Nishida T, Adamian MG et al. Bifurcation lesions: two stents versus one stent–immediate and follow-up results. J Am Coll Cardiol 2000;35:1145–51.

53. Iakovou I, Schmidt T, Bonizzoni E et al. Incidence, predictors, and outcome of thrombosis after successful implantation of drug-eluting stents. JAMA 2005;293:2126–30.

54. Brambilla N, Repetto A, Bramucci E et al. Directional coronary atherectomy plus stent implantation vs. left internal mammary artery bypass grafting for isolated proximal stenosis of the left anterior descending coronary artery. Cathet Cardiovasc Intervent 2005;64:45–52.

55. Chieffo A, Stankovic G, Bonizzoni E et al. Early and mid-term results of drug-eluting stent implantation in unprotected left main. Circulation 2005;111:791–5.

56. Lefkovits J, Blankenship JC, Anderson KM et al. Increased risk of non-Q wave myocardial infarction after directional atherectomy is platelet dependent: evidence from the EPIC trial. Evaluation of c7E3 for the Prevention of Ischemic Complications. J Am Coll Cardiol 1996;28:849–55.

57. Karvouni E, Di Mario C, Nishida T et al. Directional atherectomy prior to stenting in bifurcation lesions: a matched comparison study with stenting alone. Cathet Cardiovasc Intervent 2001;53:12–20.

10

Embolic protection devices and complications during percutaneous coronary interventions

Stéphane Carlier, Xuebo Liu and Gregg Stone

Distal protection devices • **Proximal protection devices** • **Distal embolic protection for saphenous vein graft percutaneous cardiovascular interventions** • **Distal protection on primary percutaneous cardiovascular intervention in myocardial infarction with and without ST segment elevation** • **Limitations** • **Conclusion**

Distal embolization of plaque debris and thrombus complicates percutaneous coronary interventions (PCI). This results in diminished blood flow to the distal vascular bed and is associated with periprocedural ischemia and infarction, as demonstrated by perfusion defects and serum cardiac enzyme elevation. Distal embolization of large particles at the time of balloon inflation or stent deployment may obstruct large epicardial vessels. However, microvascular obstruction due to very small particles, as little as 15–100 microns, may also lead to microinfarcts and left ventricular dysfunction. It is likely that mechanical microvascular obstruction is commonly aggravated by secondary spasm and edema due to release of humoral factors by platelets, and endothelial injury and dysfunction.

Periprocedural myocardial infarction (MI) is associated with a worse prognosis, particularly when it is large, as demonstrated in saphenous vein bypass graft interventions. This was demonstrated by Hong et al who studied 1056 consecutive patients after angiographically successful PCI of 1693 saphenous bypass grafts.[1] One-year mortality was significantly increased in patients with periprocedural creatine kinase-MB elevation, even among patients without any apparent procedural or in-hospital complication. Only limited therapeutic success has been reported in observational studies involving the use of calcium channel blockers, adenosine, and sodium nitroprusside with partial resolution of the 'no-reflow' phenomenon.

Consequently, a number of distal protection devices have been developed, using either an expandable filter mounted on the angioplasty guidewire to facilitate entrapment of particles and safe removal or a balloon occlusion combined with thromboaspiration (Figures 10.1, 10.2). The most recently introduced concept has been proximal protection with the major advantage that the lesion will not be crossed before the protection becomes active.

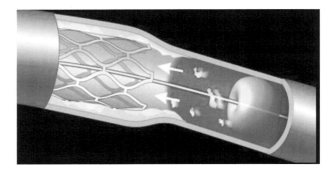

Figure 10.1   Distal occlusion device.

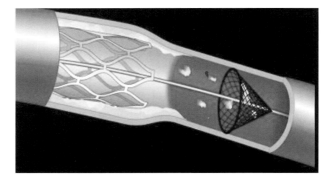

Figure 10.2   Distal filter.

DISTAL PROTECTION DEVICES

Over the past few years, several embolic protection devices have been developed and introduced into clinical practice. Three basic concepts have emerged and devices are summarized in Table 10.1. One is a flow-occlusive balloon that was the first FDA-approved device for the saphenous vein graft (SVG) interventions. The second is a distal filter that does not occlude antegrade flow. Advantages of a filtering device include continued myocardial perfusion throughout the interventional procedure. However, incomplete occlusion could potentially lead to some embolized material reaching the distal vascular bed. In contrast, balloon occlusive devices theoretically prevent the embolization of all particles. However, the cessation of regional myocardial perfusion may result in hemodynamic instability.

Balloon occlusion device

There are two devices of this type approved for use by the FDA in SVG: the PercuSurge GuardWire (Medtronic, Santa Rosa, CA, USA) and the TriActiv System (Kensey Nash, Exton, PA). They are based on a wire containing a central lumen that

Table 10.1 Distal embolic protection devices

Coronary device	Type	FDA approved	Company
1. Balloon occlusion			
GuardWire®	Temporary occlusion and aspiration system	Y (SVG)	Medtronic, Inc.
TriActiv	Temporary occlusion and distal saline infusion	Y (SVG)	Kensey Nash
2. Filter			
AngioGuard	Embolic protection filter	No (CE Mark)	Cordis/J&J
FilterWire EX™	Embolic protection filter	Yes	Boston Scientific
FilterWire EZ™	Embolic protection filter	No (CE Mark)	Boston Scientific
IntraGuard™	Embolic protection filter	No	INTRATHERAPEUTICS
Cardioshield	Embolic protection filter	No	Abbott Vascular
MedNova Emboshield	Embolic protection filter	Yes (Carotid)	Abbott Vascular
Interceptor Plus	Embolic protection filter (nitinol mesh)	No (CE Mark)	Medtronic, Inc
RX Accunet™	Embolic protection filter	Yes (Carotid)	Guidant
SpideRX	Embolic protection filter using any wire	Yes (Carotid)	eV3
TRAP	Embolic protection filter (nitinol mesh)	No	eV3
Rubicon	Embolic protection filter (sheathless)	No	Boston Scientific
3. Proximal protection			
Proxis®	Proximally deployed, temporary occlusion and aspiration system	No	St Jude Medical Sciences, Inc
PARODI	Proximal occlusion for carotid	No	Arteria Medical Science
Mo.Ma	Double balloons for proximal occlusion	No	Invatec

communicates with a low-pressure distal occlusion balloon incorporated into the tip. The wire both serves as the angioplasty guidewire and provides protection from distal embolization (Figure 10.3). An inflation device controls expansion and sizing of the occlusion balloon in the treated vessel. An aspiration catheter is used to remove the debris from the treated vessel before the balloon is deflated and antegrade flow in the treated vessel is restored (Guardwire).

In the TriActiv system there will be infusion of saline in the interrupted column of blood and there is aspiration from the guiding catheter.

One of the most important limitations of this distal balloon occlusion device is that it may cause distal ischemia that may not be tolerated by some patients. The preparation of the wire might be cumbersome. Finally, angiography cannot be performed while the distal balloon is inflated, and the assessment of the artery and stent placement are more difficult. Unless used in conduits without side-branches such as a SVG, debris can also potentially be embolized proximally.

Filter devices

The number of filter devices is increasing and several are currently undergoing clinical investigation.

AngioGuard

The AngioGuard™ (Cordis Corp., Minneapolis, MN, USA) (Figure 10.4) is a distal protection device that has recently received approval for marketing in Europe, but is not yet FDA approved. The AngioGuard's technology incorporates an angioplasty guidewire with a filter that expands to 6 mm. The AngioGuard filter has multiple, 100 micron, laser-drilled holes that allow perfusion during device deployment. This has been proposed as a major advantage. In contrast to balloon occlusion devices, complete cessation of antegrade flow does not occur during the treatment of the lesion and aspiration of the debris (typically 2–3 minutes in the hands of experienced

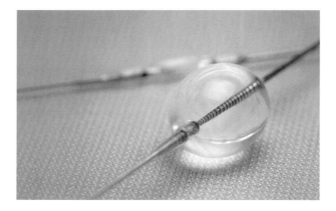

Figure 10.3   PercuSurge GuardWire temporary occlusion and aspiration system.

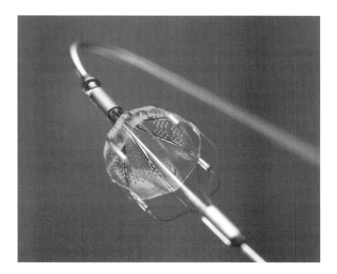

Figure 10.4 AngioGuard™ XP/AngioGuard™ RX emboli capture guidewire systems.

operators). This is very important in patients with a reduced left ventricular function or when the lesion is in an artery that supplies a large amount of myocardium. Conversely, it has been proposed that incomplete vessel occlusion with the filter devices allows passage of debris through the holes of the devices. Analysis of debris retrieved by aspiration after balloon occlusion in the SAFE trial found that 80% of the particulate matter was less than 100 microns in diameter.[2] The clinical significance of such small embolic particles is unclear, and difficult to resolve since the completeness of debris entrapment by any distal protection device is impossible to determine in clinical practice.

FilterWire EX

The FilterWire EX™ embolic protection system (Boston Scientific, Natick, MA, USA) was the first embolic protection filter to receive clearance by the FDA for use in SVG interventions. Similar to the AngioGuard, it is a low-profile (<3.5 F) filter mounted on a 0.014″ angioplasty wire with pore holes of 80 microns, allowing antegrade blood flow while providing distal protection. The filter design is characterized by an off-center position with a 'fish-mouth' opening. It can be used with any standard angioplasty balloon. A radiopaque nitinol framework provides filter support and facilitates fluoroscopic visualization (Figure 10.5).

New Comers

It is beyond the scope of this chapter to review all the technical details of the latest filters; Cardioshield, Emboshield, Interceptor, Accunet, SpideRX, and TRAP. They are listed in Table 10.1 with their principal characteristics and approved indication.

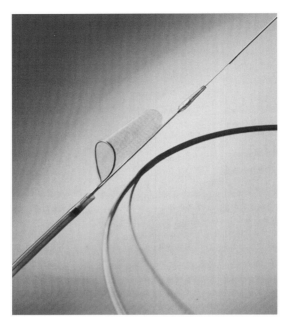

Figure 10.5   FilterWire EX™ embolic protection system.

PROXIMAL PROTECTION DEVICES

The Proxis® embolic protection system (Figure 10.6) is the first proximal embolic protection device designed for coronary application. A balloon is inflated proximally around a delivery catheter that allows wires, balloons, and stents to be advanced through the lesion. The interruption of the blood flow while injecting contrast will block a column of contrast that will offer visualization of the target lesion and

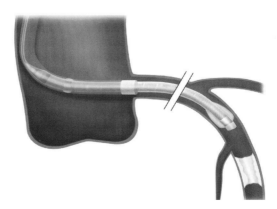

Figure 10.6   Proxis® embolic protection system.

stenting can be performed more easily. The loose debris will be aspirated before the proximal occlusion balloon is deflated. The major advantage of this approach is that no device has to cross the lesion before protection is secured.

A similar concept is applied in devices used for carotid interventions only: the PARODI (Arteria Medica Science, Inc., San Francisco, CA) and Mo.Ma (Invatec, Roncadelle, Italy). Mo.Ma protects the brain from embolization by two highly compliant atraumatic balloons, blocking antegrade blood flow from the common carotid artery and retrograde blood flow from the external carotid artery: protection is established before the critical phase of lesion crossing.

DISTAL EMBOLIC PROTECTION FOR SAPHENOUS VEIN GRAFT PERCUTANEOUS CARDIOVASCULAR INTERVENTIONS

The development of atherosclerosis in SVGs is the major limiting factor of coronary artery bypass surgery. Approximately one half of vein conduits are significantly diseased or occluded at ten years.[3] A new surgical revascularization strategy has associated incremental risks so that percutaneous treatment of SVG disease is often the first option. In addition, the novel drug-eluting stents show promise in reducing the occurrence of restenosis, one of the major problems associated with the PCI of SVG. However, catheter-based treatment of SVG disease is associated with increased morbidity and mortality compared with native coronary arterial percutaneous intervention, often the result of distal embolization of atherothrombotic material.

The Saphenous vein graft Angioplasty Free of Emboli (SAFE) trial[2] evaluated the feasibility, safety, and efficacy of distal protection using the PercuSurge GuardWire occlusion and aspiration system. A total of 103 consecutive patients undergoing planned stenting of 105 SVG lesions were prospectively enrolled in a multinational, multicenter study. Before angioplasty, protection of the distal circulation was achieved with the PercuSurge GuardWire distal balloon occlusion system, followed by stenting and debris aspiration. Mean graft age was 8.9±4.0 years. The duration of distal balloon inflation was 5.4±3.7 minutes; premature balloon deflation for ischemia was not required in any patient. Macroscopically visible red and/or yellow debris was extracted in 91% of patients. Postprocedural TIMI-III flow was present in 98.9% of grafts (vs 83.5% before intervention). No patient developed angiographic evidence of no-reflow or distal embolization. Postprocedural creatine phosphokinase MB isozyme levels were elevated to >3 times normal in only five patients (5%), and 97 patients (94%) were free of major adverse events at 30 days.

Following these encouraging results, the randomized (SAFER) trial was conducted in the United States[4] in 47 sites and enrolled 801 patients undergoing SVG PCI. Inclusion criteria were stenoses of 50–99% in SVGs 3–6 mm in diameter, more than 5 mm from the ostium and 20 mm from the distal anastomosis, with at least TIMI-I flow at baseline. Exclusion criteria were acute MI, ejection fraction <25%, creatinine >2.5 mg/dL (unless on hemodialysis), and planned use of an atherectomy device. The primary end-point was the occurrence of major adverse clinical events at 30 days, including death, MI, emergency bypass surgery, and repeat target vessel revascularization. Prespecified secondary end-points were the frequency with which TIMI-III flow was achieved, and clinically apparent no-flow occurred. The GuardWire was superior to 'standard care'. There was a 50% relative reduction in cumulative 30-day major adverse cardiac events (17.8% to 9.0%, P=0.001), a 68% relative reduction in mortality (2.8% to 0.9%, P=0.086), and a 49% relative reduction in MI (17.3% to 8.8%, P=0.003). Interestingly, although GP IIb/IIIa inhibitors were used in >60% of all patients, predominantly before intervention, major adverse clinical events were more common amongst those receiving the drug. However, no definitive conclusion could be made from this nonrandomized, retrospective analysis. Nevertheless, the reduction in major adverse clinical events in the GuardWire arm was independent of the use of GP IIb/IIIa inhibitors.

Stone et al evaluated the clinical, angiographic, and technical factors related to successful stenting of diseased SVGs using a FilterWire EX distal protection device. PCI was performed in 60 lesions in 48 patients undergoing SVG intervention with the FilterWire EX distal protection system in a phase I experience at six sites. A larger phase II study was then performed in 248 lesions in 230 SVGs at 65 US centers. Cumulative adverse events at 30 days occurred in 21.3% of patients in phase I, including a 19.1% rate of MI. Numerous anatomic, device-specific, and operator-related contributors to these adverse events were identified, resulting in significant changes to the protocol and instructions for use. Subsequently, despite similar clinical and angiographic characteristics to the phase I patients, the 30-day adverse event rate in phase II was reduced to 11.3% (P=0.09), due primarily to a lower incidence of periprocedural Q-wave and non Q-wave MI.[5]

The FilterWire during Transluminal Intervention of Saphenous Vein Graft (FIRE) trial was a randomized, multicenter study comparing this filter-based device with the PercuSurge GuardWire system.[6] This trial showed similar clinical efficacies of filter protection and balloon occlusion. Major adverse cardiac events occurred in 9.9% of FilterWire patients and 11.6% of GuardWire patients. This was statistically significant (0.0008) for proving noninferiority of the FilterWire embolic protection device.

On the basis of the results of the FIRE trial, filter-based embolic protection devices have become the preferred modality for SVG intervention. However, despite the FIRE trial data, there has been some concern whether filter-based systems can provide complete protection. In the FIRE trial, the nominal pore size of the FilterWire EX device was 110 μm. Since equivalent clinical efficacy was demonstrated in FIRE, it appears that embolization material <110 μm is unimportant clinically. However, Grube et al reported that >80% of the particles retrieved with the PercuSurge AngioGuard were <96 μm in diameter.[2] This observation conflicts with the notion that filter-based systems offer sufficient embolic protection. A recent analysis by Rogers et al[7] compared microparticle size retieved from SVG intervention with both the AngioGuard and a filter-based device. The results demonstrated that the vascular filter device was capable of trapping particulate material <100 μm, which was the average distal pore size. Explanations included the possibility that the composite of debris, platelets, and fibrin may reduce the functional pore size of the filter. These microparticle analyses may shed light on the results reported in the FIRE trial. In addition, these data will be instrumental in the development of an optimal embolic protection device for SVG intervention. The complications of distal embolic protection are listed in Tables 10.2 and 10.3. More recent trials comparing the FilterWire or the GuardWire to newcomers have been extensively reviewed recently by Mauri et al.[8]

Table 10.2   SAFER trial: cath lab outcomes

	GuardWire 1997	Control	*P*
No. of patients	395	406	
Final TIMI-III flow	97.8%	95.1%	0.04
No-reflow	3.2%	8.3%	0.001
Distal emboli	2.2%	3.2%	0.40
Perforation	0.2%	1.5%	0.05
Subacute closure	1.7%	0.5%	0.18
Dissection	4%	1%	0.12

Table 10.3   FIRE trial: device failure

	FilterWire	GuardWire	*P*
FilterWire EX any failure	4.5%	2.8%	NS
Failure to deliver	3.9%	0.6%	0.005
Failure to deploy filter	0.6%	–	–
Failure to inflate balloon	–	0.9%	–
Occlusion lost or rupture	–	1.3%	–

DISTAL PROTECTION ON PRIMARY PERCUTANEOUS CARDIOVASCULAR INTERVENTION IN MYOCARDIAL INFARCTION WITH AND WITHOUT ST SEGMENT ELEVATION

In acute myocardial infarction, primary PCI is highly successful in the restoration of epicardial blood flow, achieving full angiographic patency (TIMI grade III flow) in >90% of the patients. Despite restoration of large-vessel flow, tissue perfusion in areas at risk frequently continues to be compromised, as shown by myocardial contrast echocardiography, flow velocity measurements, and assessment of TIMI frame counts or myocardial blush. Persistent microcirculatory impairment is associated with poor recovery of contractile function and adverse clinical outcome.

The ability of the FilterWire to capture emboli has been demonstrated repeatedly from the early experience. The safety and feasibility of the FilterWire in acute myocardial infarction were recently confirmed by Limbruno and co-workers.[9] When a filter device is used in acute myocardial infarction, the possibility has to be considered that, in a vessel with a number of side branches, the device may simply shift the path of embolic material down the branches despite adequate use of the filter. Moreover, material may be embolized during crossing of the device or predilatation, when needed. Nevertheless, in the study of Limbruno and co-workers, captured debris was found in every filter that was examined microscopically, and macroscopic particles were present in 34% of the filters. Angiographically visible distal embolization occurred in only 2% of patients with FilterWire protection but in 15% of a matched case–control group (*P*=0.03). In our study, the filter wire was similarly effective in the prevention of distal embolization.

Gick et al[10] enrolled 200 patients who had angina within 48 hours after onset of pain plus at least one of three additional criteria: ST segment elevation, elevated myocardial marker proteins, and angiographic evidence of thrombotic occlusion. Among the patients included (83% men; mean age 62±12 years), 100 were randomly assigned to the FilterWire group and 100 to the control group (PROMISE trial). The primary end-point was the maximal adenosine-induced Doppler flow velocity in the recanalized infarct artery; the secondary end-point was infarct size estimated by the volume of delayed enhancement on nuclear MRI. ST segment elevation myocardial infarction was present in 68.5% of the patients; the median time from onset of pain was 6.9 hours. In the FilterWire group, maximal adenosine-induced flow velocity was 34±17 compared with 36±20 cm/s in the control group (P=0.46). Infarct sizes, assessed in 82 patients in the FilterWire group and 78 patients in the control group, were 11.8±9.3% of the left ventricular mass in the FilterWire group and 10.4±9.4% in the control group (P=0.33). Thirty-day mortality was 2% in the FilterWire group and 3% in the control group. The FilterWire as an adjunct to primary PCI in myocardial infarction with and without ST segment elevation did not improve reperfusion or reduce infarct size.

It appears more likely that the distal embolization during primary PCI that can be prevented by protection devices exerts only minor effects compared with the consequences of ischemic microvascular damage or spontaneous distal embolization arising from ruptured or eroded plaques during the natural course of an acute coronary syndrome. This inference is supported by the Enhanced Myocardial Efficacy and Recovery by Aspiration of Liberalized Debris (EMERALD) study on an alternative distal protection system, distal balloon occlusion and aspiration (GuardWire).[11] EMERALD randomized 501 patients to distal protection with balloon occlusion and aspiration or usual care. Visible debris that otherwise would have entered the distal circulation could be removed in 73% of the patients of the study group. Nevertheless, neither the primary end-point of ST segment resolution nor any of the secondary end-points, including myocardial blush or adverse cardiac events, showed any significant benefit of distal protection compared with usual care. EMERALD, PROMISE and other studies suggest that, regardless of the technology, distal protection does not improve reperfusion after primary PCI in myocardial infarction, but they might still have 'niche' applications.[12]

LIMITATIONS AND COMPLICATIONS

In general, each system has its own intrinsic limitations, and protection provided by these devices is far from 'complete'. Causes of incomplete embolic protection include device crossing profile (larger profiles may lead to embolization), incomplete filter apposition or conduit occlusion (especially in bending segments of the vessel), lack of protection of secondary branches, incomplete aspiration, filter pore size (either too large or small), device-mediated vessel wall trauma, side branches ('backwash' during occlusion versus siphoning of debris during filter), and delayed platelet–white cell embolization from the target site. In addition, balloon occlusion-type devices may cause distal ischemia that may not be tolerated by some patients, and an aspiration catheter may not retrieve all the particles trapped in the artery. Finally, filter devices have a finite lower limit in the size of particles that can be captured and smaller particles can still get through the filter.

The incidence and the type of complications in the two large SAFER and FIRE trials are given in tables 10.2 and 10.3. Another mistake to avoid when using two wires is to stent and trap the protection device: its removal would be very problematic.

CONCLUSION

Controversies about the clinical significance of the procedural infarctions that occur in approximately 10% of percutaneous interventions in the native coronary arteries, and particularly the small subclinical enzyme rises that occur during otherwise successful procedures. On the other hand, many of the embolic infarctions that occur during vein graft or carotid interventions can be prevented with these protection devices. Neither the approved device nor the devices under investigation are, at present, perfect. Doubtless all will undergo improvements in the future, and offer hope for further increasing the safety of high-risk percutaneous interventions. One must remain aware that they also increase the complexity of the procedures and must avoid bringing a serious complication by inappropriate use.

REFERENCES

1. Hong MK, Mahran R, Dangas G et al. Creatine kinase-MB enzyme elevation following successful saphenous vein graft intervention is associated with late mortality. Circulation 1999;100:2400–5.
2. Grube E, Schofer JJ, Webb J et al. Evaluation of a balloon occlusion and aspiration system for protection from distal embolization during stenting in saphenous vein grafts. Am J Cardiol 2002;89(8):941–5.
3. Fitzgibbon GM, Kafka HP, Leach AJ et al. Coronary bypass graft fate and patient outcome: angiographic follow-up of 5,065 grafts related to survival and reoperation in 1,388 patients during 25 years. J Am Coll Cardiol 1996;28(3):616–26.
4. Baim DS, Wahr D, George B et al. Randomized trial of a distal embolic protection device during percutaneous intervention of saphenous vein aorto-coronary bypass graft. Circulation 2002;105:1285.
5. Stone GW, Rogers C, Ramee S et al. Distal filter protection during saphenous vein graft stenting: technical and clinical correlates of efficacy. J Am Coll Cardiol 2002;40(10):1882–8.
6. Stone GW, Rogers C, Hermiller J et al. Randomized comparison of distal protection with a filter-based distal protection with a filter-based catheter and a balloon occlusion and aspiration system during percutaneous intervention of diseased saphenous vein aorto-coronary bypass grafts. Circulation 2003;108:548–53.
7. Rogers R, Huynh R, Seifert P et al. Embolic protection with filtering or occlusion balloons during saphenous vein graft stenting retrieves identical volumes and sizes of particulate debris. Circulation 2004;109:1735–40.
8. Mauri L, Rogers C, Bairn DS. Devices for distal protection during percutaneous coronary revascularization. Circulation 2006;113:2651–56.
9. Limbruno U, De Carlo M, Pistolesi S et al. Distal embolization during primary angioplasty: histopathologic features and predictability. Am Heart J 2005;150(1):102–8.
10. Gick M, Jander N, Bestehorn HP et al. Randomized evaluation of the effects of filter-based distal protection on myocardial perfusion and infarct size after primary percutaneous catheter intervention in myocardial infarction with and without ST-segment elevation. Circulation 2005:112:1462–9.
11. Stone GW, Webb J, Cox DA. Distal microcirculatory protection during percutaneous coronary intervention in acute ST-segment elevation myocardial infarction: a randomized controlled trial. JAMA 2005;293(9):1116–18.
12. Limbruno U, De Caterina R. EMERALD, AIMI, and PROMISE: is there still a potential for embolic protection in primary PC1? Evr Heart J 2006;27:1139–45.

11

Management and prevention of complications during specific interventions: intravascular ultrasound, intracoronary Doppler

Manel Sabaté, Eulogio García and Carlos Macaya

General complications related to invasive procedures • Specific complications related to the use of intravascular ultrasound • Specific complications related to the use of Doppler • Conclusion

GENERAL COMPLICATIONS RELATED TO INVASIVE PROCEDURES

In interventional cardiology, the saying 'practice makes perfect' applies to any individual operator performing invasive cardiac procedures that include both diagnostic and interventional approaches. In this regard, there is an inverse correlation between the caseload of an operator and the incidence of major complications.[1] Both intravascular ultrasound (IVUS) and intracoronary Doppler have to be considered as invasive interventions, and as such, they may be subject to any general complication related to these procedures[2] (Table 11.1). These complications may range from minor problems with no long-term sequelae (i.e. transient bradycardia or ST changes) to major problems that may require immediate percutaneous or surgical attention or cause irreversible damage (i.e. stroke, myocardial infarction, renal failure or even death). We can classify the general

---

Table 11.1 Complications related to percutaneous coronary interventions

Extracardiac complications
- *Located at vascular access*: hemorrhage, hematoma, arteriovenous fistulas, thrombotic occlusion, dissection, spasm
- *Systemic complications*: contrast nephropathy, hypersensibility reaction, neurologic complication, other rare complications: lactic acidosis, cholesterol microemboli, infection

Cardiac complications
- *Thrombotic complications*: thrombotic vessel occlusion, stent thrombosis, no-reflow phenomenon, myocardial infarction (Q-wave, non Q-wave)
- *Mechanical complications*: coronary dissection, side branch occlusion, coronary perforation, aortic dissection, complications related to specific techniques: Rotablator, atherectomy

complications during invasive procedures into two categories: extracardiac and cardiac (Table 11.1). Although the prevention and management of the overall complications go beyond the scope of this chapter, one should keep in mind the risk stratification during percutaneous coronary interventions (PCI) proposed by the Mayo Clinic in order to select those patients in whom an invasive morphologic (i.e. IVUS) or physiologic assessment (i.e. Doppler) has to be performed (Table 11.2).[3]

SPECIFIC COMPLICATIONS RELATED TO THE USE OF INTRAVASCULAR ULTRASOUND

IVUS is being used in clinical practice to study the natural history of coronary artery disease and to assess the effects of intracoronary, catheter-based interventions. There are two different types of IVUS transducers: the mechanically rotating transducer and the electronically switched multielement array system.[4] Mechanical systems include a single rotating transducer driven by a flexible drive cable at 1800 rpm (30 revolutions per second) to sweep a beam almost perpendicular to the catheter. At approximately 1° increments, the transducer sends and receives ultrasound signals. The time delay and amplitude of these pulses provide 256 individual radial scans for each image. Mechanical transducer catheters require flushing with saline to provide a

Table 11.2   Risk stratification for major complications following PCI (accepted from reference 2)

Risk score	Integer coefficient	
Age:		
90–99	6	
80–89	5	
70–79	4	
60–69	3	
50–59	2	
40–49	1	
Cardiogenic shock	5	
Left main coronary artery disease	5	
Serum creatinine >265 µmol/L	3	
Urgent or emergent procedure	2	
NYHA ≥3	2	
Intracoronary thrombus	2	
Multivessel disease	2	
Range	**0–25**	

Categories	Score	Percentages at risk for major complication (%)
Very low	0–5	≤2
Low risk	6–8	>2 to 5
Moderate risk	9–11	>5 to 10
High risk	12–15	>10 to 25
Very high risk	≥15	>25

NYHA: New York Heart Association classification.

fluid pathway for the ultrasound beam, because even small air bubbles can degrade image quality. In most mechanical systems, the transducer spins within a protective sheath while the imaging transducer is moved proximally and distally. This facilitates smooth and uniform mechanical pullback. Electronic systems use an annular array of small crystals rather than a single rotating transducer. The array can be programmed so that one set of elements transmits while a second set receives simultaneously. The co-ordinated beam generated by groups of elements is known as a synthetic aperture array. The image can be manipulated to focus optimally at a broad range of depths. The currently available electronic system provides simultaneous colorization of blood flow.

Despite the growing popularity of this imaging technique, its safety has been addressed in retrospective studies from multicenter surveys.[5,6] Among 2208 IVUS examinations from 28 domestic and international centers,[5] a total of 86 complications (3.9%) occurred. Of these, coronary spasm was most often related to the use of IVUS as it occurred in 63 patients (2.9%). Other complications with certain relation to IVUS examination (0.4%) included acute procedural events in six patients (three acute occlusion, one embolism, one dissection, and one thrombus) and major events in three patients (two occlusion and one dissection, all resulting in myocardial infarction). Additionally, 14 patients (0.6%) experienced complications with uncertain relation to IVUS. The complication rate was higher in patients with unstable angina or acute myocardial infarction (2.1%) as compared with patients with stable angina pectoris and asymptomatic patients (0.8% and 0.4%, respectively; χ^2 =10.9; $P<0.01$). These complications were also more frequent in patients undergoing interventions (1.9%) as compared with transplant and nontransplant patients undergoing diagnostic IVUS imaging (0% and 0.6%, respectively; χ^2=13.5; $P<0.001$).[4] Data from a multicenter European registry[6] reported eight complications (1.1%) from 718 examinations. All of them occurred in patients in whom percutaneous transluminal angioplasty was planned. These complications included spasm in four patients, guidewire entrapment in two, and possible dissection in the remaining two patients. Finally, data from a single center experience of 209 procedures revealed three minor complications (1.4%) related to the use of IVUS and five additional complications (2.4%) uncertainly related to IVUS.[7] These data are summarized in Table 11.3. Case examples of coronary spasm and distal vessel occlusion following IVUS examinations are depicted in Figures 11.1–11.3.

Other complications have been described anecdotally as case reports in the literature. Among them, IVUS catheter tip entrapment within a stent[8] or kinking, entanglement, and entrapment of sensor-tipped guidewires during intravascular examinations[9] are of potential interest as they may be related to serious major adverse events (i.e. myocardial infarction, urgent coronary surgery).

Additionally, there are some technical issues that may be inherent to the device characteristics (i.e. short monorail) or to inappropriate IVUS preparation (i.e. lack of flushing). The former may induce difficulties in accessing the lesion as the probe may be prolapsed in tortuous vessels. In this regard and due to its anatomic characteristics, the left circumflex artery is more prone to this complication (Figure 11.4). The latter may provoke air embolism during the pullback that has a characteristic pattern on the IVUS screen (Figure 11.5) followed by transient ischemia on ECG, chest pain or even bradycardia and hypotension. An IVUS pattern of slow flow (Figure 11.6) is commonly seen during complications that induce ischemia such as embolism, spasm, imaging of severe stenosis, and bradyarrhythmia, among others.

Table 11.3   Summary of reported complications during intracoronary ultrasound examinations

	Certain/uncertain complications		
	Hausmann et al (ref 5) **(n=2207)**	**Batkoff et al (ref 6)** **(n=718)***	**López-Palop et al (ref 7)** **(n=209)**
Spasm	63 (2.9%)/0	4 (0.6%)/0	1 (0.5%)/0
Acute procedural complication			
Occlusion	3/5	0/0	0/4
Dissection	1/3	2/0	1/1
Thrombus	1/0	0/0	0/0
Embolism	1/0	0/0	0/0
Arrhythmia	0/1	0/0	1/0
Total	6 (0.3%)/9 (0.4%)	2 (0.3%)/0	2 (1%)/5 (2.4%)
Major complications			
MI	3/2	0/0	0/0
CABG	0/3	0/0	0/0
Death	0/0	0/0	0/0
Total	3 (0.1)/5 (0.2%)	0/0	0/0

MI, myocardial infarction; CABG, coronary artery bypass graft.

* Batkoff et al reported two additional acute complications (wire entrapment) that were successfully resolved without sequelae.

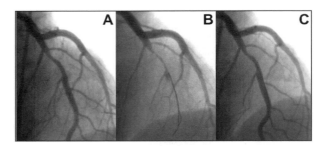

Figure 11.1   IVUS interrogation of mid segment of the left anterior descending artery (A) that induced a coronary spasm (B) resolved by intracoronary nitroglycerin administration (C).

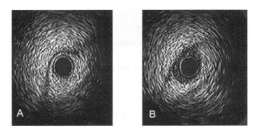

Figure 11.2   IVUS imaging during coronary spasm (A) resolved by intracoronary administration of nitroglycerin (B).

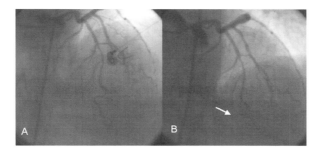

Figure 11.3   Distal occlusion of the left anterior descending coronary artery during IVUS interrogation (arrowhead).

Figure 11.4   Prolapse of the IVUS probe during interrogation of left circumflex coronary artery (arrow).

Finally, some concerns existed about potential endothelial disruption/injury leading to an acceleration of the atherosclerosis progression. This issue has been addressed in longitudinal studies involving either nontransplanted, nonintervened individuals or heart transplant patients.[10-12] At two-year follow-up, patients included

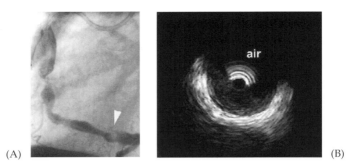

Figure 11.5 Air embolism evidenced in the right coronary artery (A). IVUS image of intracoronary air (B).

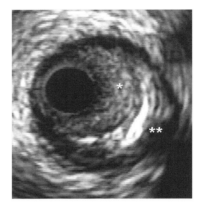

Figure 11.6 Slow flow detected during IVUS pullback induced by a transient severe bradyarrhythmia. Note the difference between the plaque burden (**) and the slow flow patterns (*).

in the Avasimibe and Progression of coronary Lesions assessed by intravascular UltraSound (A-PLUS) trial presented a similar incidence of lesion progression in nonintervened coronary arteries between those assessed by IVUS or not (11.6% vs 9.6%, P=0.27).[10] Similarly, the coronary change score, defined as the per-patient mean of minimal luminal diameter changes for all lesions measured, was comparable between IVUS-related and non-IVUS arteries (–0.06±0.23 mm vs –0.05±0.21 mm, P=0.35). In 86 heart transplant patients,[11] noninstrumented arteries evidenced a similar decrease in lumen dimensions during follow-up compared to instrumented arteries. In the same way, in 226 heart transplant patients, the development of new stenoses was observed in 16.2% of nonimaged arteries and 19.5% of imaged arteries (P=0.38).[12] Besides, the magnitude of the diameter decrease was not significantly different between the two groups.

Manipulation of IVUS: tips and tricks

Do not perform any IVUS examination if you do not have either experience in interventional cardiology or the material (i.e. coronary stent) to solve any complication related to the procedure. Good selection of guiding catheter and guidewire may help avoid problems of accessing the target coronary segment. As with any invasive procedure, IVUS imaging requires an adequate anticoagulation regimen before guidewire insertion. Guidewires that supply more stiffness near the distal tips are recommended. Always administer 0.1–0.3 mg intracoronary nitroglycerin before every IVUS interrogation in order to avoid coronary spasm. Specifically, mechanical systems need good flushing to prevent air being introduced into the catheter lumen. Try to avoid interrogation of very small, very tortuous or heavily calcified vessels. Be careful when examining recently implanted stents or stents that may not be completely apposed over the vessel wall due to the risk of IVUS probe entrapment. Never advance the distal tip of the imaging catheter near the very floppy end of the guidewire. This part of the wire will not adequately support the catheter. A catheter advanced to this position may not follow the guidewire when it is retracted and cause the guidewire to buckle into a loop which the catheter may drag along the inside of the vessel and catch on the guide catheter tip. If this occurs, it will be necessary to remove the catheter assembly, guidewire, and guide catheter together. In order to avoid coronary thrombosis, keep the IVUS catheter within the artery the minimum amount of time necessary to successfully carry out the vessel interrogation.

SPECIFIC COMPLICATIONS RELATED TO THE USE OF DOPPLER

With the introduction of Doppler-tipped guidewires, intracoronary Doppler flow measurement has been increasingly accepted as an additional diagnostic approach in the catheterization laboratory. Both pressure and flow measurements may now be obtained by the use of the same guidewire (ComboWire™ XT, Volcano Therapeutics Inc., Rancho Cordova, CA, USA). The main features of this wire are depicted in Figure 11.7. As with all catheterization procedures, complications may be encountered with the use of a Doppler wire (see Tables 11.1 and 11.2).

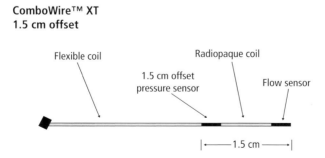

Figure 11.7   Main components of the ComboWire™ XT that combines the flow sensor (tip) and a pressure sensor (1.5 cm more proximal) (courtesy of Volcano Therapeutics Inc., Rancho Cordova, CA, USA).

Additionally, the infusion of intracoronary or intravenous adenosine presents few contraindications but may cause adverse events. Adenosine is an endogenous nucleoside occurring in all cells of the body. It is chemically 6-amino-9-b-D-ribofuranosyl-9-H-purine and has a molecular formula $C_{10}H_{13}N_5O_4$ with a molecular weight of 267.24. Its structural formula is depicted in Figure 11.8. Table 11.4 lists the reactions related to the use of intravenous adenosine as an antiarrhythmic agent in controlled US clinical trials. In postmarket clinical experience with adenosine, cases of prolonged asystole, ventricular tachycardia and ventricular fibrillation, transient increase in blood pressure, bradycardia, hypotension, atrial fibrillation, and bronchospasm have been reported. The half-life of adenosine is less than ten seconds so adverse effects are generally rapidly self-limiting. Treatment of any prolonged adverse effects should be individualized and be directed toward the specific effect. Methylxanthines, such as caffeine and theophylline, are competitive antagonists of adenosine. Intravenous adenosine is contraindicated in second- or third-degree AV block (except in patients with a functioning artificial pacemaker), sinus node disease, such as sick sinus syndrome or symptomatic bradycardia (except in patients with a functioning artificial pacemaker), history of severe bronchospasm, and, known hypersensitivity to adenosine.

Table 11.4   Summary of reactions reported with the use of intravenous adenosine

- *Cardiovascular*: facial flushing (18%), headache (2%), sweating, palpitations, chest pain, hypotension (less than 1%)
- *Respiratory*: shortness of breath/dyspnea (12%), chest pressure (7%), hyperventilation, head pressure (less than 1%)
- *Central nervous system*: light-headedness (2%), dizziness, tingling in arms, numbness (1%), apprehension, blurred vision, burning sensation, heaviness in arms, neck and back pain (less than 1%)
- *Gastrointestinal*: nausea (3%), metallic taste, tightness in throat, pressure in groin (less than 1%)

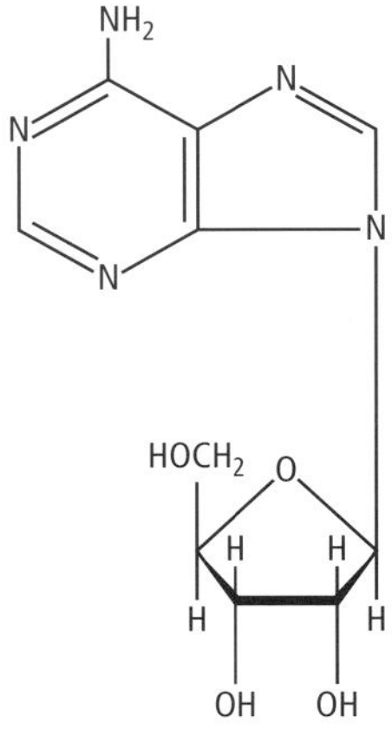

Figure 11.8   Structural formula of adenosine.

The safety of intracoronary Doppler flow measurement has been investigated in a single-center study of 906 patients.[13] For coronary flow reserve measurement, intracoronary injection of adenosine or papaverine was used. Of the patients studied, 77 were cardiac transplant recipients and 829 were patients who had not received a transplant, of whom 617 had undergone diagnostic coronary procedures and 212 had coronary interventions. In 27 (3%) of 906 patients, adverse cardiac events were observed. Fifteen (1.7%) of 906 patients had severe transient bradycardia (asystole or second- to third-degree atrioventricular block) after intracoronary administration of adenosine, 14 of which occurred in the right coronary artery and one in the left anterior descending artery. Nine (1%) of 906 patients had coronary spasm during the passage of the Doppler wire (five in the right coronary artery, four in the left anterior descending artery). Two (0.2%) of 906 patients had ventricular fibrillation during the procedure. Hypotension with bradycardia and ventricular extrasystole each occurred in one (0.1%) of 906 patients. The incidence of complications was significantly higher in transplant recipients than in patients who underwent either diagnostic or interventional procedures (13% vs 2.4% vs 0.9%, $P<0.001$). The Doppler measurements in the right coronary artery were associated with a higher incidence of complications, especially bradycardia, compared with the left anterior descending and the left circumflex arteries (right coronary 5.9% vs left anterior descending 1.1% vs left circumflex 0.2%, $P<0.001$). All complications were cured medically.

Manipulation of Doppler wire: tips and tricks

As for any invasive procedure, do not perform a Doppler examination if you do not have either experience in interventional cardiology or the material (i.e. coronary stent) to solve any complication related to the procedure. Administer 0.1–0.3 mg intracoronary nitroglycerin before the insertion of the Doppler guidewire. The proximal end of the guidewire (proximal 4.7 cm) surface needs to remain clean and dry before being attached to the connector cable assembly. Be careful when shaping the guidewire tip as the flow sensor is located at that spot and may be damaged (Figure 11.7). Manipulation of the wire has to be performed with care in an attempt to obtain good Doppler signal both at baseline and following adenosine infusion. Perform ECG and pressure recordings during adenosine infusion. If a secondary event occurs (i.e. hypotension, extreme bradycardia), stop adenosine infusion. In a few seconds, heart rate and pressure will be normalized. If bradycardia and hypotension persist, initiate supportive measures such as atropine or liquid infusion, among others. In this instance, other causes of complications have to be ruled out (i.e. coronary dissection, abrupt vessel closure, etc.). In the event of severe bronchospasm, theophyline as a competitive antagonist of adenosine must be given, in addition to other standard supportive measures.

CONCLUSION

Both IVUS and Doppler assessments have to be considered as invasive procedures and, as such, must be performed by experienced interventional cardiologists. Overall, the complication rates related to these procedures are rather low. The acute adverse events that occur are commonly transient, well tolerated and present *ad integrum* recovery in most cases. However, the interventional cardiologist must be aware of all potential complications and be able to prevent, recognize, and treat those serious and rare events that may occur during physiologic or anatomic coronary examinations.

REFERENCES

1. Ellis SG, Weintraub W, Holmes D, Shaw R, Block PC, King SB 3rd. Relation of operator volume and experience to procedural outcome of percutaneous coronary revascularization at hospitals with high interventional volumes. Circulation 1997;95:2479–84.
2. Cequier A, Jara F, Iráculis E, Gómez-Hospital JA, Ariza A, Esplugas E. Prevención y tratamiento de las complicaciones durante el intervencionismo coronario percutáneo. In: Hernandez JM, ed. Manual de Cardiología Intervencionista. Publicación Oficial de la Sección de Hemodinámica y Cardiología Intervencionista. Sociedad Española de Cardiología, Madrid 2005;37–54.
3. Singh M, Rihal CS, Lennon RJ, Garratt KN, Holmes DR Jr. Comparison of Mayo Clinic risk score and American College of Cardiology/American Heart Association lesion classification in the prediction of adverse cardiovascular outcome following percutaneous coronary interventions. J Am Coll Cardiol 2004;44:357–61.
4. Mintz GS, Nissen SE, Anderson WD et al. American College of Cardiology Clinical Expert Consensus Document on Standards for Acquisition, Measurement and Reporting of Intravascular Ultrasound Studies (IVUS). A report of the American College of Cardiology Task Force on Clinical Expert Consensus Documents. J Am Coll Cardiol 2001;37(5):1478–92.
5. Hausmann D, Erbel R, Alibelli-Chemarin MJ et al. The safety of intracoronary ultrasound: a multicenter survey of 2207 examinations. Circulation 1995;91:623–30.
6. Batkoff BW, Linker DT. Safety of intracoronary ultrasound: data from a multicenter European registry. Cathet Cardiovasc Diagn 1996;38:238–41.
7. Lopez-Palop R, Botas J, Elizaga J et al. Feasibility and safety of intracoronary ultrasound: experience of a single center. Rev Esp Cardiol 1999;52:415–22.
8. Sasseen BM, Burke JA, Shah R et al. Intravascular ultrasound catheter entrapment after coronary artery stenting. Cathet Cardiovasc Intervent 2002;57:229–33.
9. Alfonso F, Flores A, Escaned J et al. Pressure wire kinking, entanglement, and entrapment during intravascular ultrasound studies: a potentially dangerous complication. Cathet Cardiovasc Intervent 2000;50:221–5.
10. Guedes A, Keller PF, L'Allier PL, Lesperance J, Gregoire J, Tardif JC. Long-term safety of intravascular ultrasound in nontransplant, nonintervened, atherosclerotic coronary arteries. J Am Coll Cardiol 2005;45:559–64.
11. Son R, Tobis JM, Yeatman LA, Johnson JA, Wener LS, Kobashigawa JA. Does use of intravascular ultrasound accelerate arteriopathy in heart transplant recipients? Am Heart J 1999;138:358–63.
12. Ramasubu K, Schoenhagen P, Balghith MA et al. Repeated intravascular ultrasound imaging in cardiac transplant recipients does not accelerate transplant coronary artery disease. J Am Coll Cardiol 2003;41:1739–43.
13. Qian J, Ge J, Baumgart D et al. Safety of intracoronary Doppler flow measurement. Am Heart J 2000;140:502–10.

12

Percutaneous left ventricular assist devices in the high-risk patient

Stephan Windecker and Bernhard Meier

Principle of action • Implantation technique • Indications for percutaneous left ventricular assist devices • Hemodynamic effects of left ventricular assist devices • Clinical results • Conclusion

The incidence of cardiogenic shock has not declined during the past 20 years despite significant progress in the management of acute myocardial infarction.[1,2] Thus, up to 7% of acute ST segment elevation and 2.5% of non-ST segment elevation myocardial infarctions are still complicated by cardiogenic shock.[3,4] Expeditious definition of coronary artery anatomy by coronary angiography followed by appropriate percutaneous or surgical revascularization of patients with cardiogenic shock has been shown to improve survival in randomized clinical trials.[5,6] Although mortality rates of patients with cardiogenic shock declined during the 1990s, this syndrome remains fatal despite reperfusion therapy in approximately one half of patients (50–70%) within the first month.[4,7] Irreversible pump failure with compromise of the systemic circulation and vital organ perfusion is one explanation (Figure 12.1). In addition, there is a large body of evidence pointing to a systemic inflammatory reaction with activation of the complement system and expression of cytokines and nitric oxide (NO) synthase, which result in inappropriate vasodilatation and myocardial depression, thus aggravating the already compromised circulation.[8]

The immediate therapeutic benefit of left ventricular assist devices (LVADs) in patients with cardiogenic shock is the restoration of normal hemodynamics and vital organ perfusion even in cases of complete myocardial pump failure. In addition, protagonists of the 'ventricular unloading' hypothesis claim that LVADs positively affect long-term outcome by reducing ventricular strain and improving remodeling of the acute failing ventricle. Indeed, experimental studies showed a reduced infarct size and improved microcirculatory perfusion in dogs supported by a ventricular assist device as opposed to control animals supported by an intra-aortic balloon pump.[9] Since the extent of microcirculatory perfusion correlates with left ventricular remodeling, this could be one possible explanation for the reduced infarct size.[10] Further evidence of improved remodeling with the use of LVADs stems from isolated human specimens. Thus, failing ventricles harvested at the time of heart transplantation demonstrated reduced left ventricular size as well as myocyte diameter when a LVAD was in place prior to transplantation compared to unassisted hearts.[11] Of note, the beneficial effect was dependent on the duration of ventricular assist device support and was more pronounced if support was provided for more than 30 days.

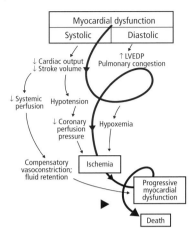

Figure 12.1 Cardiogenic shock is a syndrome characterized by decreased cardiac output, increased cardiac filling pressures, and ineffective tissue perfusion. Left ventricular failure resulting from ischemia or other causes perpetuates the downward spiral, leading to progressive myocardial failure and death. Reproduced with permission.[16]

PRINCIPLE OF ACTION

Left ventricular assist devices maintain partial or total circulatory support in cases of severe left ventricular failure. While the intra-aortic balloon pump (IABP) solely decreases preload and afterload, LVADs actively augment cardiac output and may even completely replace left ventricular function. As opposed to the traditional extracorporeal circulation pumps, LVADs aspirate freshly oxygenated blood from the left atrium or ventricle, thus avoiding the need for an oxygenator.

Currently, two percutaneous left ventricular assist devices are available. The TandemHeart™ (Cardiac Assist Inc, USA)[12] utilizes an outflow cannula placed via transseptal puncture in the left atrium to aspirate oxygenated blood from there, which is then injected by means of a centrifugal pump into the femoral artery, establishing a left atrial-to-femoral arterial bypass (Figure 12.2). The Impella Recover® system (Impella Cardiosystems, AG, Aachen, Germany) has a caged blood flow inlet, which is placed retrogradely into the left ventricle to aspirate oxygenated blood from there, which is then injected by means of a microaxial pump into the ascending aorta, establishing a left ventricular-to-aortic bypass (Figure 12.3).

IMPLANTATION TECHNIQUE

Prior to implantation of either percutaneous LVAD system, angiography of the abdominal aorta, iliac, and femoral vessels is advised to delineate significant obstruction of these vessels possibly prohibiting insertion of the large-caliber cannulas and to assess for excessive tortuosity. In case of the TandemHeart, venous and arterial femoral access are necessary, whereas the Impella Recover system requires only femoral arterial access.

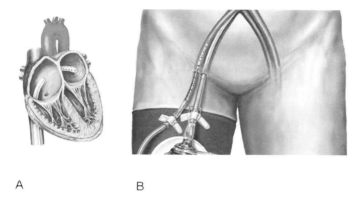

A   B

Figure 12.2 A 21 F inflow cannula is placed into the left atrium via transseptal puncture (A). Oxygenated blood is aspirated from the left atrium through a centrifugal pump and injected via outflow cannulas into the femoral arteries, establishing a left atrial-to-femoral bypass (B). The in- and outflow cannulas are carefully secured by suture at the vascular access site to avoid dislocation. Reproduced with permission.[17]

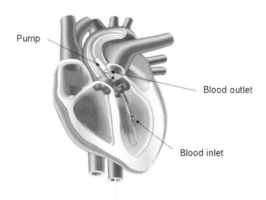

Pump

Blood outlet

Blood inlet

Figure 12.3 Retrograde placement of the Impella Recover® LP 2.5 device through the aortic valve into the left ventricle. Reproduced with permission from Impella Cardiosystems AG, Aachen, Germany.

Implantation of the TandemHeart

Using femoral venous access, transseptal puncture is performed using standard techniques. Following access to the left atrium, systemic anticoagulation is achieved with an intravenous bolus of 5000 IE heparin. Then the interatrial septum is dilated with the supplied dilator sheath to accommodate the 21 French (F) inflow cannula (Figure 12.4). It is important to ensure that the inflow cannula with all of its aspiration holes is deployed within the left as opposed to the right atrium to avoid an inadvertent right-to-left shunt. On the other hand, care should be taken not to advance the cannula too far towards the left atrial roof or into the left atrial

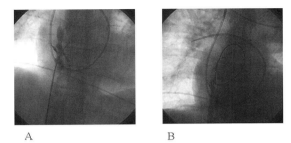

A   B

Figure 12.4 A. Transseptal puncture with a Brockenbrough catheter using dye injections through the transseptal needle to localize the fossa ovalis. B. Following transseptal puncture, the Brockenbrough catheter is exchanged over a stiff guidewire with a distal soft wire look (Toray Europe, Inc.) as commonly used for mitral valvuloplasty. The transseptal puncture site is then dilated with a two-stage dilator to finally accommodate the 21 F inflow cannula.

appendage to avoid laceration of the thin-walled atrial structures and suction of the cannula against the atrial walls.

Using the Seldinger technique, a 15–17 F outflow cannula is placed retrogradely into the femoral artery. In small-sized femoral arteries or significant peripheral vascular disease prohibiting placement of these large cannulas, insertion of two smaller 12 F cannulas into the left and right femoral artery is an alternative option. They are then fused via a Y-connector to accommodate sufficient blood flow. The inflow and outflow cannulas are subsequently connected to the centerpiece of the TandemHeart, the centrifugal pump, with careful evacuation of any air within the tubing (Figure 12.5). The centrifugal pump consists of two chambers: the top chamber accommodates the turbine through which in- and outflow of blood are ensured; the bottom chamber houses the rotor and tiny channels which allow infusion of heparinized saline into the top chamber. The centrifuge is powered by a microprocessor-controlled electromechanical unit which enables rotation at 3500–7000 rpm with a blood flow of up to four liters per minute.

Both inflow and outflow cannulas have to be carefully secured by suture at the entrance site to avoid dislocation. Inadvertent dislocation of the inflow cannula from the left into the right atrium is detrimental, since it cannot easily be corrected and

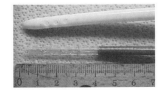
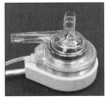

Figure 12.5 Components of the TandemHeart™ consisting of a 21 F inflow cannula, a 15–17 F outflow cannula, and the continuous flow centrifugal pump. Following placement of the inflow cannula into the left atrium and of the outflow cannula into the femoral artery, both cannulas are connected to the centrifugal pump with careful evacuation of any air within the tubing.

aspiration of oxygenated blood immediately subsides. Displacement of the outflow cannula from the femoral artery is equally detrimental since left atrial-to-femoral artery bypass is immediately interrupted, with severe bleeding from the access site. Following successful weaning from circulatory support, the cannulas can be removed and hemostasis achieved by either manual compression or surgical access site closure. Manual compression is to be preferred in all cases free from access site complications during implantation.

Implantation of the Impella Recover system

Implantation of the Impella Recover system requires femoral arterial but no venous access. Currently there are two LVAD types available: the Impella Recover LP 2.5 and LP 5.0 models. The Impella Recover LP 2.5 is a 12 F catheter (Figure 12.6) suitable for percutaneous implantation, whereas the larger Impella Recover LP 5.0 catheter requires surgical cutdown for device insertion. The following description is limited to the Impella Recover LP 2.5 system, but implantation of the larger LP 5.0 system is similar except for the surgical cutdown.

Following local anesthesia, a 13 F peel-away sheath is placed into the right or left femoral artery and systemic anticoagulation is achieved with administration of an intravenous bolus of heparin. First, a 5 F pigtail or right coronary artery catheter serves to intubate the left ventricle. This catheter is then exchanged over a 0.014″ guidewire for the 12 F Impella Recover LP 2.5 catheter inserted through the 13 F hemostatic sheath. The correct position of the device is verified by fluoroscopy (Figure 12.7) and an electronic placement signal which appears on the console. Device position can be adjusted by advancing or withdrawing the catheter assembly through the intra-arterial sheath. Circulatory support is initiated and can be adjusted to nine different positions (P 1–9, maximal flow approximately 2.5 L/min). Notably, as soon as the LP 2.5 catheter has been introduced into the left ventricle, the minimum pump speed (P1) must be initiated to overcome the catheter-mediated aortic regurgitation (Figure 12.7).

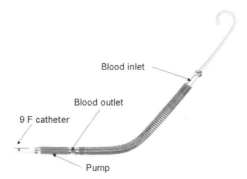

Blood inlet

Blood outlet

9 F catheter

Pump

Figure 12.6 Components of the Impella Recover® LP 2.5 pump. The caged blood flow inlet is placed retrogradely into the left ventricle from where it aspirates oxygenated blood by means of a low-profile, 12 F microaxial pump, which rotates the impeller at high speed. Thus, blood is aspirated from the inlet through the hollow, nitinol tube and ejected past the impeller into the ascending aorta, establishing a left ventricular-to-aortic bypass.

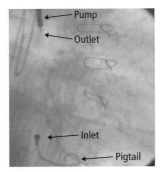 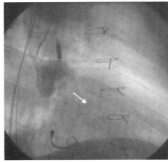

Figure 12.7 Fluoroscopic appearance of the Impella Recover® LP 2.5 pump following placement into the left ventricle (left). Angiographic evidence of mild aortic regurgitation during aortography engendered by the 12 F catheter traversing the aortic valve (right). Reproduced with permission.[18]

Following successful weaning of the patient from circulatory support, the LP 2.5 catheter is withdrawn from the left ventricle into the abdominal aorta, and then both catheter and intra-arterial sheath are removed together, allowing for some back bleeding.

INDICATIONS FOR PERCUTANEOUS LEFT VENTRICULAR ASSIST DEVICES

Three principal categories can be considered for percutaneous LVAD support.

- *Reversible, severe left ventricular failure*: temporary circulatory support until recovery has ensued or revascularization has been performed.
- *Large ischemic area at risk*: temporary circulatory support during high-risk percutaneous or surgical revascularization procedures.
- *Bridging therapy*: temporary circulatory support as bridge to a permanent (surgical) assist device or heart transplantation.

In general, any cause of cardiogenic shock qualifies as a potential indication for percutaneous LVAD support. A high therapeutic benefit is to be expected in potentially reversible causes of severe left ventricular failure such as acute myocarditis, drug overdose, hypothermia, and incessant ventricular tachycardia or fibrillation (electrical storm). Patients evaluated for percutaneous LVAD support typically fulfill the hemodynamic criteria of cardiogenic shock (cardiac index <2 L/min/m², systolic blood pressure <90 mmHg, pulmonary capillary wedge pressure ≥20 mmHg, left atrial pressure ≥20 mmHg, urine output ≤20 mL/Std, systemic vascular resistance >2100 dynes/sec cm⁻⁵). The exception to this rule is patients without cardiogenic shock but a large ischemic area at risk, who undergo high-risk percutaneous or surgical revascularization. In such circumstances, the percutaneous LVAD is implanted prophylactically and provides circulatory support during the intervention to bridge time periods of insufficient myocardial perfusion during the intervention or during complications (revascularization of the left main coronary artery or a last remaining vessel).[13]

Table 12.1   Indications for percutaneous left ventricular assist devices

Cardiogenic shock
- Consequence of an extensive myocardial infarction
- Mechanical complications of myocardial infarction (severe mitral regurgitation due to papillary muscle rupture, rupture of the ventricular septal wall)
- Acute myocarditis
- Primary valvular catastrophe
- Postcardiotomy syndrome
- Chronic heart failure with acute hemodynamic deterioration
- Hemodynamically unstable, refractory ventricular arrhythmias (incessant VT, electrical storm)
- Myocardial depression due to drug overdose
- Myocardial depression due to hypothermia

High-risk revascularization procedures
- Percutaneous coronary interventions (PCI) of left main coronary artery or equivalent (last remaining vessel supplying viable myocardium)
- Percutaneous closure of ventricular septal defect due to myocardial infarction
- Coronary artery bypass surgery (CABG) in high-risk patients

Bridge therapy
- Bridge to permanent (surgically implanted) assist devices
- Heart transplantation

Percutaneous LVAD implantation as a bridge to a definitive therapy such as a permanent (surgical) assist device or heart transplantation is another evolving indication. The advantage of this so-called bridging therapy is the possibility to gain time in the acute phase of ventricular failure to perform additional diagnostic procedures and to determine the suitability of patients for the financially and technically more demanding therapy options. Table 12.1 provides a summary of the indications for percutaneous LVAD support.

Contraindications for percutaneous LVAD therapy are severe right heart failure, severe peripheral vascular disease prohibiting device implantation, and severe bleeding diathesis.

HEMODYNAMIC EFFECTS OF LEFT VENTRICULAR ASSIST DEVICES

The hemodynamic effects of percutaneous LVAD support using the TandemHeart have been investigated by Thiele and colleagues[12] in 18 patients with cardiogenic shock due to myocardial infarction. Cardiac output (without support: 3.5±0.8 L/min vs with support: 4.8±1.1 L/min, $P<0.001$) and mean arterial blood pressure (without support: 63.1±7.8 mmHg vs with support: 80.2±8.9 mmHg, $P<0.001$) significantly increased. This circulatory support of vital organ perfusion was accompanied by a decrease in preload with a significant decrease of pulmonary capillary wedge pressure (without support: 20.8±3.6 mmHg vs with support: 14.2±3.5 mmHg, $P<0.001$), mean pulmonary arterial pressure (without support: 31.2±8.1 mmHg vs with support: 23.2±6.3 mmHg, $P<0.001$), and central venous pressure (without support: 12.7±3.7 mmHg vs with support: 9.3±3.0 mmHg, $P<0.001$). The impressive effects on hemodynamic parameters in individual patients are summarized in Figure 12.8.

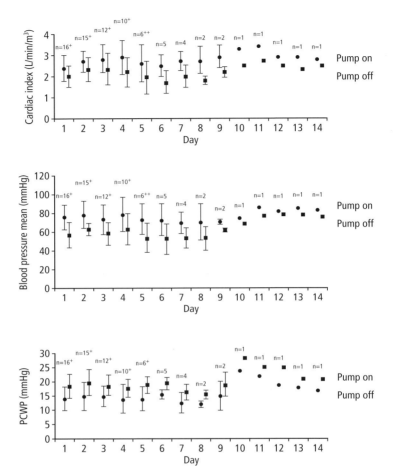

Figure 12.8   Hemodynamic parameters (cardiac output, blood pressure, pulmonary capillary wedge pressure) with and without TandemHeart™ assisted circulation. The increase in cardiac output and blood pressure in individual patients is accompanied by a salutary decline in pulmonary capillary wedge pressure. Reproduced with permission.[12]

Differences between the TandemHeart and the Impella Recover systems

In the case of the TandemHeart, oxygenated blood is bypassed from the left atrium into the systemic circulation. In contrast to surgically implanted LVADs and the Impella Recover system, which aspirate oxygenated blood directly from the left ventricle with ejection into the ascending aorta (i.e. in flow direction), systemic blood flow with the TandemHeart is directed retrogradely through the femoral artery towards the heart. Accordingly, the left ventricle must eject against the flow provided by the assist device, which may lead to an undesirable increase in afterload. Therefore, it remains to be shown whether the TandemHeart provides unloading of the left ventricle with reduced myocardial strain and improved myocardial energetics. On the other hand, the Impella Recover system engenders some aortic regurgitation by the catheter traversing the aortic valve (see Figure 12.7).

The principal advantage of the Impella Recover LP 2.5 device over the TandemHeart[12] is its ease of implantation and the smaller catheter size (13 F vs 17 F). Moreover, there is no need for a transseptal puncture and the retrograde insertion of the device over a guidewire through the aortic valve into the LV is familiar to all cardiologists. There is no extracorporeal blood and the central portion of the microaxial pump avoids the friction problem of the drive shaft of the Hemopump, the predecessor of the Impella device.[14] The motor of the Hemopump was outside the body and overheating of the device shaft was one of its major drawbacks. The circulatory support provided by the Impella Recover LP 2.5 is limited to 2.5 L/min, which does not suffice in patients without at least some LV function. The TandemHeart may deliver up to 3.5 L/min and completely replace LV function.

CLINICAL RESULTS

We used the TandemHeart in 24 patients between November 2000 and November 2004. The indication for LVAD support was ischemic cardiomyopathy in 19 patients (79%), endstage dilated cardiomyopathy in three patients (13%), acute myocarditis in one patient and chemotherapy-induced cardiomyopathy in another patient. Implantation of the TandemHeart was successful in all but one patient, where the left atrial cannula dislodged from the left into the right atrium during ongoing mechanical resuscitation. The mean implantation time was 3±4 days (1–18 days) during which 15 (63%) patients underwent percutaneous coronary intervention, three (13%) patients had coronary artery bypass surgery, three (13%) patients were bridged to heart transplantation, and three (13%) patients were managed medically. Severe complications included lower limb ischemia or amputation (14% of patients), sepsis (5%), cerebrovascular accident (5%), and intracranial hemorrhage (10%). In-hospital mortality was 44% in the overall population. Mortality was exceedingly high in patients implanted with a LVAD during ongoing mechanical resuscitation (78%), whereas patients not requiring mechanical resuscitation during LVAD implantation had a lower 30-day mortality (13%) (Figure 12.9).

Currently more than 160 patients undergoing percutaneous LVAD implantation have been followed in a worldwide registry. The mean duration of LVAD support was 3.3±3.6 days. Severe complications comprised lower limb ischemia (4%), dislocation of the inflow cannula (3%), arterial vessel dissection (3%), cardiac tamponade (1%), and infection (1%). The mortality rate was 24% at the time of cessation of LVAD support, and in-hospital mortality was 40%.

The TandemHeart has been compared with IABP support in patients with cardiogenic support due to acute myocardial infarction undergoing primary percutaneous coronary intervention in a recent single-center report.[15] A total of 41 patients were randomly assigned treatment with the TandemHeart (21 patients), and IABP (20 patients), with a mean support duration of 3.5 days in the LVAD and of 4.0 days in the IABP group. The primary end-point of cardiac power index was more effectively improved by the TandemHeart (0.37 W/m^2) compared with IABP support (0.22 W/m^2, $P=0.004$), and this was accompanied by a more rapid decrease in serum lactate and improved renal function. However, there were no significant differences with respect to 30-day mortality (43% in the TandemHeart group, 45% in the IABP

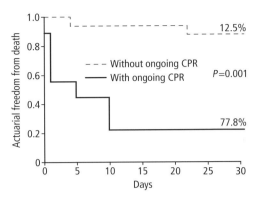

Figure 12.9 Actuarial freedom from death in patients undergoing implantation of the TandemHeart™ stratified according to the need for cardiopulmonary resuscitation (CPR) during device placement. While survival of patients without ongoing CPR is relatively low at 30 days, mortality rate for patients undergoing TandemHeart™ implantation during ongoing CPR is exceedingly high.

group, $P=0.86$) and complications including limb ischemia and severe bleeding were more frequent with LVAD than IABP balloon support.

Currently, a multicenter study in the United States is comparing LVAD support in 100 patients with cardiogenic shock with standard care including IABP support. Endpoints of the study are safety and survival six weeks after device removal. Another randomized trial intended to assess the effect of percutaneous LVAD support with the TandemHeart on left ventricular modeling compared to standard care in patients with large anterior myocardial infarction but was prematurely stopped due to slow recruitment.

CONCLUSION

The introduction of easily manageable percutaneous LVADs constitutes an important advance in the practice of interventional cardiology.[13] It provides a new armamentarium in the management of patients with severe left ventricular dysfunction and cardiogenic shock and may serve as a bridge to recovery or heart transplantation in carefully selected patients. In addition, it may provide a safety net during high-risk surgical or percutaneous coronary interventions in patients undergoing revascularization of lesions subtending a large area at risk. Further clinical trials are clearly needed to more precisely identify the risks and benefits associated with this new procedure before it can be embraced widely.

REFERENCES

1. Goldberg RJ, Samad NA, Yarzebski J, Gurwitz J, Bigelow C, Gore JM. Temporal trends in cardiogenic shock complicating acute myocardial infarction. N Engl J Med 1999;340:1162–8.
2. Rogers WJ, Canto JG, Lambrew CT et al. Temporal trends in the treatment of over 1.5 million patients with myocardial infarction in the US from 1990 through 1999: the National Registry of Myocardial Infarction 1, 2 and 3. J Am Coll Cardiol 2000;36:2056–63.

3. Holmes DR Jr, Berger PB, Hochman JS et al. Cardiogenic shock in patients with acute ischemic syndromes with and without ST-segment elevation. Circulation 1999;100:2067–73.
4. Hasdai D, Harrington RA, Hochman JS et al. Platelet glycoprotein IIb/IIIa blockade and outcome of cardiogenic shock complicating acute coronary syndromes without persistent ST-segment elevation. J Am Coll Cardiol 2000;36:685–92.
5. Hochman JS, Sleeper LA, Webb JG et al. Early revascularization in acute myocardial infarction complicated by cardiogenic shock. SHOCK Investigators. SHould we emergently revascularize Occluded Coronaries for cardiogenic shocK? N Engl J Med 1999;341:625–34.
6. Hochman JS, Sleeper LA, White HD et al. One-year survival following early revascularization for cardiogenic shock. JAMA 2001;285:190–2.
7. Hochman JS, Buller CE, Sleeper LA et al. Cardiogenic shock complicating acute myocardial infarction – etiologies, management and outcome: a report from the SHOCK Trial Registry. SHould we emergently revascularize Occluded Coronaries for cardiogenic shocK? J Am Coll Cardiol 2000;36:1063–70.
8. Hochman JS. Cardiogenic shock complicating acute myocardial infarction: expanding the paradigm. Circulation 2003;107:2998–3002.
9. Laschinger JC, Grossi EA, Cunningham JN Jr et al. Adjunctive left ventricular unloading during myocardial reperfusion plays a major role in minimizing myocardial infarct size. J Thorac Cardiovasc Surg 1985;90:80–5.
10. Gerber BL, Rochitte CE, Melin JA et al. Microvascular obstruction and left ventricular remodeling early after acute myocardial infarction. Circulation 2000;101:2734–41.
11. Barbone A, Holmes JW, Heerdt PM et al. Comparison of right and left ventricular responses to left ventricular assist device support in patients with severe heart failure: a primary role of mechanical unloading underlying reverse remodeling. Circulation 2001;104:670–5.
12. Thiele H, Lauer B, Hambrecht R, Boudriot E, Cohen HA, Schuler G. Reversal of cardiogenic shock by percutaneous left atrial-to-femoral arterial bypass assistance. Circulation 2001; 104:2917–22.
13. Lemos PA, Cummins P, Lee CH et al. Usefulness of percutaneous left ventricular assistance to support high-risk percutaneous coronary interventions. Am J Cardiol 2003;91:479–81.
14. Panos A, Kalangos A, Urban P. High-risk PTCA assisted by the Hemopump 14F: the Geneva experience. Schweiz Med Wochenschr 1999;129:1529–34.
15. Thiele H, Sick P, Boudriot E et al. Randomized comparison of intra-aortic balloon support with a percutaneous left ventricular assist device in patients with revascularized acute myocardial infarction complicated by cardiogenic shock. Eur Heart J 2005;26:1276–83.
16. Hollenberg SM, Kavinsky CJ, Parrillo JE. Cardiogenic shock. Ann Intern Med 1999; 131:47–59.
17. Windecker S, Meier B. Perkutane linksventrikuläre Unterstützungssysteme. Kardiovaskuläre Medizin 2004;7:26–32.
18. Windecker S, Meier B. Impella assisted high risk percutaneous coronary intervention. Kardiovaskuläre Medizin 2005;8:187–9.

Section E
Specific issues

13

How to prevent and manage complications during primary percutaneous cardiovascular interventions

David Antoniucci and Dariusz Dudek

Thrombus removal and prevention of microvessel embolism • Definition of the anatomy of the target vessel and lesion in persistently occluded infarct artery after wiring • Infarct artery stenting technique • Glycoprotein IIb/IIIa inhibition • Subsets at high risk of primary percutaneous cardiovascular intervention complications

The prevention and treatment of percutaneous cardiovascular intervention (PCI) complications in the setting of acute myocardial infarction (AMI) are largely similar to those in other clinical settings. Thus, in order to avoid overlapping and repetition of arguments already extensively treated in other sections, this chapter will focus on PCI complications that are more specific to AMI patients, and are subsequent to the more important characteristics of this setting. These include the thrombotic component of the target lesion that is invariably present, the emergent treatment of patients with a wide spectrum of coronary anatomy complexity and clinical status, from focal single vessel disease in asymptomatic patients to complex multivessel disease in patients with cardiogenic shock, and the need for mechanical and pharmacologic adjunctive treatments for the restoration of an effective reperfusion at the microcirculatory level.

THROMBUS REMOVAL AND PREVENTION OF MICROVESSEL EMBOLISM

Thrombectomy

A strong rationale supports the use of devices that may decrease the risk of embolism during PCI for AMI. It has been shown that embolism may lead to microvessel disruption resulting from direct mechanical obstruction and activation of a complex inflammatory cascade by thromboembolic material, causing further obstruction and ultimately an ineffective myocardial reperfusion.

The rheolytic thrombectomy system (AngioJet, Possis Medical Inc., Minneapolis, MN) consists of a dual-lumen catheter with an external pump providing pressurized saline solution via the effluent lumen to the catheter tip. Multiple saline jets from the distal part of the catheter travel backwards at 390 mph, and create a localized negative pressure zone that draws thrombus from where the jets fragment it and propel the small particles to the evacuation lumen of the catheter. The first 5 F generation catheter for coronary use (LF 140) was associated with a substantial device failure rate due to the inability of the large and poorly trackable catheter to cross the lesion, embolization, and vessel perforation. In a *post hoc* analysis in a series of 70 patients with AMI enrolled in the VEGAS 1 and 2 trials, the device failure rate was 22%.[1]

The second-generation AngioJet catheter for coronary use (XMI) is a 4 F catheter with improved design of the profile and of the opening of the jets, allowing easy and nontraumatic navigation through the coronary vessels and more thrombectomy power. The results of a randomized trial from the Florence investigators comparing rheolytic thrombectomy before direct infarct artery stenting with direct stenting alone in 100 patients with AMI showed that rheolytic thrombectomy using the second-generation catheter provided a more effective myocardial reperfusion, as shown by the more frequent early ST segment resolution, the lower cTFC values, and smaller infarcts as assessed by scintigraphy in patients randomized to thrombectomy as compared to patients randomized to stenting alone.[2] The efficacy of the rheolytic thrombectomy system in removal of thrombus and atherosclerotic debris from the disrupted plaque was proved by the re-establishment of a TIMI grade 3 flow before stenting in most patients. In this study, the new thrombectomy catheter directly crossed the target lesion in nearly all treated patients without any mechanical complication (device success rate 96%). Conversely, a concluded unpublished trial, the AngioJet Rheolytic Thrombectomy in Patients Undergoing Primary Angioplasty for Acute Myocardial Infarction (AIMI) trial based on 480 patients, has produced negative results: no differences in infarct size between patients randomized to thrombectomy and control, and increased one-month mortality in patients randomized to thrombectomy (4.6% vs 0.8%, *P*<0.02) (Alì A., at TCT 2004, Washington DC, September 2004, unpublished). The negative results of this study have suggested several concerns about study design, biased patient selection, and thrombectomy technique used.

The ev3-X-SIZER (EndiCor Medical Inc., San Clemente, CA) thrombectomy device provides direct mechanical thrombus ablation using a distal helical cutter and vacuum-assisted debris removal. The device is available in 1.5, 2.0, and 2.3 mm cutter sizes and is compatible with 7 F to 9 F guide catheters according to the cutter diameter. The device works mostly within the same radius of the catheter and efficacy in thrombectomy is dependent on the mismatch between the diameter of the vessel and the size of the device. This limitation is more evident in large or aneurysmal vessels. The first reported randomized clinical experience with this device in the setting of acute coronary syndromes was based on a cohort of 66 patients.[3] Patients randomized to the X-SIZER catheter had a better corrected TIMI frame count and ST segment elevation resolution as compared to patients randomized to placebo, and multivariate analysis showed randomization to X-SIZER thrombectomy as the single independent predictor of ST segment elevation resolution (OR 4.35, *P*<0.04). Another randomized study based on 92 patients with ST segment elevation AMI has shown better ST segment elevation resolution and blush grade in patients randomized to X-SIZER thrombectomy before infarct artery stenting.[4] Complete (>70%) ST segment resolution rate was 58.7% in patients randomized to thrombectomy and 32.6% in patients randomized to placebo (*P*=0.001), while a blush grade 3 was achieved in 71.7% and 36.9% of patients, respectively (*P*=0.006). The X-AMINE trial, based on a sample of 201 patients, reported similar results, confirming that thrombectomy before infarct artery stenting may provide an enhanced myocardial reperfusion (ST segment elevation resolution >50% in 68% of patients randomized to thrombectomy and 53% in the control group, $P=0.037$).[5]

The Rescue (SCIMED Boston Scientific, Maple Grove, MN) and the Export catheters (Medtronic, Santa Rosa, CA) are catheter-based aspiration systems. The efficacy of the Rescue catheter in the removal of thrombus and atherosclerotic debris was demonstrated in a small series of patients with AMI.[6,7] The Rescue system is safe and effective in thrombus removal from the coronary lumen. However, shortcomings include difficulties with complex coronary anatomy proximal to the culprit lesion. Some small studies showed improved ST segment resolution at 60 minutes after PCI and trends to improved myocardial perfusion.[1,2] An additional limitation in comparison to the X-SIZER and AngioJet is lack of active defragmentation of thrombus before removal. This seems to be the main reason why the Rescue system is less effective than the other two devices in handling massive thrombi in large coronary vessels.[3]

The major limitations of this device, and others based on the same principle, are the high profile, the relatively poor trackability, and the unpredictable aspiration power. Moreover, an overly high negative pressure may result in the collapse of the vessel, preventing any aspiration. A first randomized study by Dudek et al showed the device to be effective in thrombus removal.[8] Conversely, a second concluded randomized study including 215 patients did not show any benefit of this type of thrombectomy, and patients randomized to Rescue catheter thrombectomy had larger infarct size as compared to controls (Kaltoft AK at TCT 2005, Washington DC, October 2005, unpublished).

Thrombectomy devices using alternative energies such as laser or ultrasounds have produced negative results due to the high profile of the devices, their poor trackability, and the potential for vessel injury and perforation.[9–12]

Thus, in conclusion, the AngioJet and the X-SIZER device have the potential for improvement in myocardial reperfusion in patients undergoing PCI for AMI, decreasing embolization into the microvessel network. However, large-scale trials should provide additional meaningful insight into whether the use of these devices before infarct artery stenting represents a major breakthrough in the mechanical treatment of patients with AMI.

Emboli protection devices

There are two types of antiembolic systems: the nonocclusive system based on filters that trap embolic debris, and the occlusive system based on the occlusion of the vessel distal to the target lesion, and subsequent retrieval of the embolic debris after the procedure by aspiration catheters. Both systems have the potential major disadvantage that emboli protection may be complete only if the device can be placed beyond the occlusion in a segment without major branches. Otherwise, debris from the target lesion may embolize into the branches.

The filter devices consist of a guidewire with an integrated filter at the distal end of the device. The basket travels in a closed position into a delivery sheath and is deployed after crossing the target lesion. After the interventional procedure, another shaft allows the retrieval of the device by collapsing and capturing the basket. The device must oversize the vessel diameter by 0.5–1.0 mm in order to provide the right apposition to the vessel wall of the filter in the open position. Otherwise, a poor circumferential wall apposition between the struts of the basket allows embolization. A potential disadvantage of this type of device is embolization during wiring or during collapse of a basket full of embolic debris that may extrude from the device.

A randomized study including 200 patients with AMI did not reveal any benefit from the use of this device. Patients randomized to the FilterWire had microvascular function, ST segment elevation resolution, and infarct size similar to the control group.[13]

The GuardWire (Medtronic, Santa Rosa, CA) is the prototype of the occlusive protection systems. The system consists of a 0.014″ balloon wire, a microseal adapter for inflation and deflation the balloon, and a 5 F aspiration catheter (Export catheter). The balloon wire has a very low profile (2.1 F), allowing good trackability and a relatively low risk of embolization during wiring of the target lesion.

The efficacy of this device in protection from embolization was shown in patients with diseased saphenous vein grafts. In the SAFER trial, 801 patients with diseased saphenous vein grafts underwent percutaneous intervention with or without the protection of the GuardWire system in a randomized fashion.[14] The device success rate was 90.1% and patients randomized to the GuardWire had a significant reduction in the rate of adverse events related to embolization as compared to the control group (9.6% vs 16.5%, P=0.004). The major advantages of this system are the good support of the wire, no limit to the amount of retrieved material, and the low profile as compared to the available filter devices.

The correct use of the device for coronary vessels is not as easy and simple as in venous grafts or carotid vessels. The correct placement of the tip of the GuardWire and the right occlusive balloon diameter are relatively simple in an already open infarct artery. In persistently occluded vessels, after passage of the GuardWire, repeat passages of a low-profile balloon angioplasty or direct aspiration with the Export catheter may restore the flow, but with a high risk of significant embolization (Figure 13.1). Oversizing the diameter of the balloon is advisable, since after stenting and restoration of good flow, the balloon diameter originally selected may no longer be occlusive, frustrating the entire protection procedure. However, excessive balloon oversizing may result in vessel trauma and disruption of the intimal tear.

The high support of the GuardWire may produce pseudonarrowing of a tortuous infarct artery, preventing any aspiration and retrieval by the Export catheter (Figure 13.2). Aspiration by the Export catheter of blood and debris may be difficult or impossible; in this case a large piece of debris may have obstructed the lumen of the catheter. The catheter must be retrieved immediately under negative pressure; the debris may be easily removed by pushing it out of the catheter with a forced saline injection. Excessive negative pressure on the Export catheter may result in collapsing of the vessel and prevention of aspiration. Finally, the GuardWire must be handled very carefully, avoiding any damage to the wire by an excessively tight torque or any kinking that may prevent inflation of the balloon, or, much worse, its deflation.

The efficacy of this device in AMI was assessed by the Enhanced Myocardial Efficacy and Recovery by Aspiration of Liberalized Debris (EMERALD) trial. EMERALD randomized 501 patients and despite the fact that visible debris was retrieved in 73% of patients randomized to the GuardWire, no differences in ST segment resolution, infarct size, and clinical outcome between the GuardWire group and the control group were found.[15] Another randomized study based on the use of the GuardWire, the ASPARAGUS trial, including 341 patients with AMI, showed that

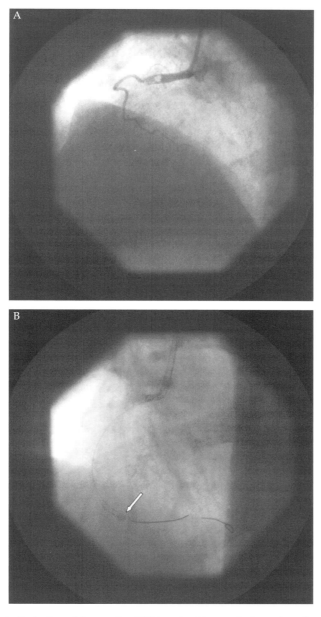

Figure 13.1 A. Occlusion of the proximal RCA and evidence of a large thrombus. B. Placement of a coronary wire in the retroventricular branch and an antiembolic occlusive device (the arrow indicates the inflated balloon of the antiembolic device; GuardWire, Medtronic). C. Stenting of the proximal RCA. D. Occlusive embolization into the posterior descending artery. E. Rheolytic thrombectomy (AngioJet, Possis) of the posterior descending artery (the two radiopaque markers indicate the thrombectomy device). F. Effective removal of the embolus by thrombectomy; no further intervention.

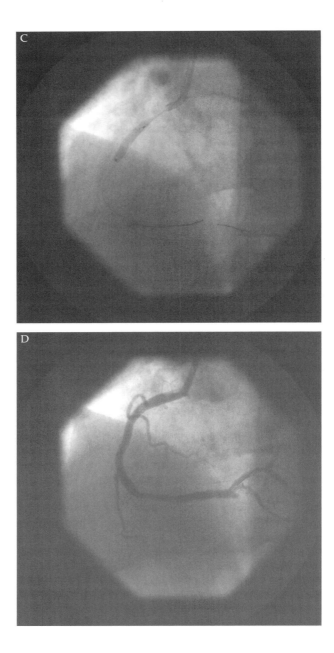

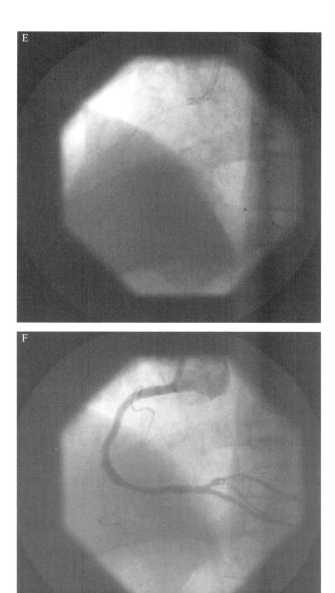

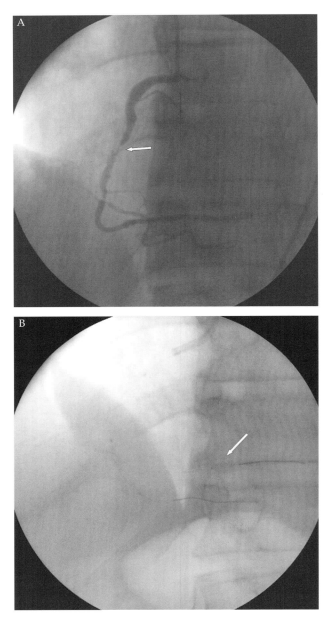

Figure 13.2 A. Multiple subocclusive lesions within RCA and evidence of a small thrombus in the mid portion of the vessel (arrow). B. Placement of a coronary wire and an antiembolic occlusive device in the distal portion of the vessel; the arrow indicates the inflated balloon of the antiembolic device (GuardWire, Medtronic). C. After stenting, diffuse pseudonarrowing is evident at the third portion of the RCA, which prevented aspiration of blood by the Export catheter. D. Reversal of the pseudonarrowing after removal of the coronary wire and restoration of a normal epicardial flow.

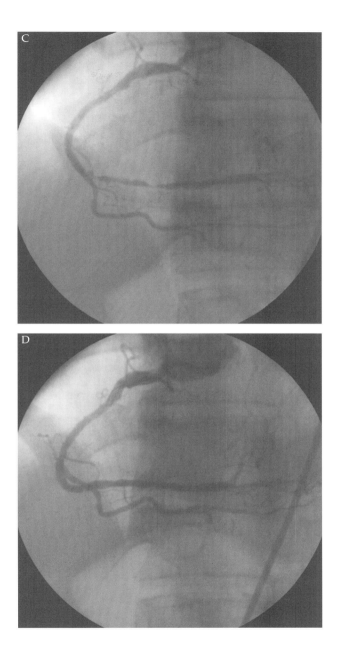

patients randomized to distal protection had a lower incidence of slow flow and embolization, and a higher incidence of postprocedure blush grade 3 as compared to controls, while there were no differences in major adverse event rates between groups (Muramatsu T at TCT 2004, Washington DC, September 2004, unpublished).

Thus, concluded randomized studies do not show that distal occlusive protection devices and filters provide a better clinical outcome.

An innovative concept for protection from embolization during intervention is based on proximal occlusion of the vessel. This system (Proxis, Velocimed, Minneapolis, MN) has the potential for complete protection of the vessel and branches before any intervention device crosses the target lesion. The stagnating blood distal to the proximally occluded device or its reversal prevents any embolization to the distal bed and an easy retrieval of atherothrombotic debris after the stenting procedure. Moreover, the large lumen of the occlusive catheter provides excellent visualization of the target vessel. The revascularization procedure is performed through the large lumen of the Proxis catheter that can easily accommodate the coronary wire and any delivery stent system. A randomized study including 600 patients with diseased venous grafts compared the proximal occlusion device with the distal occlusive GuardWire or FilterWire. The one-month major adverse cardiac event rate was lower in the PROXIS arm as compared to the filter arm (6.2% vs 11.2%) (Rogers C, at TCT 2005, Washington DC, October 2005, unpublished). The feasibility and safety of the system in the left coronary system, with unfavorable take-off of the left anterior descending artery or circumflex artery, are unknown.

DEFINITION OF THE ANATOMY OF THE TARGET VESSEL AND LESION IN PERSISTENTLY OCCLUDED INFARCT ARTERY AFTER WIRING

In a substantial minority of patients, passage of the coronary wire is not followed by the re-establishment of infarct artery flow. A persistent TIMI grade 0–1 flow after passage of the wire prevents the angiographic definition of the anatomy of the vessel, and of the characteristics of the target lesion. In this case, an ultraselective dye injection beyond the occlusion may be extremely useful for judgment on the right placement of the wire, the need for a second wire if a major branch is involved in the target lesion, the thrombotic burden, the length of the lesion, and other significant lesions within the infarct artery.

The more convenient approach to this problem is the use of a dual-lumen catheter (Multifunctional Probing, Boston Scientific, Maple Grove, MN). One lumen is used for transport of the catheter beyond the occlusion with the monorail system, while the second lumen can be used for dye injection (Figure 13.3). The multiple functions of the device include ultraselective administration of drugs, exchange of the coronary wire, and support for the placement of a second wire into a branch with an unfavorable take-off.

An alternative device is an over-the-wire balloon catheter but its use has several disadvantages, such as the need for removal of the coronary wire for dye injection and ultimately a more time-consuming procedure.

An alternative technique to the ultraselective dye injection is the re-establishment of flow, avoiding embolization. This goal may be achieved with a thrombectomy device, since in most cases of a wired infarct artery that is persistently occluded, the thrombus is a large component of the occlusion.

Other techniques with the potential for major embolization, such as repeat passages of a deflated angioplasty balloon through the occlusion or angioplasty using undersized balloons, should be avoided.

INFARCT ARTERY STENTING TECHNIQUE

The stent size should match the vessel diameter proximally to the occlusion, since in most cases the postocclusion vessel diameter may underestimate the actual vessel size due to low pressure or spasm. An undersized stent is associated with a high incidence of thrombosis and restenosis due to incomplete stent apposition and disturbed flow.

For occlusion involving the ostium, or the very proximal portion, of the left anterior descending artery or circumflex artery, the most relevant technical problem is the prevention of retrograde shift of atherothrombotic material after angioplasty or stenting of the target vessel. The risk of retrograde plaque shift is very high in patients with AMI, and this fact may be explained by the characteristics of the occlusive plaque, that in most cases is a low-density, large-volume mass with the potential for high strain under low stress. Thrombectomy is the best primary mechanical approach if the thrombotic component of the plaque is prominent. Conversely, plaque debulking is indicated as the more effective treatment if the residual stenosis after thrombectomy is severe, suggesting a prominent atherosclerotic component of the occlusion. In all cases the placement of a protection wire into the nontarget vessel is indicated and should be considered mandatory when the characteristics of take-off of the nontarget vessel suggest a potentially difficult bail-out engagement of the vessel by a coronary wire.

For occlusion involving a major branch, it is mandatory to obtain a correct definition of the geometry of the disrupted atherosclerotic plaque before stenting. The occlusion may be a true bifurcation lesion or the branch may be involved only by the thrombotic component of the plaque. In the first case, as in patients with angina, the more effective approach includes the placement of two wires, angioplasty of both vessels, elective stenting of the main vessel, and provisional stenting of the branch. In the second case, the more effective strategy includes thrombectomy of the main vessel, followed by thrombectomy of the branch if necessary, and stenting of the main vessel. Also, in the drug-eluting stent era, elective bifurcation stenting is contraindicated due to the higher risk of macro- and microembolization and late restenosis. For a branch that is not too large, the goal is the re-establishment of a good flow whatever the residual stenosis, since a late positive remodeling is relatively frequent, while the risk of in-stent restenosis is high.

The increased invasiveness of the conventional stenting technique, with repeat balloon dilatations, as compared to the direct stenting technique, may be considered a risk factor for embolization. Paradoxically, the advantage of the direct stenting technique in the reduction of embolization could be superior in those anatomic settings currently considered unfavorable, such as long lesions or multiple lesions within the infarct artery, since the atherosclerotic burden of the target vessel is related to the risk of embolization during stenting.[16,17] Again, the use of very high pressure for stent deployment and expansion may result in a deterioration of flow due to embolization. As a consequence, direct stenting and the use of the right pressure for the characteristics of the lesion and the stent are advisable.

A randomized study based on 206 patients with AMI comparing direct stenting with conventional stenting confirmed a better reperfusion after direct stenting with

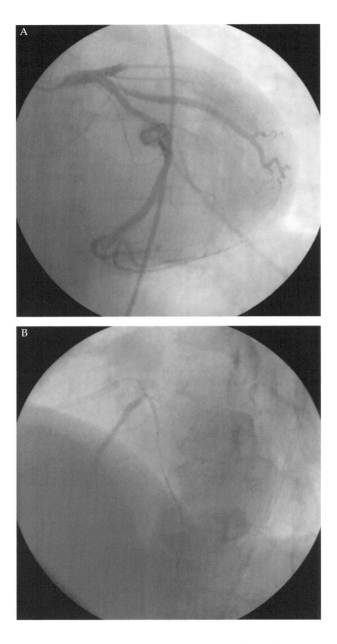

Figure 13.3   A. Proximal LAD occlusion. B. After crossing the occlusion, ultraselective dye injection beyond the occlusion shows that the wire is placed in a first large diagonal branch, and the target lesion involves also a large septal branch (trifurcation). C. Placement of the other two wires into the main vessel and first septal branch and restoration of the flow after rheolytic thrombectomy (AngioJet); no evidence of involvement of the ostia of the branches by the culprit lesion. D. After direct stenting of the main vessel.

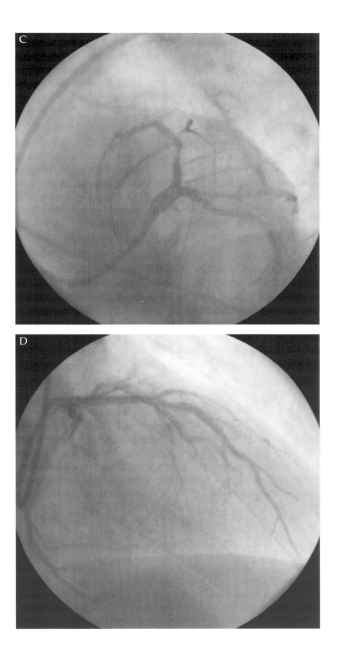

decreased incidence of the no-reflow phenomenon and macroembolization, and a higher rate of early ST segment resolution, which is a marker of effectiveness of reperfusion.[18] Direct stenting was associated with a better clinical outcome, but the improvement in outcome did not reach significance due to the small size of the studied population. Direct stenting was associated with a decreased incidence of the no-reflow phenomenon as compared to conventional stenting in two other nonrandomized studies.[19,20] However, the patient selection bias should be taken into account in order to correctly assess the potential advantages of direct stenting, since patients with more complex anatomy and the potential for a high risk of embolism during stenting are generally deemed nonsuitable for direct stenting.

Direct infarct artery stenting should be considered as a valuable approach in patients who undergo thrombectomy. The removal of thrombus allows the correct definition of the length of the disrupted plaque and of the proper stent.

The safety and efficacy of bare metal stents in AMI have been shown by several controlled randomized trials comparing infarct artery stenting with conventional balloon angioplasty.[21–26] Conversely, there are very few data on drug-eluting stents in the setting of AMI. Preliminary data from registries suggest that stent thrombosis is not a concern, while the effect in decreasing late restenosis is similar to that in other clinical settings.[27] Ongoing trials will assess the safety and efficacy of drug-eluting stents in the setting of AMI.

GLYCOPROTEIN IIB/IIIA INHIBITION

Several studies have shown that abciximab, the prototypic GP IIb/IIIa inhibitor, as adjunctive therapy to infarct-related artery stenting provides a significant decrease in the incidence of major cardiac adverse events that is not attributable exclusively to the reduction of ischemic events related to early target vessel failure but also to an enhanced reperfusion at the microcirculatory level.[28–31] The effects of abciximab may be related to the prevention or reduction of platelet microvascular plugging by inhibition of glycoprotein IIb/IIIa receptors, as well as neutrophil activation by inhibition of alfaMbeta2 receptors and Bbeta3 receptors that are present on granulocytes and monocytes.[32] The inhibitory effects of abciximab also include one of the most important platelet mediators, the CD40 ligand, which is principally expressed in monocytes, macrophages, and endothelial cells and plays a major role in the unleashing of inflammation and production of interleukins and chemokines.[33]

The benefit of abciximab parallels the risk of the patient, and is decreased in low-risk patients.[26]

The evidence of a strong benefit of IIb/IIIa receptor inhibition in the setting of PCI for AMI is limited only to abciximab, while the appropriateness of the use of IIb/IIIa inhibitors other than abciximab in the setting of coronary stenting for AMI has not been shown.

SUBSETS AT HIGH RISK OF PRIMARY PERCUTANEOUS CARDIOVASCULAR INTERVENTION COMPLICATIONS

Elderly patients

There are no technical aspects of AMI PCI that are specific to the elderly. However, several technical aspects are more frequently encountered with increasing age, and most are subsequent to the increased diffusion of the atherosclerotic process in the coronary system as well as in the other vascular districts.

Femoral access may be difficult or even impossible in patients with diffuse atherosclerosis and tortuosity of the iliac–femoral axes. The use of hydrophilic wires and long shafts under fluoroscopic guidance may solve the access problem. Extremely tortuous aortoiliac trees may prevent advancement of the guide catheter over a long shaft; the more direct solution for this problem is the use of guide catheters smaller than the size of the shaft (typically a 6 F guiding catheter on an 8 F shaft) and of a 0.63 wire for the guiding catheter. The radial and brachial access are alternatives to the femoral access. However, it should be highlighted that in nearly all patients with a tortuous aortoiliac axis, the tortuosity will also be a problem using the alternative brachial approach.

For patients who need intra-aortic balloon counterpulsation, the balloon assistance should be stopped as soon as possible due to the increased risk in elderly patients of device-related fatal complications (retroperitoneal hematoma, visceral embolism).

Anatomic coronary characteristics that are more frequently associated with increasing age are diffuse calcification and tortuosity of coronary arteries. Both these characteristics suggest the use of very trackable and high support coronary wires, as well as a guiding catheter with high back-up (Voda, Amplatz left, and hockey stick may be considered the first choice for guiding catheters). Predilatation of the target lesion should be considered mandatory in patients with diffusely calcified and tortuous vessels in order to decrease the risk of coronary stent deployment failure.

It should be remembered that in elderly patients a substantial minority of in-hospital deaths are due to noncardiac causes[34] and great attention should be paid to the correct use of heparin and contrast medium in order to decrease the risk of hemorrhagic complications and renal insufficiency.

No specific contraindication exists to the use of abciximab in elderly patients, and the safety profile of the drug in the elderly is similar to that in younger patients.[35]

Spontaneous coronary artery dissection

Spontaneous coronary artery dissection is a rare cause of AMI and in the majority of cases occurs in women, frequently in the postpartum period.[36,37] However, AMI complicating spontaneous coronary artery dissection may occur also in postmenopausal women, and in men. Despite the low incidence, the correct recognition and treatment of this condition may be difficult and challenging. Recognition is easy when baseline angiography clearly shows nonocclusive dissection, or the occlusion occurring distally to a dissected coronary artery segment, or the dissection process involves more than one coronary artery (exceptionally all three coronary arteries may be involved in the dissection process).[38,39] Recognition by angiography is difficult or even impossible when the occlusion complicates the dissection at the same level as the beginning of the dissection, or the dissection planes are distal and long, and result in a diffuse and uniform reduction of the vessel lumen due to the thrombosis of the dissecting hematoma in the false lumen which prevents contrast medium penetration. The right diagnosis may be indirectly suggested by clinical data, such as gender, postpartum period, and the absence of angiographic evidence of coronary atherosclerosis, or directly, by ultraselective angiography, using a dual-lumen catheter or an over-the-wire catheter, or by intravascular ultrasound interrogation after placement of a coronary wire in the true lumen of the vessel.

The goal of PCI is the re-establishment of a brisk flow with minimal aggressiveness in order to avoid extension of the dissection, coronary perforation or rupture. A global 'soft' interventional approach includes careful manipulation of the guiding catheter and the coronary wire, and the use of long balloons at low pressure. If conventional angioplasty, even with long inflation times, is unsuccessful, stenting remains the only effective therapeutic option. For long dissections involving major branches, typically in the dissections of the left coronary system, spot stenting should be considered the first stenting technique, since a short stent may be effective in re-establishment of a good flow, avoiding the complications related to long or multiple stent implantation, such as loss of major branches, and proximal or distal extension of dissection. Stent placement should be accomplished with the minimum inflation pressure sufficient to expand the stent, since high inflation pressure may be complicated by extension of the dissection. The indication for the use of IIb/IIIa inhibitors should be matched with the risk of coronary perforation or rupture, and these drugs should be administered only after the correct placement of the coronary wire in the true lumen of the vessel. Residual nonocclusive dissection, even long, should not be treated, since a normal flow may be spontaneously maintained and contribute to the spontaneous healing of the dissection.

Right ventricular infarction and cardiogenic shock

Isolated right ventricular infarction is a rare occurrence, but this condition may be associated with a severe low-output state and shock that may be unresponsive to fluid administration, inotropic agents, and intra-aortic balloon pumping. Conversely, involvement of the right ventricle in inferior myocardial infarction is relatively frequent and associated with a poor prognosis. Percutaneous recanalization of the occluded coronary artery has a strong impact on mortality in patients with right ventricular infarction. A key study using direct angioplasty showed that restoration of normal flow in right ventricular branches resulted in dramatic recovery of right ventricular function and a mortality rate of only 2%, whereas unsuccessful reperfusion of the right ventricle was associated with persistent hemodynamic compromise and a mortality rate of 58%.[40]

REFERENCES

1. Rinfret S, Katsiyiammis PT, Ho KK et al. Effectiveness of rheolytic coronary thrombectomy with the AngioJet catheter. Am J Cardiol 2002;90:470–6.
2. Antoniucci D, Valenti R, Migliorini A et al. A randomized trial comparing rheolytic thrombectomy before infarct artery stenting with stenting alone in patients undergoing percutaneous coronary intervention for acute myocardial infarction. Am J Cardiol 2004; 93:1033–5.
3. Beran G, Lang I, Schreifer W et al. Intracoronary thrombectomy with the X-Sizer catheter system improves epicardial flow and accelerates ST-segment resolution in patients with acute coronary syndromes. Circulation 2002;105:2355–60.
4. Napodano M, Reimers B, Pasquetto G et al. Intracoronary thrombectomy improves myocardial reperfusion in patients undergoing direct angioplasty for acute myocardial infarction. J Am Coll Cardiol 2003;42:1395–402.

5. Lefevre T, Garcia E, Reimers B et al. X-sizer for thrombectomy in acute myocardial infarction improves ST-segment resolution: results of the X-sizer in AMI for Negligible Embolization and optimal ST resolution (X AMINE ST) trial. J Am Coll Cardiol 2005;46:246–52.

6. Ito Y, Muramatsu T, Tsukahara R et al. Efficacy of suction thrombectomy for acute myocardial infarction. Am J Cardiol 2002;90 (Suppl 6A):187H (TCT-487).

7. Ito Y, Muramatsu T, Tsukahara R et al. Success or lack of success of suction thrombectomy using Rescue catheter system in acute myocardial infarction and findings of intravascular ultrasound. Am J Cardiol 2002;90 (Suppl 6A):187H (TCT-488).

8. Dudek D, Mielecki W, Legutko J et al. Percutaneous thrombectomy with the RESCUE system in acute myocardial infarction. Kardiol Pol 2004;61:523–33.

9. Topaz O, Minisi AJ, Bernardo N, Alimar K, Ereso A, Shah R. Comparison of effectiveness of excimer laser angioplasty in patients with acute coronary syndromes in those with versus without normal left ventricular function. Am J Cardiol 2003;91:797–802.

10. Rosenchlin U, Roth A, Rassin T et al. Analysis of coronary ultrasound thrombolysis end point in acute myocardial infarction (ACUTE) trial. Results of the feasibility phase. Circulation 1997;95:1411–16.

11. Halkin A, Rosenchein V. Catheter-delivered ultrasound therapy for native coronary arterial thrombosis and occluded saphenous vein grafts. Echocardiography 2001;18:225–31.

12. Singh M, Rouseschen U, Kalon KL et al. Treatment of saphenous vein bypass grafts with ultrasound thrombolysis. A randomized study (ATLAS). Circulation 2003;107:2331–6.

13. Gick M, Jander N, Bestehorn H-P et al. Randomized evaluation of the effects of filter-based distal protection on myocardial perfusion and infarct size after primary percutaneous catheter intervention in myocardial infarction with and without ST-segment elevation. Circulation 2005;112:1462–9.

14. Baim D, Wahr D, George B et al. Randomized trial of distal embolic protection device during percutaneous intervention of saphenous vein aortocoronary bypass grafts. Circulation 2002; 105:1285–90.

15. Stone GW, Webb J, Cox D et al. Distal microcirculatory protection during percutaneous coronary intervention in acute ST-segment elevation myocardial infarction: a randomized controlled trial. JAMA 2005;293:1063–72.

16. Topol EJ, Yadav JS. Recognition of the importance of embolization in atherosclerotic vascular disease. Circulation 2000;101:570–80.

17. Rogers C, Parikh S, Seifert P et al. Remnant endothelium after stenting enhances vascular repair. Circulation 1996;94:2909–14.

18. Loubeyre C, Morice MC, Lefevre T, Piechaud JF, Louvard Y, Dumas P. A randomized comparison of direct stenting with conventional stent implantation in selected patients with acute myocardial infarction. J Am Coll Cardiol 2002;39:15–21.

19. Herz I, Assali A, Solodoky A et al. Coronary stent deployment without predilation in acute myocardial infarction: a feasible, safe, and effective technique. Angiology 1999;50:901–8.

20. Antoniucci D, Valenti R, Migliorini A et al. Direct infarct artery stenting without predilation and no-reflow in patients with acute myocardial infarction. Am Heart J 2001;142:684–90.

21. Rodriguez A, Bernardi V, Fernandez M et al. In-hospital and late results of coronary stents versus conventional balloon angioplasty in acute myocardial infarction (GRAMI trial). Am J Cardiol 1998;81:1286–91.

22. Suryapranata H, van't Hof AWJ, Hoorntje JCA, de Boer MJ, Zijlstra F. Randomized comparison of coronary stenting with balloon angioplasty in selected patients with acute myocardial infarction. Circulation 1998;97:2502–5.

23. Antoniucci D, Santoro GM, Bolognese L, Valenti R, Trapani M, Fazzini PF. A clinical trial comparing primary stenting of the infarct-related artery with optimal primary angioplasty for acute myocardial infarction. J Am Coll Cardiol 1998;31:1234–9.

24. Saito S, Hosokawa G, Tanaka S, Nakamura S. Primary stent implantation is superior to balloon angioplasty in acute myocardial infarction: final results of the Primary Angioplasty versus Stent Implantation in Acute Myocardial Infarction (PASTA) trial. Cathet Cardiovasc Intervent 1999;48:262–8.

25. Grines CL, Cox DA, Stone GW et al. Coronary angioplasty with or without stent implantation for acute myocardial infarction. N Engl J Med 1999;341:1949–56.
26. Stone GW, Grines CL, Cox DA et al. Comparison of angioplasty with stenting, with or without abciximab, in acute myocardial infarction. N Engl J Med 2002;346:957–66.
27. Lemos PA, Lee CH, Degertekin M et al. Early outcome after sirolimus-eluting stent implantation in patients with acute coronary syndromes. Insights from Rapamycin Eluting Stent Evaluated At Rotterdam Cardiology Hospital (RESEARCH) registry. J Am Coll Cardiol 2003;41:2093–9.
28. Montalescot G, Barragan P, Wittenberg O et al. Platelet glycoprotein IIb/IIIa inhibition with coronary stenting for acute myocardial infarction. N Engl J Med 2001;344:1895–903.
29. Neumann F-J, Kastrati A, Schmitt C et al. Effect of glycoprotein IIb/IIIa receptor blockade with abciximab on clinical and angiographic restenosis rate after the placement of coronary stents following acute myocardial infarction. J Am Coll Cardiol 2000;35:915–21.
30. Neumann FJ, Blasini R, Schmitt C et al. Effect of glycoprotein IIb/IIIa receptor blockade on recovery of coronary flow and left ventricular function after the placement of coronary-artery stents in acute myocardial infarction. Circulation 1998;98:2695–701.
31. Antoniucci D, Migliorini A, Parodi G et al. Abciximab-supported infarct artery stent implantation for acute myocardial infarction and long-term survival: a prospective multicenter, randomized trial comparing infarct artery stenting plus abciximab with stenting alone. Circulation 2004;109:1704–6.
32. Neumann FJ, Zohlnhofer D, Fakhoury L, Ott I, Gawaz M, Schomig A. Effect of glycoprotein IIb/IIIa receptor blockade on platelet-leukocite interaction and surface expression of the leukocyte integrin Mac–1 in acute myocardial infarction. J Am Coll Cardiol 1999;34:1420–6.
33. Reininger AJ, Agneskirchner J, Bode PA, Spannagl M, Wurzinger LJ. c7E3 Fab inhibits low shear flow modulated platelet adhesion to endothelium and surface-absorbed fibrinogen by blocking platelet GP IIb/IIIa as well as endothelial vitronectin receptor – results from patients with acute myocardial infarction and healthy controls. Thromb Haemost 2000;83:217–23.
34. Sakai K, Nakagawa Y, Kimura T et al. Comparison of results of coronary angioplasty for acute myocardial infarction in patients ≥ 75 years of age versus patients < 75 years of age. Am J Cardiol 2002;89:797–800.
35. Antoniucci D, Valenti R, Migliorini A et al. Abciximab therapy improves one-month survival rate in unselected patients with acute myocardial infarction undergoing routine infarct artery stent implantation. Am Heart J 2002;144:315–22.
36. De Maio SJ, Kinsella SH, Silverman ME. Clinical course and long-term prognosis of spontaneous coronary artery dissection. Am J Cardiol 1989;64:471–4.
37. Bac DJ, Lotgering FK, Verkaaik APK et al. Spontaneous coronary artery dissection during pregnancy and post partum. Eur Heart J 1995;16:136–8.
38. Antoniucci D, Diligenti M. Spontaneous dissection of three major coronary arteries. Eur Heart J 1990;11:1130–4.
39. Eltchaninoff H, Cribier A, Letac B. Multiple spontaneous coronary artery dissection in young women. Lancet 1995;346:310–11.
40. Bowers TR, O'Neill WW, Grines CL, Pica MC, Safian RD, Goldstein JA. Effect of reperfusion on biventricular function and survival after right ventricular infarction. N Engl J Med 1998; 338:933–40.

14

Chronic total occlusion: potentials for serious adverse events

Kenichi Fujii, Etsuo Tsuchikane, Tetsuo Matsubara and Takahiko Suzuki

Coronary perforation • **Dissection and acute closure** • **Radiation-induced skin injury** • **Contrast-induced nephropathy** • **Other complications**

Since the introduction of percutaneous coronary intervention (PCI), revascularization of chronic total occlusion (CTO) has been recognized as a true challenge. The first patients of Andreas Grüntzig with CTO were those whose coronary arteries had silently occluded while waiting for a PCI procedure initiated while the lesions were still patent. Their primary success rate was 62%. Subsequently, patients with documented short, and presumably recent, total occlusions were accepted. Despite remarkable advances in the procedural and clinical outcomes of percutaneous revascularization of CTO,[1-3] the primary success rate was still low, mainly owing to an inability to cross the occlusion with the guidewire.

Procedural success rates have shown only modest improvement in the past 20 years, from 50–60%[4] in the 1980s to 60–70% in the 1990s.[5] Although CTO lesions present in 20–40% of patients with angiographically documented coronary artery disease,[6] revascularization attempts account for less than 8% of all PCI.[7] Moreover, the presence of a CTO was the most common reason for referral to bypass surgery or for persisting with medical therapy. Technical challenges, high restenosis rates, and fears of procedural complication due to the procedural difficulty of the CTO PCIs may contribute to this response to CTO.

Recently, drug-eluting stents releasing sirolimus or paclitaxel have been shown to reduce dramatically the risk of angiographic and clinical restenosis compared with bare metal stents,[8,9] and their efficacy in reducing the incidence of restenosis and the need for further revascularization without increasing the risk of MI or death in CTO applications has been proven.[10,11] However, interventionalists must first be able to recanalize total occlusions before even considering which type of stent to implant. PCI of a CTO is generally considered a low-risk procedure. As shown in Table 14.1, the major acute clinical complication rate of CTO procedures is somewhere between that of diagnostic coronary angiography and that of PCI of nonoccluded lesions.[12-16] Although additional minor complications would cause a slight increase in the overall complication rate, it would still be in the acceptable range. However, major procedural complications may occur more frequently with more aggressive approaches.

Table 14.1   PCI of CTO: acute clinical complications

Series	N	Non Q-MI	Q-MI	CABG	Death	Combined
Stone[5]	905		0.6	0.8	0.8	1.9
Bell[13]	354		1.7	2.5	1.7	5.6
Maiello[14]	365		0.6	1.6	0.3	1.9
Tan[28]	433		0.6	0.6	0	1.2
Noguchi[16]	226		1.3	0	0	1.7
Suero[2]	2007	1.9	0.5	0.7	1.3	3.8
Olivari[3]	376	4.3	0.3	0.5	0.3	5.1

Data are indicated as percentages.
CABG, coronary artery bypass graft; MI, myocardial infarction.

CORONARY PERFORATION

Coronary perforation has been reported in 0.2–0.6% of all patients who undergo PCI[17,18] and has a higher incidence when new atheroablative devices are used.[19,20]

Coronary perforation occurs when a dissection or intimal tear propagates far enough outward to penetrate the arterial wall completely. A significant risk factor for perforation during percutaneous transluminal coronary angioplasty (PTCA) is the balloon-to-artery ratio. Ajluni et al reported that coronary perforations occurred from a measured balloon-to-artery ratio of 1.3±0.3, significantly larger than the ratio for other lesions in which perforation did not occur ($P<0.001$).[17] There are no data reporting that coronary perforation occurs more frequently during CTO procedures than during procedures involving nonoccluded lesions.

Recently, however, new PCI guidewires specifically designed for CTO lesions, which have stiff or tapered tips, have been introduced in order to cross the CTO lesions. Coronary perforation may occur frequently when using these special guidewires in the CTO procedures (Figure 14.1). However, guidewire-induced coronary perforation usually does not have clinical sequelae, and is usually recovered by prolonged balloon inflation with low pressure or reverse of the anticoagulated state. On the other hand, coronary perforation after debulking and stenting is associated with poor clinical outcome. However, in most cases, the perforation involves the distal portion of a vessel and can be managed by various percutaneous techniques, including prolonged balloon inflations (Figure 14.2), placement of covered stents[21] or Gelfoam embolization.[22] For a perforation involving a large proximal vessel, another option is intravascular coil embolization[23] (Figure 14.3). If these percutaneous techniques are suboptimal to manage the perforation, the next therapeutic option is urgent surgical intervention.

DISSECTION AND ACUTE CLOSURE

Coronary dissection and intramural hematoma formation leading to acute coronary closure was one cause of in-hospital major adverse cardiac events. This occurred in 2–10% of elective PCIs in the pre-stent era,[24] usually in the catheterization laboratory or within six hours of case completion. In one report, acute coronary closure within 24 hours of successful angioplasty occurred in 8% of CTO procedures compared with 1.8% of non-CTO procedures, although reocclusion was silent in 87% of cases.[25] In

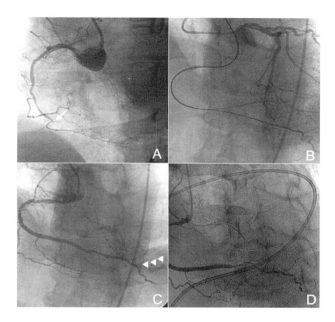

Figure 14.1   Coronary perforation type I. A. Angiogram showed a CTO in the distal RCA (white arrow). B. The tapered-tip guidewires (Conquest Pro 12 and Conquest Pro 20, Asahi Intec, Japan) could be penetrated into the distal true lumen using the parallel wire technique. C. After the deployment of two stents in the mid RCA, angiogram showed coronary perforation with contrast staining of perivascular tissue but no contrast jet in the distal right posterolateral artery (arrowheads). D. This perforation was sealed without any specific management.

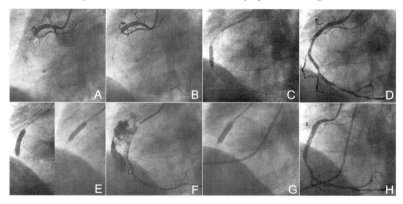

Figure 14.2   Coronary perforation type II. A. Angiogram showed a CTO in the proximal RCA. B. The guidewire could be penetrated into the distal true lumen. C. After predilation using a 1.5 mm PTCA balloon, a 4.0 × 15 mm cutting balloon was inflated to 6 atm. D. Subsequent angiogram showed a type D1 dissection in the mid RCA. E. Two 4.0 mm Bx Velocity stents (Cordis) were deployed in the mid and proximal left anterior descending artery (LAD) to 18 atm. F. Angiogram showed coronary perforation with contrast staining of pericardial tissue and contrast jet. G. Prolonged balloon inflation with the use of a 4.0 × 20 mm perfusion balloon (RX Esprit, Guidant, California) was performed. H. Final angiogram showed complete sealing of the perforation.

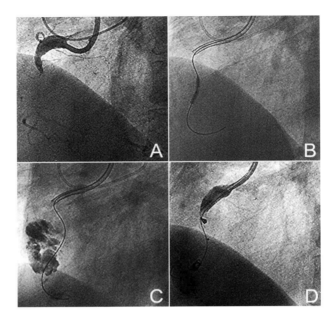

Figure 14.3   Coil embolization for coronary perforation of CTO. A. Angiogram showed a CTO in the proximal RCA. B. After a stiff guidewire (Miracle 12, Asahi Intec) penetrated into the distal lumen, a 2.5 × 15 mm PTCA balloon (Ranger, Boston Scientific) was inflated. C. Angiogram showed coronary perforation with contrast staining of pericardial tissue and contrast jet. D. Because of persistence of the bleeding from the proximal RCA perforation after prolonged balloon inflation and reverse of the anticoagulated drug, a decision was made to proceed with coil embolization at the site of the perforation. Coronary perforation was sealed completely after the coil embolization.

contrast to other devices, stents reduced the incidence of acute coronary closure to less than 1.0%.[26] Although subacute stent thrombosis has been reported to occur within 30 days after stent deployment, the incidence was usually less than 1%, which is lower than that of acute coronary closure after balloon angioplasty. In the stent era, there have been no reports that the incidence of acute coronary closure and stent thrombosis is higher in CTO lesions than in non-CTO lesions.

Risk factors for acute coronary closure

Previous clinical and angiographic studies reported that the most powerful predictor of acute coronary closure is the presence of a complex coronary dissection.[27,28] In the balloon angioplasty era, coronary dissection was detected by angiography in 20–40% of cases[29] and by intravascular ultrasound (IVUS) in 70% of cases.[30] In the stent era, IVUS still detects edge dissection in 10–20% of cases.[31] The mechanism of lumen enlargement after balloon angioplasty is plaque fracture, intimal splitting, and localized dissection. These therapeutic dissections may have the appearance of minor intraluminal radiolucencies. In contrast, complex dissections are characterized by deep medial tears that may create long or spiral dissections. These complex dissections have the angiographic appearance of contrast staining. Complex dissections also expose collagen and tissue factor to circulating platelets and other blood elements, increasing the risk of thrombosis and acute coronary closure.

Prevention of acute coronary closure

Anticoagulation by heparin has been shown to reduce the risk of acute closure after balloon angioplasty.[32] Although bolus intravenous administration of 10,000 units of heparin is widely used for anticoagulation before coronary intervention, this dose results in suboptimal prolongation of the activated clotting time (ACT) in 5% of patients with stable angina and 15% of patients with unstable angina.[33] In addition, procedure time for CTO is relatively longer than that for nonoccluded lesions. Because a low ACT is a powerful predictor of acute coronary closure, repetition of ACT measurements every 30 minutes during the procedure, once a therapeutic ACT has been achieved, is recommended.

A previous study reported that preprocedural administration of aspirin reduces the risk of acute coronary closure by 50%.[34] Although the optimal dose and timing are unknown, elective intervention should be postponed if the patient has not received aspirin for at least one day prior to the procedure. Ticlopidine and clopidogrel may also be administered to reduce the stent thrombosis.

RADIATION-INDUCED SKIN INJURY (FIGURE 14.4)

Radiation doses received by patients during PCI are relatively high, especially in the CTO procedure, compared with those received during diagnostic radiography

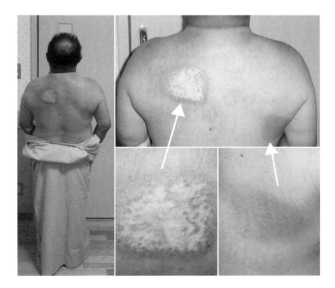

Figure 14.4 Radiation-induced skin injury. A middle-aged man with obesity and two CTO lesions in the RCA and left circumflex artery (LCX) who underwent two PCI and stent placements within three months. Radiation exposure times are unknown; procedure times were 4 hours 15 minutes and 3 hours 55 minutes, respectively. Photograph of left back obtained six months after last PTCA shows area of hyper- and hypopigmentation and skin atrophy.

procedures.[35] Doses from the prolonged use of fluoroscopy can be very high and place the skin at risk for injury. Even though some modern x-ray equipment uses dose-saving measures, such as added filtration and dose-reducing variable-pulsed fluoroscopy, it should be kept in mind that a high dose may produce unacceptable skin damage and should be avoided.[36,37]

Skin injury is a deterministic effect of radiation: once a threshold dose has been exceeded on a portion of the patient's skin, the severity of injury at that point increases with increasing dose.[37] The threshold doses for transient skin injuries are typically 2 Gy for erythema and 3 Gy for hair loss. However, these are arbitrary numbers. The threshold needed to cause injury in a particular patient varies owing to factors that include individual biologic variation in radiation sensitivity and the presence of co-existing diseases such as diabetes mellitus and connective tissue disorders.[38] The injury threshold is also reduced in previously irradiated skin. For these reasons, some patients will show signs of deterministic injury at a relatively low dose. In addition, sensitive patients are likely to experience more severe injury than typical patients at higher doses. The threshold doses for various types of skin injuries are summarized in Table 14.2. A previous study reported that high doses are likely to occur under the following circumstances: fluoroscopy time >60 minutes; gantry positioning unchanged throughout the procedure; and irradiation occurring through a highly attenuating (e.g., bone), thick body mass, requiring a high radiation quality during fluoroscopy and cinematography (>110 kVp).[39]

Minimization of radiation exposure

Dose reduction requires attention to several basic principles, including control of fluoroscopy time, control of the number of images obtained, and control of technical factors that affect dose. Control of fluoroscopic time is the direct responsibility of the operator. Fluoroscopic time can be minimized by means of the judicious use of intermittent fluoroscopy and last-image hold. Control of the number of images obtained during a procedure requires awareness and planning. With modern digital subtraction angiography units, it is a simple matter to set the unit to acquire images at a rate of two or more images per second and then perform the entire angiographic run at that rate.

Although biplane cineangio systems are used by many interventional cardiologists for CTO procedures in order to understand the orientation of the CTO lesions, total

Table 14.2	Threshold skin entrance doses for various skin injuries	
Effect	**Radiation dose (Gy)**	**Onset**
Early transient erythema	2	Hours
Main erythema	6	~10 days
Temporary epilation	3	~3 weeks
Permanent epilation	7	~1 week
Dry desquamation	14	~4 weeks
Moist desquamation	18	~4 weeks
Secondary ulceration	24	>6 weeks
Late erythema	15	~8–10 weeks
Ischemic dermal necrosis	18	>10 weeks

dose can also be minimized through optimization of technical factors. Some of these are under the operator's direct control and can be optimized with any fluoroscopic device. These include maximizing source-to-skin distance, minimizing the air gap between the patient and the image intensifier, and limiting the use of electronic magnification. The assistance of a medical physicist may be required for optimization of other technical factors, including beam filtration, grid removal (when appropriate), and adjustment of fluoroscopic voltage (kVp) and fluoroscopic and digital imaging dose settings. These settings should not be changed in a way that impairs image quality to the point where it is inadequate for diagnosis and guidance of interventions. In addition, changing the position of the radiation field on the patient's skin by using gantry angulation, table movement or both, and collimation use, can reduce the peak skin dose and the area of skin subjected to the peak skin dose.

CONTRAST-INDUCED NEPHROPATHY

Contrast-induced nephropathy is a recognized iatrogenic complication after coronary angiography and intervention that has been associated with prolonged hospitalization and adverse clinical outcomes.[40,41] It is reported that 14.5% of patients develop a 25% increase in serum creatinine levels following cardiac catheterization.[41] Risk factors for contrast-induced nephropathy include pre-existing renal dysfunction, particularly that caused by diabetic nephropathy; congestive heart failure; reduced effective arterial volume; intracardiac injection; and the use of concomitant drugs that impair renal responses, such as angiotensin converting enzyme inhibitors.[42,43] High-dose administration of a contrast agent during the CTO procedure is also recognized as a risk factor for contrast-induced nephropathy. Nonoliguric creatinine elevation peaking within 1–2 days and returning to baseline by seven days is the usual clinical setting of contrast nephrotoxicity. Nonionic contrast agents are associated with less volume overload than ionic agents, but previous studies indicate that they do not decrease the risk of contrast-induced nephropathy.[44]

The clinical outcomes of patients with advanced renal insufficiency undergoing PCI are poor. Previous studies have reported significant higher cumulative one-year mortality and cardiac events in patients with creatinine clearance <30 mL/min (0.5 mL/s) than those with moderate renal disease (25% vs 10%, $P<0.001$).[45]

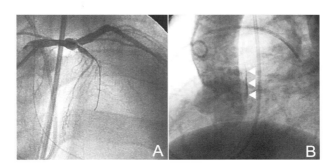

Figure 14.5 Ascending aorta dissection. A. Angiogram showed a CTO in the middle LAD. The guidewire could not get to the distal lumen. B. Aortography showed a dissection (Stanford A) in the ascending aorta wall that might be induced by the guiding catheter (arrowheads).

Prevention of contrast-induced nephropathy

Contrast nephropathy is potentially preventable because the administration of radiocontrast agent is predictable and because high-risk populations have been identified. Hydration with half-normal saline for 12 hours before and after the procedure provides better protection against creatinine rise.[46] Recently, in addition, it was reported that antioxidant acetylcysteine attenuates contrast-induced nephropathy in patients with chronic renal insufficiency undergoing PCI.[47,48] However, other than the use of intravenous hydration and antioxidant acetylcysteine, no previous strategies have been shown convincingly to prevent contrast nephropathy in high-risk patients.

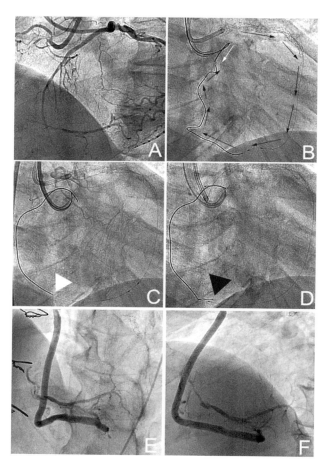

Figure 14.6   Guidewire broken in the collateral artery. A. Angiogram showed a CTO in the proximal RCA. B. Because the guidewire could not get to the distal lumen (white arrow), the retrograde approach technique was performed from the LCX through the collateral artery (black arrow). D. When removal of the guidewire from the LCX was attempted, the guidewire broke and remained in the coronary artery (black arrowhead). E, F. Because retrieval of the guidewire from the coronary artery failed, it was removed surgically.

Diuretics do not protect against contrast-induced nephrotoxicity.[49] Two prospective trials have demonstrated that mannitol also does not reduce contrast nephropathy.[50,51]

OTHER COMPLICATIONS

In general, a support microcatheter is used for back-up during the CTO procedure. Recently, various complex techniques have been introduced to increase the success rate of CTO procedures, including guiding catheter deep engagement, anchor balloon technique, and guidewire retrograde approach. However, these complex techniques may be associated with higher complication rates. Guiding catheter deep engagement can cause left main or ostial right coronary artery (RCA) dissection and intramural hematoma formation, and is also associated with subsequent abrupt vessel closure or ascending aortic dissection (Figure 14.5). The retrograde approach can lead to coronary perforation or breaking of the guidewire or PTCA balloon in the coronary (Figure 14.6), because collaterals are usually bent at their distal portion. Therefore, removal of the guidewire and balloon from the collateral artery must be done with care, especially when these techniques are used.

REFERENCES

1. Warren RJ, Black AJ, Valentine PA, Manolas EG, Hunt D. Coronary angioplasty for chronic total occlusion reduces the need for subsequent coronary bypass surgery. Am Heart J 1990;120:270–4.
2. Suero JA, Marso SP, Jones PG et al. Procedural outcomes and long-term survival among patients undergoing percutaneous coronary intervention of a chronic total occlusion in native coronary arteries: a 20-year experience. J Am Coll Cardiol 2001;38:409–14.
3. Olivari Z, Rubartelli P, Piscione F et al. Immediate results and one-year clinical outcome after percutaneous coronary interventions in chronic total occlusions: data from a multicenter, prospective, observational study (TOAST-GISE). J Am Coll Cardiol 2003;41:1672–8.
4. Ellis SG, Shaw RE, Gershony G et al. Risk factors, time course and treatment effect for restenosis after successful percutaneous transluminal coronary angioplasty of chronic total occlusion. Am J Cardiol 1989;63:897–901.
5. Stone GW, Rutherford BD, McConahay DR et al. Procedural outcome of angioplasty for total coronary artery occlusion: an analysis of 971 lesions in 905 patients. J Am Coll Cardiol 1990;15:849–56.
6. Baim DS, Ignatius EJ. Use of percutaneous transluminal coronary angioplasty: results of a current survey. Am J Cardiol 1988;61:3G–8G.
7. Srinivas VS, Brooks MM, Detre KM et al. Contemporary percutaneous coronary intervention versus balloon angioplasty for multivessel coronary artery disease: a comparison of the National Heart, Lung and Blood Institute Dynamic Registry and the Bypass Angioplasty Revascularization Investigation (BARI) study. Circulation 2002;106:1627–33.
8. Moses JW, Leon MB, Popma JJ et al. Sirolimus-eluting stents versus standard stents in patients with stenosis in a native coronary artery. N Engl J Med 2003;349:1315–23.
9. Stone GW, Ellis SG, Cox DA, et al. A polymer-based, paclitaxel-eluting stent in patients with coronary artery disease. N Engl J Med 2004;350:221–31.
10. Ge L, Iakovou I, Cosgrave J et al. Immediate and mid-term outcomes of sirolimus-eluting stent implantation for chronic total occlusions. Eur Heart J 2005;26:1056–62.
11. Werner GS, Krack A, Schwarz G, Prochnau D, Betge S, Figulla HR. Prevention of lesion recurrence in chronic total coronary occlusions by paclitaxel-eluting stents. J Am Coll Cardiol 2004;44:2301–6.

12. Stone GW, Rutherford BD, McConahay DR et al. Procedural outcome of angioplasty for total coronary artery occlusion: an analysis of 971 lesions in 905 patients. J Am Coll Cardiol 1990;15:849–56.

13. Bell MR, Berger PB, Bresnahan JF, Reeder GS, Bailey KR, Holmes DR Jr. Initial and long-term outcome of 354 patients after coronary balloon angioplasty of total coronary artery occlusions. Circulation 1992;85:1003–11.

14. Maiello L, Colombo A, Gianrossi R et al. Coronary angioplasty of chronic occlusions: factors predictive of procedural success. Am Heart J 1992;124:581–4.

15. Tan KH, Sulke N, Taub NA, Watts E, Karani S, Sowton E. Determinants of success of coronary angioplasty in patients with a chronic total occlusion: a multiple logistic regression model to improve selection of patients. Br Heart J 1993;70:126–31.

16. Noguchi T, Miyazaki S, Morii I, Daikoku S, Goto Y, Nonogi H. Percutaneous transluminal coronary angioplasty of chronic total occlusions. Determinants of primary success and long-term clinical outcome. Cathet Cardiovasc Intervent 2000;49:258–64.

17. Ajluni SC, Glazier S, Blankenship L, O'Neill WW, Safian RD. Perforations after percutaneous coronary interventions: clinical, angiographic, and therapeutic observations. Cathet Cardiovasc Diagn 1994;32:206–12.

18. Topaz O, Cowley MJ, Vetrovec GW. Coronary perforation during angioplasty: angiographic detection and demonstration of complete healing. Cathet Cardiovasc Diagn 1992;27:284–8.

19. Ellis SG, Ajluni S, Arnold AZ et al. Increased coronary perforation in the new device era. Incidence, classification, management, and outcome. Circulation 1994;90:2725–30.

20. van Suylen RJ, Serruys PW, Simpson JB, de Feyter PJ, Strauss BH, Zondervan PE. Delayed rupture of right coronary artery after directional atherectomy for bail-out. Am Heart J 1991;121:914–16.

21. Caputo RP, Amin N, Marvasti M, Wagner S, Levy C, Giambartolomei A. Successful treatment of a saphenous vein graft perforation with an autologous vein-covered stent. Cathet Cardiovasc Intervent 1999;48:382–6.

22. Dixon SR, Webster MW, Ormiston JA, Wattie WJ, Hammett CJ. Gelfoam embolization of a distal coronary artery guidewire perforation. Cathet Cardiovasc Intervent 2000;49:214–17.

23. Mahmud E, Douglas JS Jr. Coil embolization for successful treatment of perforation of chronically occluded proximal coronary artery. Cathet Cardiovasc Intervent 2001;53:549–52.

24. Lincoff AM, Popma JJ, Ellis SG, Hacker JA, Topol EJ. Abrupt vessel closure complicating coronary angioplasty: clinical, angiographic and therapeutic profile. J Am Coll Cardiol 1992;19:926–35.

25. Favereau X, Corcos T, Guerin Y. Early reocclusion after successful coronary angioplasty of chronic total occlusions. J Am Coll Cardiol 1995;25:139A.

26. Carrozza JP Jr, Kuntz RE, Levine MJ et al. Angiographic and clinical outcome of intracoronary stenting: immediate and long-term results from a large single-center experience. J Am Coll Cardiol 1992;20:328–37.

27. Detre KM, Holmes DR Jr, Holubkov R et al. Incidence and consequences of periprocedural occlusion. The 1985–1986 National Heart, Lung, and Blood Institute Percutaneous Transluminal Coronary Angioplasty Registry. Circulation 1990;82:739–50.

28. Tan K, Sulke N, Taub N, Sowton E. Clinical and lesion morphologic determinants of coronary angioplasty success and complications: current experience. J Am Coll Cardiol 1995;25:855–65.

29. Hermans WR, Foley DP, Rensing BJ et al. Usefulness of quantitative and qualitative angiographic lesion morphology, and clinical characteristics in predicting major adverse cardiac events during and after native coronary balloon angioplasty. CARPORT and MERCATOR Study Groups. Am J Cardiol 1993;72:14–20.

30. Kovach JA, Mintz GS, Pichard AD et al. Sequential intravascular ultrasound characterization of the mechanisms of rotational atherectomy and adjunct balloon angioplasty. J Am Coll Cardiol 1993;22:1024–32.

31. Sheris SJ, Canos MR, Weissman NJ. Natural history of intravascular ultrasound-detected edge dissections from coronary stent deployment. Am Heart J 2000;139:59–63.

32. Laskey MA, Deutsch E, Hirshfeld JW Jr, Kussmaul WG, Barnathan E, Laskey WK. Influence of heparin therapy on percutaneous transluminal coronary angioplasty outcome in patients with coronary arterial thrombus. Am J Cardiol 1990;65:179–82.
33. Ogilby JD, Kopelman HA, Klein LW, Agarwal JB. Adequate heparinization during PTCA: assessment using activated clotting times. Cathet Cardiovasc Diagn 1989;18:206–9.
34. Barnathan ES, Schwartz JS, Taylor L et al. Aspirin and dipyridamole in the prevention of acute coronary thrombosis complicating coronary angioplasty. Circulation 1987;76:125–34.
35. Okkalides D, Fotakis M. Patient effective dose resulting from radiographic examinations. Br J Radiol 1994;67:564–72.
36. Shope TB. Radiation-induced skin injuries from fluoroscopy. Radiographics 1996;16:1195–9.
37. Koenig TR, Wolff D, Mettler FA, Wagner LK. Skin injuries from fluoroscopically guided procedures: part 1, characteristics of radiation injury. AJR Am J Roentgenol 2001;177:3–11.
38. Wagner LK, McNeese MD, Marx MV, Siegel EL. Severe skin reactions from interventional fluoroscopy: case report and review of the literature. Radiology 1999;213:773–6.
39. den Boer A, de Feijter PJ, Serruys PW, Roelandt JR. Real-time quantification and display of skin radiation during coronary angiography and intervention. Circulation 2001;104:1779–84.
40. Levy EM, Viscoli CM, Horwitz RI. The effect of acute renal failure on mortality. JAMA 1996;275:1489–94.
41. McCullough P, Wolyn R, Rocher LL, Levin RN, O'Neill WW. Acute renal failure after coronary intervention. Am J Med 1997;103:368–75.
42. Weisberg LS, Kurnik PB, Kurnik BRC. Risk of radiocontrast nephropathy in patients with and without diabetes mellitus. Kidney Int 1994;45:259–65.
43. Barrett BJ. Contrast nephrotoxicity. J Am Soc Nephrol 1994;5:125–37.
44. Davidson CJ, Hlatky M, Morris KG et al. Cardiovascular and renal toxicity of a nonionic radiographic contrast agent after cardiac catheterization: a prospective trial. Ann Intern Med 1989;110:119–24.
45. Best P, Lennon R, Ting H et al. The impact of renal insufficiency on clinical outcomes in patients undergoing percutaneous coronary interventions. J Am Coll Cardiol 2002;39:1113–19.
46. Solomon R, Werner C, Mann D, D'Elia J, Silva P. Effects of saline, mannitol and furosemide on acute decreases in renal function induced by radiocontrast agents. N Engl J Med 1994;331:1416.
47. Kay J, Chow WH, Chan TM et al. Acetylcysteine for prevention of acute deterioration of renal function following elective coronary angiography and intervention: a randomized controlled trial. JAMA 2003;289:553–8.
48. Goldenberg I, Shechter M, Matetzky S et al. Oral acetylcysteine as an adjunct to saline hydration for the prevention of contrast-induced nephropathy following coronary angiography. A randomized controlled trial and review of the current literature. Eur Heart J 2004;25:212–18.
49. Weinstein JM, Heyman S, Brevis M. Potential deleterious effects of furosemide in radiocontrast nephropathy. Nephron 1992;62:413–15.
50. Rudnick M, Goldfarb S, Wexler L et al. Nephrotoxicity of ionic and nonionic contrast media in 1196 patients: a randomized trial. Kidney Int 1995;47:254–61.
51. Stevens MA, McCullough PA, Tobin KJ et al. A prospective randomized trial of prevention measures in patients at high risk for contrast nephropathy. J Am Coll Cardiol 1999;33:403–11.

15

Left main interventions: treatment of serious potential complications

Seung-Jung Park, Young-Hak Kim, Seung-Whan Lee and Seong-Wook Park

Left main dissection during angiography or intervention • **Left main coronary artery spasm: catheter-induced spasm** • **Left main coronary artery perforation** • **Thrombotic occlusion of left main coronary artery during catheter-based procedure** • **Aortocoronary dissection during left main coronary artery intervention** • **Stent loss during stenting procedure** • **Aneurysm or pseudoaneurysm formation after left main coronary artery intervention** • **Mortality related to left main stem disease before the stent era**

The introduction of stents and advances in percutaneous techniques and equipment allow patients with severe narrowing of the left main coronary artery (LMCA) to be safely treated by percutaneous intervention. However, percutaneous intervention on an unprotected left main stem requires careful manipulation of the catheter or device used in the angiography or interventional procedure because occurrence of catheter- or procedure-related complications (including dissection, perforation, and thrombotic occlusion) may culminate in disastrous outcomes. In this chapter, we review the LMCA intervention-related complications and their management.

LEFT MAIN DISSECTION DURING ANGIOGRAPHY OR INTERVENTION

Left main coronary artery dissection is a rare complication during a catheter-based procedure. It is usually the result of injury related to manipulation of the catheter and the coronary artery during an intervention for treatment of a lesion in other vessels. Previous reports have described the incidence of such LMCA dissection as being from 0.03% to 0.1%.[1,2] If prompt action is not taken before development of hemodynamic deterioration, LMCA dissection may result in a fatal outcome. The major risk factors of this life-threatening complication remain to be identified. Reported risk factors include the presence of atherosclerotic obstructive disease in the LMCA and an unusual location or anatomy of the LMCA that necessitates extensive catheter manipulation for entry.[3,4]

Treatment options for this complication include intracoronary stenting and emergency coronary artery bypass grafting (CABG). Although CABG can be successfully performed, prolonged periods of ischemia often culminate in severe left ventricular dysfunction and death. Stent implantation could be the fastest technique to achieve vessel patency and stabilize hemodynamic status in this circumstance. A previous study of ten patients with LMCA dissection demonstrated that all were successfully treated with stent implantation. There was no in-stent restenosis at six-months follow-up, and no major adverse cardiac events during a mean follow-up of 31 ± 25 months.[2] In several case reports of LMCA dissection, intracoronary stent placement has been demonstrated to be effective in repairing major epicardial coronary artery dissection complicating catheter-based procedures.[2,5–7] Thus, prompt stent deployment may be a valuable procedure in patients with LMCA dissection, and may reduce mortality.

LEFT MAIN CORONARY ARTERY SPASM: CATHETER-INDUCED SPASM

Catheter-induced coronary artery spasm may occur during coronary cannulation and angiography. The incidence of spasm (0.26–3%) varies with the type of approach, the catheter used, the skill of the angiographer, and medication received by the patient prior to the procedure.[8–10]

Several local vasoconstrictor mechanisms have been postulated. They include a myogenic stimulus, i.e. mechanical irritation or stress receptor activation,[11] and platelet aggregation at the catheter tip with release of vasoactive agents.[12] While often producing vasodilatation, angiographic dye has also been reported to cause coronary vasoconstriction.[13] Catheter-induced spasm is thought by some researchers to relate to vasospastic angina, since such patients are more likely to have spontaneous spasm.[14,15]

The right coronary artery is usually more prone to catheter-induced spasm than the left coronary artery.[15] Patients with catheter-induced spasm typically demonstrate short, concentric, smooth areas of narrowing just at the location of the catheter tip. Usually there are no associated symptoms or electrocardiographic changes. Administration of nitroglycerin and/or repositioning of the catheter usually leads to prompt resolution of the spasm.[16] Very rarely, the spasm may be prolonged.[17,18]

Interventional cardiologists should always keep this phenomenon in mind during every procedure, in order to avoid misdiagnosing the spasm as a fixed stenosis, and thereby preventing an unnecessary intervention.

LEFT MAIN CORONARY ARTERY PERFORATION

There are few data available regarding perforation of the LMCA. However, it could be possible because of the expanded use of stents in LMCA interventions. Perforation in other coronary arteries, with an incidence of 0.1%, has usually been associated with high-pressure post-stenting dilatation to achieve optimal stent expansion.[19] Previous studies have shown that high-pressure dilatation using appropriately sized balloons (balloon-to-artery ratio, 1.1) was safe, but that the use of oversized balloons (balloon-to-artery ratio, ≥1.2) carried a 1.2% risk of perforation and vessel rupture.[20] Although small perforations can be successfully managed with prolonged balloon dilatation and reversal of heparin anticoagulation with protamine, larger perforations may require emergency bypass surgery or a covered stent. If cardiac tamponade follows perforation, emergency pericardiocentesis may be needed. These findings in other coronary artery interventions may be extrapolated to interventions in the LMCA, but the relatively large size of the LMCA may offer a protective effect for high-pressure balloon dilatation. Only one case report describing LMCA perforation after stenting, followed by large pseudoaneurysm formation, has been published.[21] However, interventional cardiologists should be aware of this complication that may occur during adjunctive high-pressure dilatation.

THROMBOTIC OCCLUSION OF LEFT MAIN CORONARY ARTERY DURING CATHETER-BASED PROCEDURE

Thrombus formation in the LMCA during coronary angiography or during intervention procedures in other coronary arteries has rarely occurred. To our knowledge, there were only a few case reports regarding thrombus formation associated with intervention for other coronary vessel disease[22] or angiography.[23] These thrombotic complications are one of the more common causes of abrupt closure of the LMCA, which may end fatally if prompt action is not taken.

The most plausible explanation of thrombus formation in the LMCA during angiography is that the deposition of platelets and fibrin, even in heparinized patients, can occur in the catheter and arterial sheath. This may occlude the LMCA during angiography or during catheter exchange with a guidewire, although co-existing circumstance, such as the use of nonionic contrast dyes or a transient hypercoagulable state, might also have an influence. Careful technique and precautions are probably the most effective preventive measures. These include shortening the procedure time as much as possible; avoiding guidewires for catheter exchange; flushing catheters away from coronary ostia; not allowing contrast media and blood to remain stagnant together in catheters or syringes; and flushing the side arm of the arterial sheath before any new catheter is inserted.

During an intervention in other coronary arteries, the cardiologist should also be careful to avoid damage of the LMCA due to a traumatic intimal tear by the balloon, stent or guidewire, which are the most plausible causes of LMCA thrombosis formation. The balloon catheter pulling back the initial thrombus inside the original lesion (other than the LMCA) is another possible source of thrombotic occlusion of the LMCA during an intervention. Therefore, occurrence of intracoronary thrombi should be checked before every percutaneous coronary intervention. It should also be kept in mind that thrombus formation after balloon angioplasty is a possible complication even during antiplatelet therapy, including heparin and glycoprotein IIb/IIIa receptor blockers, and an acute coronary arterial closure can develop during the stenting procedures.

Thrombotic occlusion of the LMCA can occur during catheter-based procedures, caused by several factors, and can result in a fatal complication. Treatment options for this complication include intracoronary thrombolysis; angioplasty with a coronary stent, using aggressive antiplatelet aggregation drugs; emergency bypass surgery; and intracoronary transcatheter aspiration,[24,25] which may be life-saving. Therefore, prompt recognition of this complication and appropriate and rapid treatment are very important during any catheter-based procedure.

AORTOCORONARY DISSECTION DURING LEFT MAIN CORONARY ARTERY INTERVENTION

Coronary artery dissection is a well-recognized complication of angioplasty. However, aortic dissection has rarely been reported, with an incidence of 0.02% for coronary angiography and 0.07% for coronary angioplasty.[26] Such dissection usually is accompanied by LMCA or right coronary artery ostial dissection, a potentially life-threatening complication.

The primary mechanism of aortic dissection during coronary artery manipulation remains unclear. A previously published study suggested that forceful manipulation of the catheter may be the trigger for coronary dissection, resulting in aortic dissection.[27] Anatomically, the entry point of aortic dissection originates within the coronary artery dissection and leads to progressive retrograde dispersion of the subintimal space into the aortic root.[28] Another study reported that aortic dissection usually developed in the setting of acute myocardial infarction (AMI).[29] However, the relationship between development of aortic dissection and AMI needs to be further defined.

One of the above studies suggested that sealing of the entry point within the LMCA by stent implantation was effective management for aortic dissection.[28] In some cases, a covered stent might be another useful option if the entry point is not occluded by the stent implantation.

Dunning et al classified coronary dissection with retrograde aortic root dissection according to the extent of aortic involvement by dissection.[29] Class 1 was defined as a focal dissection restricted to the coronary cusp; Class 2 extends up the aorta but is less than 40 mm long. Class 3 is the most extensive dissection, extending from the coronary cusp up the ascending aorta more than 40 mm. These authors suggested that the best treatment in Class 1 and Class 2 dissection was stenting of the intracoronary entry point when possible, and close clinical follow-up. Class 3 dissection usually requires an open surgical approach. They also showed that most patients with Class 1 or 2 dissections were successfully managed with intracoronary stenting. Therefore, in Class 1 and 2 dissections, imaging studies usually were not required except in unstable patients; progression of the dissection after index stenting is unlikely. However, in Class 3 cases, the patients undergoing surgery sometimes died.

Dissection into the aorta is an exceedingly rare but potentially fatal complication of coronary angiography and coronary intervention. It is usually associated with coronary dissection, with communication via the entry point in the coronary artery; therefore, the interventional cardiologist should not hesitate to insert a stent at the entry point of coronary dissection, especially in patients with limited aortic involvement. It may reduce the mortality of the complication.

STENT LOSS DURING STENTING PROCEDURE

Stent loss during the stenting procedure is an infrequent but potentially harmful complication, which might result from the inability to cross the target lesion with the stent. Previous clinical studies have described the incidence of stent loss as 0.9–8.4% during treatment for all coronary interventions.[30-35] Bolte et al reported that the incidence of stent loss or stent embolization during LMCA intervention (5.8%) was higher than that during other coronary artery interventions (LAD 1.4%, LCX 2.3%, RCA 2.2%, graft vessel 2.4%).[35] The higher prevalence of stent loss during LMCA intervention is partially explained by the weak position of the guiding catheter in the LMCA ostium, thereby providing insufficient back-up support.

Stent loss during LMCA intervention usually results in systemic embolization. The site of stent embolization is a clinically important issue because systemically embolized stents may produce symptoms of arterial insufficiency, depending on the embolized site. The most common systemic embolization sites are femoral artery 92%, brachial artery 6%, and radial artery 0.5%.[35] Uncommonly, involvement of the vertebral artery,[35] tibial artery,[36] renal artery,[31] and mitral valve leaflet[35] has been reported. Bolte et al[35] and Alfonso et al[29] reported that, in contrast to intracoronary stent embolization, extracoronary stent embolization did not cause a serious ischemic symptom even if the lost stent could not be retrieved. But there has been a case report showing that a stent lodged in the right posterior tibial artery caused subsequent vascular insufficiency and required a surgical approach for stent retrieval.[36] Therefore, if stent dislodgment and embolization occur, interventional cardiologists must make an effort to document and retrieve the lost stent. Unfortunately, previous studies have reported that the exact embolization site could be documented in only 55–65% of all lost stents.[29,35] Among those, about 50% of the systemically embolized stents could be retrieved with a snaring device.

In summary, although extracoronary stent embolization during LMCA intervention is an uncommon complication and has a relatively benign prognosis, every effort should be made to find and retrieve the lost stent, even if it is not possible to observe whether or not it produces vascular insufficiency.

ANEURYSM OR PSEUDOANEURYSM FORMATION AFTER LEFT MAIN CORONARY ARTERY INTERVENTION

Coronary aneurysms other than LMCA have been reported to occur in 3.9–7.0% of cases after balloon angioplasty, 3.9% after stenting, and 10% after directional atherectomy.[37,38] It is known that postintervention coronary aneurysms are the result of coronary injury, weakening, and stretching of the arterial wall.[38] However, to our knowledge, there are no data regarding occurrence of aneurysms related to LMCA intervention. There is only one case report describing large pseudoaneurysm formation following LMCA perforation after stenting, which was successfully managed with a covered stent.[39] In coronary beds, pseudoaneurysm formation following perforation or dissection even after stenting has been reported.[21,40,41] The covered stent has been shown to be a valuable therapeutic strategy to seal the perforation and prevent aneurysms. Therefore, in this unexpected situation, the immediate use of a covered stent should be considered.

MORTALITY RELATED TO LEFT MAIN STEM DISEASE BEFORE THE STENT ERA

The mortality rate related to diagnostic cardiac catheterization in patients with left main stem disease has ranged from 0.7% to 1.6%,[42,43] significantly higher than that for any of the other coronary anatomy subgroups (0% to 0.068%).[40] The mechanisms of death due to procedures involving left main disease include catheter-induced spasm, thrombus, and dissection. One study reported that 90% of deaths associated with left main stem disease were related to left main dissection, in 93% of which the catheter tip abutted the lesion on the first injection.[43] Gordon et al showed that the end of catheter to lesion distance was the only procedural predictor that correlated with complications. They found that when this distance was 6 mm or less the complication rate was 24% but it was only 3% when more than 6 mm.[44]

A previous study demonstrated that in most cases with procedural deaths related to left main disease, the initial view chosen was inappropriate for visualization of the left main stem and ostium, which could be well identified in LAO, straight AP or angulated AP view. The end of the catheter contacted the left main lesion on the first injection and as a result, dissection and occlusion occurred.[43] Thus, careful technique that reduced risk included initial nonselective injection of the ostium in a LAO view; co-axial positioning of the catheter in the left main stem trunk; a shallow oblique projection for visualization of the entire left main stem, and for identification of the distance between the end of the catheter and a lesion; a limited number of injections; and a larger catheter to delineate the ostial lesion or to reduce the ostial damage due to deep seating of the catheter into a diseased left main stem.

Nowadays, these unexpected catastrophic conditions may be remedied by the prompt use of stents. However, preventing such complications is the best treatment strategy.

REFERENCES

1. Cameron J. Left main coronary artery dissection during coronary angioplasty or angiography treated by stent insertion without requirement for emergency bypass graft surgery. Aus NZ J Med 2000;20:726–8.
2. Lee SW, Hong MK, Kim YH et al. Bail-out stenting for left main coronary artery dissection during catheter-based procedure: acute and long-term results. Clin Cardiol 2004;27:393–5.
3. Slack JD, Pinkerton CA, van Tassel JW, Orr CM. Left main coronary artery dissection during percutaneous coronary angioplasty. Cathet Cardiovasc Diagn 1986;12:255–60.
4. Kovac JD, de Bono DP. Cardiac catheter complications related to left main stem disease. Heart 1996;76:76–8.
5. Garcia-Robles JA, Garcia E, Rico M, Esteban E, de Prado AP, Delcan JL. Emergency coronary stenting for acute occlusive dissection of left main coronary artery. Cathet Cardiovasc Diagn 1993;30:227–9.
6. Al-Saif SM, Liu MW, Al-Mubarak N, Agrawal S, Dean LS. Percutaneous treatment of catheter-induced dissection of the left main coronary artery and adjacent aortic wall: a case report. Cathet Cardiovasc Intervent 2000;49:86–9.
7. Connors JP, Thnavaro S, Shaw RC, Sandza JG, Ludbrook PA, Krone RJ. Urgent myocardial revascularization for dissection of the left main coronary artery. J Thorac Cardiovasc Surg 1982;84:349–52.
8. Gensini GG. Coronary artery spasm and angina pectoris. Chest 1975;68:709–13.
9. Lafia P, Dincer B. Coronary artery catheter-induced spasm. Cathet Cardiovasc Diagn 1982;8:607–10.
10. Demany A. Editorial: coronary artery spasm. Cathet Cardiovasc Diagn 1982;8:610–11.
11. Heijman J, El Gamal M, Rolf M. Catheter induced spasm in aortocoronary vein grafts. Br Heart J 1983;49:30–2.
12. Chierchia S. Pathogenetic mechanism of coronary vasospasm. Acta Med Scand 1982;660(Suppl):49–56.
13. Dodeck A, Hooper RO. Coronary spasm provoked by angiography. Am Heart J 1984;107:781–4.
14. MacAlpin RN. Relation of coronary arterial spasm to sites of organic stenosis. Am J Cardiol 1980;46:143–53.
15. Mautner RK, Cooper MD, Phillips JH. Catheter-induced coronary artery spasm: an angiographic manifestation of vasospastic angina? Am Heart J 1983;106:659–65.
16. Friedman AC, Spindola-Franco H, Nivatpumin T. Coronary spasm: Prinzmetal's variant angina vs. catheter-induced spasm; refractory spasm vs. fixed stenosis. Am J Radiol 1979;132:897–904.
17. Murphy ES, Rosch J, Boicourt W, Rahimtoola SH. Left main coronary artery spasm. Arch Intern Med 1976;136:350–1.
18. Gaspardone A, Tomai F, De-Peppo AP, Chiarfiello L, Gioffre PA. Prolonged asymptomatic catheter-induced left and right coronary artery spasm resistant to high dose of intracoronary nitroglycerin. Cardiologia 1992;37:701–4.

19. Ellis SG, Ajluni S, Arnold AZ et al. Increased coronary perforation in the new device era: incidence, classification, management and outcome. Circulation 1994;90:2725–30.
20. Colombo A, Hall P, Nakamura S et al. Intracoronary stenting without anticoagulation accomplished with intravascular guidance. Circulation 1995;91:1676–88.
21. Nameki M, Ishiwata S, Momomura SI. Large pseudoaneurysm after left main trunk stenting sealed by polytetrafluoroethylene-covered stent. Cathet Cardiovasc Intervent 2003;60:233–5.
22. Sanz AJ, Hernandez F, Tasco JC. Thrombotic occlusion of the left main coronary artery during coronary angiography. J Invasive Cardiol 2002;14:426–9.
23. Gunduz H, Akdemir R, Arine H, Ozhan H, Tamer A, Uyan C. Iatrogenic left main coronary artery thrombosis during percutaneous coronary intervention. Int J Cardiol 2005;102:345–7.
24. Shani J, Abittan M, Galarello F, Frankel R. Mechanical manipulation of thrombus: coronary thrombectomy, intracoronary clot displacement, and transcatheter aspiration. Am J Cardiol 1993;72:116–18.
25. Satyavan J. Management of left main coronary artery stenosis. Int J Cardiol 2003;2:6–12.
26. Vega MR. Aortic dissection: exceedingly rare complicating coronary intervention. Cathet Cardiovasc Diagn 1997;42:416.
27. Oda H, Hatada K, Sakai K, Takahasi K, Miida T, Higuma N. Aortocoronary dissection resolved by coronary stenting guided by intracoronary ultrasound. Circ J 2004;68:389–91.
28. Al-saif SM, Liu MW, Al-Mubarak N, Agrawal S, Dean LS. Percutaneous treatment of catheter induced dissection of the left main coronary artery and adjacent aortic wall: a case report. Cathet Cardiovasc Intervent 2000;49:86–9.
29. Dunning DW, Kahn JK, Hawkins ET, O'Neill WW. Iatrogenic coronary artery dissection extending into and involving the aortic root. Cathet Cardiovasc Intervent 2000;51:387–93.
30. Schatz RA, Baim DS, Leon M et al. Clinical experience with Palmaz-Schatz coronary stents. Initial results of a multicenter study. Circulation 1991;83:148–61.
31. Alfonso F, Martinez D, Hernandez R et al. Stent embolization during intracoronary stenting. Am J Cardiol 1996;78:833–5.
32. Elsner M, Pfeifer A, Kasper W. Intracoronary loss of balloon-mounted stents: successful retrieval with a 2 mm-'Microsnare-Device.' Cathet Cardiovasc Diagn 1996;39:271–6.
33. Cantor WJ, Lazzam C, Cohen EA et al. Failed coronary stent deployment. Am Heart J 1998;136:1088–95.
34. Eggebrecht H, Haude M, von Birgeler C et al. Nonsurgical retrieval of embolized coronary stents. Cathet Cardiovasc Diagn 2000;51:432–40.
35. Bolte J, Neumann U, Pfafferott C et al, Arbeitsgemeinschaft Leitende Kardiologische Krankenhausartze (ALKK). Incidence, management, and outcome of stent loss during intracoronary stenting. Am J Cardiol 2001;88:565–7.
36. Nguyen AH, Khan AA, Chait A, Fallahnejad M. The wandering coronary stent. J Cardiovasc Surg 1998;39:807–9.
37. Slota PA, Fishman DL, Savage MP, Rake R, Goldberg S. Frequency and outcome of development of coronary artery aneurysm after intracoronary stent placement and angioplasty: STRESS trial invastigators. J Am Coll Cardiol 1997;79:1104–6.
38. Bell MR, Garratt KN, Bresnahan JF, Edwards WD, Holmes DR. Relation of deep arterial resection and coronary artery aneurysm after directional coronary atherectomy. J Am Coll Cardiol 1992;20:1474–81.
39. Cafri C, Gilutz H, Kobal S et al. Rapid evolution from coronary dissection to pseudoaneurysm after stent implantation: a glimpse at the pathogenesis using intravascular ultrasound. J Invasive Cardiol 2002;14:286–9.
40. Briguori C, Nishida T, Anzuini A, Mario CD, Grube E, Colombo A. Emergency polytetrafluoroethylene-covered stent implantation to treat coronary ruptures. Circulation 2000;102:3028–31.
41. Briguori C, Sarais C, Sivieri G, Takagi T, Mario CD, Colombo A. Polytetrafluoroethylene-covered stent and coronary artery aneurysms. Cathet Cardiovasc Intervent 2002;55:326–30.
42. Kovac JD, de Bono DP. Cardiac catheter complications related to left main stem disease. Heart 1996;76:76–8.

43. Devlin GD, Lazzam L, Schwartz L. Mortality related to diagnostic cardiac catheterization. Int J Cardiac Imag 1997;13:379–84.
44. Gordon PR, Abrams C, Gash AK, Carabello BA. Precatheterization risk factors in the left main coronary artery stenosis. Am J Cardiol 1987;59:1080–3.

16

Specific concerns to improve the safety of drug-eluting stents

Alexandre Abizaid, Vinicius Daher, Jose de Ribamar Costa Jr and J Eduardo Sousa

Patient preparation • Lesion type and stent implantation technique • Duration of adjunctive medical therapy, stent thrombosis, and other aspects of drug-eluting stent usage • Drug-eluting stent selection

According to recent reports, nearly two million percutaneous coronary interventions (PCI) are performed annually worldwide. The most significant reason for this extensive implementation of PCI was, unquestionably, the introduction of coronary stents for the treatment of obstructive coronary artery disease. However, in-stent restenosis, with overall rates ranging from 8% to as high as 80% (in high-risk populations), has been the Achilles heel of interventional cardiology ever since stents were first used, more than 15 years ago.[1,2]

The emergence of drug-eluting stents (DES) has revolutionized the field of interventional cardiology by showing remarkable in-stent neo-intimal suppression and reducing restenosis rates to less than 10% across a wide spectrum of clinical and angiographic subsets.[3-6] With over 1.5 million Cypher stents and 1.0 million Taxus stents implanted worldwide since 2000, the safety profile of DES has been extensively demonstrated. However, only five years have past since they were first available for use in humans, and a number of concerns and questions remain without a definite answer.

Drug-eluting stents are devices that release into the bloodstream single or multiple active agents which can deposit in or affect tissues adjacent to the stent. Usually, the drug is embedded and released through a polymer linked to the surface of the stent. Although an assortment of drugs have been proven to be effective in reducing neo-intimal proliferation, only sirolimus- (Cypher™, Cordis Corp, Johnson & Johnson, Warren, NJ, USA) and paclitaxel-eluting stents (Taxus™, Boston Scientific, Natick, MA, USA) have been clinically and market approved and will be discussed here. Since the only two characteristics that differentiate bare metal stents (BMS) and DES are the presence of an embedded drug and a coating polymer, any new and unexpected adverse events should be linked to these two variables.

In the present chapter, we focus on issues related to these two DES, from patient selection and preparation to long-term adjunctive medical therapy, trying to establish practical recommendations to improve their safe use in a 'real-world' scenario.

PATIENT PREPARATION

Ever since the early balloon angioplasty, aspirin has proven to be effective in reducing the risk of abrupt coronary occlusion by 50–75% and has become an essential medicine for use before the procedure and lifelong following revascularization.[7] The optimal dose and timing of aspirin have yet to be established but typically, patients should take 75–325 mg at least one day before elective procedures, or 325–500 mg chewable aspirin at the time of urgent procedures. Higher doses of aspirin have not been shown to be more effective and have been associated with higher risk of bleeding.[8]

The addition of an adenosine diphosphate (ADP) P2Y$_{12}$ receptor antagonist (thienopyridines) to aspirin as the standard anticoagulation therapy has been shown to offer patients even greater protection against thrombotic complications following stent implantation. Both ticlopidine and clopidogrel have been demonstrated to be effective in reducing subacute thrombotic complications after stent placement to rates lower than 1%.[9]

Several randomized trials have demonstrated the benefit of ticlopidine plus aspirin over other anticoagulation therapies. However, as the onset of ticlopidine action ranges between 48 and 72 hours and full effect is evident only in 5–7 days, it should be administered at least three days prior to intervention to maximize its antiplatelet effect. A loading dose of 500 mg improves antiplatelet effects and may add some benefit in urgent situations.

Clopidogrel is another thienopyridine that has proven to be as effective as its analogue, ticlopidine, but with faster onset of action, longer half-life, and fewer collateral effects. For these reasons, the association of clopidogrel and aspirin before stent placement has been widely investigated and has largely replaced ticlopidine worldwide. The outstanding results of the aspirin/clopidogrel combination in the randomized clinical trial CLASSICS helped to set them as the first-line regimen following percutaneous intervention with BMS implantation,[9] although in this study a loading dose of 300 mg of clopidogrel was not shown to have superiority over a single dose of 75 mg. Several recent studies have investigated this issue. For instance, the CREDO trial showed a time dependence in the clinical benefit of a 300 mg clopidogrel loading dose before PCI, as ischemic adverse events were reduced only in the prespecified subgroup pretreated for at least six hours before the procedure.[10] Furthermore, an *ad hoc* analysis of the CREDO trial suggested benefit only in the subgroup of patients who received the loading dose 15 hours before the procedure.[11]

Recently, *in vitro* studies have suggested that a 600 mg loading dose of clopidogrel accelerates inhibition of platelet aggregation, when compared with 300 mg of clopidogrel, leading to two innovative clinical trials testing this higher loading dose of clopidogrel in humans.[12,13] The ISAR-REACT study has shown that in patients who undergo elective PCI, adding a glycoprotein IIb/IIIa inhibitor (abciximab) to a 600 mg loading dose of clopidogrel at least two hours before PCI was associated with no clinical benefit within 30 days.[14] In addition, a 600 mg loading dose of clopidogrel was safe, without higher bleeding complications. Moreover, the same benefit was observed whether patients had received the loading dose 2–3 hours, 3–6 hours, 6–12 hours or >12 hours before the procedure. Another landmark study, the ARMYDA-2, randomized 255 patients to a 600 mg or 300 mg loading regimen of clopidogrel given six hours before the procedure.[15] Pretreatment with a 600 mg loading dose was safe and showed a 50% risk reduction of periprocedural myocardial infarction, when compared with a 300 mg loading dose.

In light of these findings, it seems reasonable to recommend pretreatment of elective PCI patients with at least a 300 mg loading dose of clopidogrel 24 hours before the procedure. Patients who could not be pretreated with this thienopyridine should receive a 600 mg loading dose of clopidogrel at least two hours before the PCI. Aspirin should ideally be given preintervention (75–325 mg) and patients should be encouraged to take it indefinitely.

We must emphasize that preprocedure treatment for DES implantation requires no further specific medications other than the standard antiplatelet regimen adopted for BMS since several trials have shown that DES do not increase the risk of subacute stent thrombosis in patients under appropriate antiplatelet therapy (Table 16.1).

LESION TYPE AND STENT IMPLANTATION TECHNIQUE

In the BMS era, stent thrombosis rate was estimated to be around 1%, varying among published reports from only 0.2% with IVUS-guided stent deployment up to 2.8% after multiple stent deployment and/or treatment of complex lesions.[16,17] Its occurrence was almost exclusively acute (within 48 hours of the procedure) or subacute (any time between the second and the 30th day of the baseline procedure).

In a recent pooled analysis of ten randomized trials, Moreno et al reported no difference in the incidence of this complication among patients treated with BMS and either sirolimus or paclitaxel DES.[18] The overall rate of stent thrombosis remained below 1% for bare metal and drug-eluting stents. Nevertheless, considering the increasingly complex milieu of PCI in the DES era, and adding to this the highly deliverable devices and better metal stent profile available, that can extend farther into lesion settings, we are beginning to treat even more complex lesions. Hence, we are including in our daily practice more total occlusions, vein graft disease, multivessel and left main disease, bifurcations, in-stent restenosis, very long and

Table 16.1 Studies with bare metal stents (BMS), sirolimus-eluting stents (SES) and paclitaxel-eluting stents (PES) and the subacute stent thrombosis incidence (<30 days)

Study	Year	N	BMS	Stent thrombosis (%)	
				SES	PES
Wang et al[33]	2002	1191	0.92	–	–
Wenaweser et al[34]	2004	6058	1.17	–	–
RAVEL	2002	238	0	0	–
SIRIUS	2003	1058	0.19	0.18	–
E-SIRIUS	2003	352	0	1.1	–
C-SIRIUS	2004	100	0	2.0	–
TAXUS II	2003	536	0	–	0.35
TAXUS IV	2004	1314	0.8	–	0.6
Bavry et al[19]	2005	3817	0.76	–	0.75
T-SEARCH	2005	1084	–	0.4	1.0
TAXI	2005	202	–	0	0
SIRTAX	2005	1012	–	2.0	1.6
Iakouvou et al[21]	2005	2229	–	0.4	0.8
Ong et al[28]	2005	2512	1.2	1.0	1.0
Moreno et al[18]	2005	5030	0.54	0.58	0.57
Mean			**0.50**	**0.76**	**0.74**

ostial lesions, very small vessels, and diabetics. Besides, some clinical features (e.g. premature antiplatelet therapy discontinuation, renal failure, diabetes, and lower ejection fraction) have also been identified as independent predictors of DES thrombosis. In summary, we are treating more complex lesions which have naturally and independently posed a higher risk of stent thrombosis.[18,19]

Long lesions

The initial DES reports have encouraged operators to deploy longer stents (from 'normal' to 'normal' reference) to avoid the so-called 'edge restenosis'. However, lately, the relationship between longer stents and/or multiple overlapping stents for the treatment of long lesions and the increasing rates of adverse events (especially higher incidence of periprocedure non Q-wave myocardial infarction and, mainly, higher rates of stent thrombosis) has turned the current practice towards rationalizing the stent length.[20,21] This fact may be related to the risk of compromising the flow in numerous side branches and the higher risk of debris embolization. However, it is worth noting that most of these data are based on subanalysis of general studies not designed to assess this particular subject (see Table 16.1). A more liberal administration of GP IIb/IIIa inhibitors as well as a high-quality pretreatment with clopidogrel could reduce the incidence of this complication, although further consideration on this topic is still required.

Bifurcations

Generally, and more consensually, the risks of acute and subacute complications are higher when treating bifurcation lesions, especially when both main and side branch are treated with stents (Table 16.2). Stent thrombosis was as high as 4.4% following the 'crush' technique and 3.5% after the T-stenting or V-stenting technique, with an average of 3.9% in a large cohort of patients where all techniques were employed.[22–24] Final kissing balloon post dilatation following the 'crush' technique might be essential to optimize sustained stent patency, but it has not been proven to reduce thrombotic complications. Furthermore, an IVUS analysis has observed incomplete apposition of stent struts against the vessel wall in the area of the crush, and it is worth noting that this was independent of final kissing balloon dilatation and was clinically associated with a higher rate of stent thrombosis.[25]

   Although double DES deployment (main and side branch) for the treatment of bifurcation disease might decrease restenosis rates, this benefit is achieved at the expense of higher stent thrombosis risk. In this circumstance, sustained dual

Table 16.2 Bifurcation lesions and stent thrombosis					
Study	**Year**	**N**	**Technique**	**Stent thrombosis (%)**	
				BMS	**DES**
Colombo et al[22]	2004	63	Double-stent	–	6.3
Ge et al[24]	2005	181	'Crush'	–	4.4
Costa et al[25]	2005	40	'Crush'	–	2.5
Lefevre et al[44]	2005	105	Dedicated stent	0	–

antiplatelet therapy should be strongly advised. The role of GP IIb/IIIa inhibitors in this scenario is not completely elucidated and therefore they should not be recommended as mandatory adjunctive therapy.

Conversely, the implantation of a DES at the main vessel with provisional stent at the side branch is generally safe and most of the time effective; however, this is not feasible in many cases. Almost half of these patients require another stent at the side branch to achieve a good final angiographic result (due to significant residual lesion after balloon angioplasty and/or presence of flow-compromising dissection at the site of the dilatation). The best technique and pharmacologic approach for the treatment of bifurcations with DES are yet to be defined.

Diabetics

Diabetes has naturally been linked to microvascular, metabolic, platelet, and endothelial abnormalities, resulting in higher incidence of thrombosis, myocardial infarction, and death post PCI. Compared to BMS, DES have markedly reduced restenosis and target lesion revascularization in this population; however, major adverse cardiac events (e.g. death and myocardial infarction) remain an important issue among these patients.[26–28] In almost all studies with DES, the rates of major adverse events remain higher in diabetics than in nondiabetics, especially in the subset of patients requiring insulin therapy. To a certain extent, this may be linked to the higher risk of stent thrombosis, especially subacute stent thrombosis, consistently observed in large registries and in one meta-analysis. Nonetheless, it seems not to differ from the incidence of stent thrombosis in the diabetic population treated with BMS. Yet aggressive medical management in diabetics (glucose control, lipid management) should be emphasized to reduce postintervention major cardiac events (MACE). In addition, aggressive platelet inhibition during and post PCI (including GP IIb/IIIa inhibitors) should also be encouraged.

Chronic renal failure

Renal failure has been linked to an increased cardiac mortality rate despite successful revascularization. Recently, it has been related to higher rates of stent thrombosis. In one meta-analysis, renal failure was one of the most important independent predictors of subacute DES thrombosis.[21] This issue is of great concern if we take into account the increasing number of patients with renal failure who undergo PCI. Nevertheless, at present, little can be done to improve the outcome of these patients.

Other complex lesions

The remaining subset of complex lesions, such as those located at the ostial portion of the coronaries and in very small vessels, left main and saphenous vein graft disease, chronic total occlusion and in-stent restenosis, have not clearly been linked to an increase in the risk of DES thrombosis.

Hence, final good stent implantation (balloon-to-artery ratio at least 1:1), optimized, if necessary, with intravascular ultrasound-guided postdilatations (especially when treating left main and bifurcations); full lesion and dissection coverage; and careful inspection of the final result, trying to avoid these abnormalities, might also help to reduce the incidence of acute and subacute stent thrombosis.

DURATION OF ADJUNCTIVE MEDICAL THERAPY, STENT THROMBOSIS, AND OTHER ASPECTS OF DRUG-ELUTING STENT USAGE

Sirolimus- and paclitaxel-eluting stents differ in their drug release kinetics. While most of the sirolimus in the Cypher has eluted by six weeks, leaving the polymer-coated BMS, in the Taxus Express 2 only 10% of the paclitaxel is released by ten days and the rest remains in the polymer indefinitely. Based on the drug release kinetics and the design of pivotal clinical trials, dual antiplatelet therapy is recommended empirically for three months after Cypher implantation, and for six months after Taxus implantation, with life-long aspirin.

Recently a few reports, including angiographic documentation of DES late thrombosis (both sirolimus and paclitaxel), have drawn our attention to very late thrombosis after DES deployment, with special concern about those cases happening after cessation of the recommended dual antiplatelet regimen[29-32] (Table 16.3). In one large registry with sirolimus- and paclitaxel-eluting stents, early stent thrombosis occurred in 1.0%, while late angiographically proven stent thrombosis happened in 0.35%.[31] In some of them, late stent thrombosis occurred shortly after the completion of the prescribed course of clopidogrel (21–28 days). In others, who were on aspirin therapy, the events occurred late (8–23 months) after clopidogrel cessation. A few events occurred in patients who were on monotherapy with aspirin and shortly (5–7 days) after its discontinuation.

Due to the shortage of reports, it is difficult to compare the incidence of late DES thrombosis with those from BMS.[33,34] Although late BMS thrombosis was not a major concern in the pre-DES era, one single-center registry with 1191 patients treated with BMS reported nine cases of late (>30 days) stent thrombosis (0.76%), an incidence similar to the late DES thrombosis incidence related just above.[33] Therefore, until large-scale registries comparing both stents are available, we should not assume that late DES thrombosis happens more or less than with BMS.

Although the mechanisms behind the acute and subacute stent thrombosis after BMS and DES are very similar[35,36] (e.g. stent underexpansion, alone or in association with stent malapposition, inflow/outflow residual disease, residual dissection and thrombus, etc.), the reasons for late stent thrombosis in the DES population remain

Table 16.3 Studies with bare metal stents (BMS), sirolimus-eluting stents (SES) and paclitaxel-eluting stents (PES) and the late stent thrombosis incidence (>30 days)

Study	Year	N	BMS	Late stent thrombosis (%)	
				SES	PES
Wang et al[33]	2002	1191	0.76	–	–
Wenaweser et al[34]	2004	6058	0.39	–	–
RAVEL	2002	238	0	0	–
SIRIUS	2003	1058	0.57	0.18	–
E-SIRIUS	2003	352	0	0	–
TAXUS II	2003	536	0	0.7	–
C-SIRIUS	2004	100	2.0	0	–
T-SEARCH	2005	1084	–	0	0.34
Iakouvou et al[21]	2005	2229	–	0.5	0.8
Ong et al[28]	2005	2006	–	0.3	0.5
Mean			**0.53**	**0.21**	**0.54**

incompletely understood. Some clinical features (e.g. premature antiplatelet therapy discontinuation, renal failure, diabetes, and lower ejection fraction) have been identified as independent predictors of DES thrombosis (Table 16.4).

In 2004, Virmani et al published the first anatomic-pathologic report of localized vasculitis in response to a Cypher stent implanted in a human coronary artery that led to late stent thrombosis (18 months after the baseline procedure).[37] Impressive positive remodeling and late-acquired incomplete stent apposition were also noticed in the IVUS images of their case. They linked this peculiar vascular response to an interaction between the polymer and the vessel.

Recently, our group reported two cases of late stent thrombosis after DES implantation, one after Cypher implantation, occurring 40 months after the procedure (corresponding to the latest DES thrombosis case ever described) and one after Taxus implantation, occurring 12 months after percutaneous treatment of the coronary artery.[38] By means of serial angiography and IVUS images, we described a peculiar vessel response to DES (i.e. huge positive remodeling throughout the treated segment), leading to impressive late-acquired incomplete stent apposition and ultimately causing stent thrombosis and acute myocardial infarction. It is worth mentioning that the patient whose RCA was treated with the Cypher stent exhibited a volume increase in the vessel size of 35% in between the baseline and the event date, 40 months later. The patient who received one Taxus stent in the LAD and two Taxus stents in the RCA evolved with subacute stent thrombosis (SAT) 12 months after the treatment and, curiously, both the LAD (culprit vessel) and the RCA showed impressive positive remodeling at the IVUS performed at the event time (39% and 57% vessel volume increase, respectively). While most cases of incomplete stent apposition (acute or late acquired) do have a benign clinical evolution, these two cases suggest that stent malapposition secondary to an exacerbated positive remodeling might increase the risk of late events.

Although most cases of late thrombosis after DES placement have been clearly linked to the discontinuation of either aspirin or the thienopyridine, we still lack strong evidence to identify the subset of patients who might benefit from prolonged sustained dual antiplatelet therapy. Conceivably, those patients with a naturally higher risk of stent thrombosis, such as diabetics, multiple overlapping or very long stented segments, bifurcations, or in those where a thrombotic event could be catastrophic, such as percutaneously treated left main, should be kept under long-term (at least one year) dual regimen (aspirin and clopidogrel).

Table 16.4 Predictors of acute, subacute, and late stent thrombosis[21,35,36]

Variables	
Premature antiplatelet discontinuation	+++++
Renal failure	++++
Diabetes	+++
Stent underexpansion	+++
Lesion bifurcation	+++
Residual reference segment stenosis	++
Residual dissection	++
Left ventricular dysfunction	+
Stent length	+/?
In vitro resistance to aspirin	+/?

It is worth noting that some of these late events have occurred when patients were in the recommended market window of dual antiplatelet therapy, and have stopped at least one of them due to the necessity of undergoing a noncardiac surgery. Thus, it is imperative that all physicians following patients treated with DES be aware of this rare but very serious and potentially fatal complication of percutaneous treatment of coronary atherosclerosis (the estimated 30-day mortality ranges from 20% to 48% and can lead to myocardial infarction in 60–70% of patients).[39,40] Moreover, when a noncardiac surgery is scheduled for the next six months after the coronary angioplasty, a BMS should be used rather than a DES.

DRUG-ELUTING STENT SELECTION

Currently, a vast number of different platforms, with new polymers, and single or combinations of drugs, are being tested. However, only a few of these new DES have shown enthusiastic preliminary results. It is important to remember that most DES currently under study will never achieve market approval.

As pioneers, Cypher and Taxus safety and efficacy have been evaluated in several randomized trials as well as single- and multicenter registries, with very long clinical, angiographic, and ultrasonographic follow-up.[3–6,41–43]

Both stents have proven to be equally clinically safe and efficient in reducing restenosis. However, we must keep in mind that the safety profile of a new DES is far more important than its efficacy. While in-stent restenosis is almost a benign condition, stent thrombosis is a disastrous event and remains as the major cause of death after percutaneous coronary intervention.

REFERENCES

1. Serruys PW, de Jaegere P, Kiemeneij F et al. A comparison of balloon-expandable-stent implantation with balloon angioplasty in patients with coronary artery disease. Benestent Study Group. N Engl J Med 1994;331(8):489–95.
2. Serruys PW, Kay IP, Disco C, Deshpande NV, de Feyter PJ. Periprocedural quantitative coronary angiography after Palmaz-Schatz stent implantation predicts the restenosis rate at six months: results of a meta-analysis of the BElgian NEtherlands Stent study (BENESTENT) I, BENESTENT II Pilot, BENESTENT II and MUSIC trials. Multicenter Ultrasound Stent In Coronaries. J Am Coll Cardiol 1999;34(4):1067–74.
3. Morice MC, Serruys PW, Sousa JE et al, RAVEL Study Group. Randomized study with the sirolimus-coated Bx velocity balloon-expandable stent in the treatment of patients with de novo native coronary artery lesions. A randomized comparison of a sirolimus-eluting stent with a standard stent for coronary revascularization. N Engl J Med 2002;346(23):1773–80.
4. Moses JW, Leon MB, Popma JJ et al, SIRIUS Investigators. Sirolimus-eluting stents versus standard stents in patients with stenosis in a native coronary artery. N Engl J Med 2003;349(14):1315–23.
5. Stone GW, Ellis SG, Cox DA et al, TAXUS-IV Investigators. One-year clinical results with the slow-release, polymer-based, paclitaxel-eluting TAXUS stent: the TAXUS-IV trial. Circulation 2004;109(16):1942–7.
6. Dawkins KD, Grube E, Guagliumi G et al, TAXUS VI Investigators. Clinical efficacy of polymer-based paclitaxel-eluting stents in the treatment of complex, long coronary artery lesions from a multicenter, randomized trial: support for the use of drug-eluting stents in contemporary clinical practice. Circulation 2005;112(21):3306–13.
7. Lembo NJ, Black AJ, Roubin GS et al. Effect of pretreatment with aspirin versus aspirin plus

dipyridamole on frequency and type of acute complications of percutaneous transluminal coronary angioplasty. Am J Cardiol 1990;65(7):422–6.

8. Schwartz L, Bourassa MG, Lesperance J et al. Aspirin and dipyridamole in the prevention of restenosis after percutaneous transluminal coronary angioplasty. N Engl J Med 1988;318(26):1714–19.

9. Bertrand ME, Rupprecht HJ, Urban P, Gershlick AH, CLASSICS Investigators. Double-blind study of the safety of clopidogrel with and without a loading dose in combination with aspirin compared with ticlopidine in combination with aspirin after coronary stenting: the Clopidogrel Aspirin Stent International Cooperative Study (CLASSICS). Circulation 2000;102(6):624–9.

10. Steinhubl SR, Berger PB, Mann JT 3rd et al, CREDO Investigators. Clopidogrel for the Reduction of Events During Observation. Early and sustained dual oral antiplatelet therapy following percutaneous coronary intervention: a randomized controlled trial. JAMA 2002;288(19):2411–20.

11. Steinhubl SR, Topol EJ. Risk reduction with long-term clopidogrel following percutaneous coronary intervention. Eur Heart J 2004;25(23):2169–70.

12. Muller I, Seyfarth M, Rudiger S et al. Effect of a high loading dose of clopidogrel on platelet function in patients undergoing coronary stent placement. Heart 2001;85:92–3.

13. Pache J, Kastrati A, Mehilli J et al. Clopidogrel therapy in patients undergoing coronary stenting: value of a high-loading-dose regimen. Cathet Cardiovasc Intervent 2002;55:436–41.

14. Kandzari DE, Berger PB, Kastrati A et al, ISAR-REACT Study Investigators. Influence of treatment duration with a 600-mg dose of clopidogrel before percutaneous coronary revascularization. J Am Coll Cardiol 2004;44(11):2133–6.

15. Patti G, Colonna G, Pasceri V, Pepe LL, Montinaro A, Di Sciascio G. Randomized trial of high loading dose of clopidogrel for reduction of periprocedural myocardial infarction in patients undergoing coronary intervention: results from the ARMYDA-2 (Antiplatelet therapy for Reduction of MYocardial Damage during Angioplasty) study. Circulation 2005;111(16):2099–106.

16. Serruys PW, Unger F, Sousa JE et al, Arterial Revascularization Therapies Study Group. Comparison of coronary-artery bypass surgery and stenting for the treatment of multivessel disease. N Engl J Med 2001;344(15):1117–24.

17. Dangas G, Aymong ED, Mehran R et al, CADILLAC Investigators. Predictors of and outcomes of early thrombosis following balloon angioplasty versus primary stenting in acute myocardial infarction and usefulness of abciximab (the CADILLAC trial). Am J Cardiol 2004;94(8):983–8.

18. Moreno R, Fernandez C, Hernandez R et al. Drug eluting stent thrombosis. Results from a pooled analysis including 10 randomized studies. J Am Coll Cardiol 205;45:954–9.

19. Bavry A, Kumbhani D, Helton T, Bhatt D. What is the risk of stent thrombosis associated with the use of paclitaxel-eluting stents for percutaneous coronary intervention? A meta-analysis. J Am Coll Cardiol 2005;45:941–6.

20. Tsagalou E, Chieffo A, Ioannis I et al. Multiple overlapping drug eluting stents to treat diffuse disease of the left anterior descending coronary artery. J Am Coll Cardiol 2005;45:1570–3.

21. Iakovou I, Schmidt T, Bonizzoni E et al. Incidence, predictors, and outcome of thrombosis after successful implantation of drug-eluting stents. JAMA 2005;293:2126–30.

22. Colombo A, Moses JW, Morice MC et al. Randomized study to evaluate sirolimus-eluting stents implanted at coronary bifurcation lesions. Circulation 2004;109:1244–9.

23. Ge L, Airoldi F, Iakovou I et al. Clinical and angiographic outcome after implantation of drug-eluting stents in bifurcation lesions with the crush stent technique. Importance of final kissing balloon post-dilation. J Am Coll Cardiol 2005;46:613–20.

24. Ge L, Iakovou I, Cosgrave J. Treatment bifurcation lesions with two stents: crush versus T stenting – one year angiographic and clinical follow-up. Heart 2006;92(3):371–6.

25. Costa RA, Mintz GS, Carlier SG et al. Bifurcation coronary lesions treated with the 'crush' technique: an intravascular ultrasound analysis. J Am Coll Cardiol 2005;46:599–605.

26. Moussa I, Leon MB, Baim DS et al. Impact of sirolimus-eluting stents on outcome in diabetic patients: a SIRIUS (SIRolImUS-coated Bx Velocity balloon-expandable stent in the treatment of patients with de novo coronary artery lesions) substudy. Circulation 2004;109(19):2273–8.
27. Hermiller JB, Raizner A, Cannon L et al, TAXUS-IV Investigators. Outcomes with the polymer-based paclitaxel-eluting TAXUS stent in patients with diabetes mellitus: the TAXUS-IV trial. J Am Coll Cardiol 2005;45(8):1172–9.
28. Ong AT, Aoki J, van Mieghem CA et al. Comparison of short- (one month) and long- (twelve months) term outcomes of sirolimus– versus paclitaxel-eluting stents in 293 consecutive patients with diabetes mellitus (from the RESEARCH and T-SEARCH registries). Am J Cardiol 2005;96(3):358–62.
29. McFadden E, Stabile E, Regar E et al. Late thrombosis in drug-eluting coronary stents after discontinuation of antiplatelet therapy. Lancet 2004;364:1519–21.
30. Ishikawa T, Mori C, Abe Y et al. A case report of late coronary stent thrombosis manifested as acute myocardial infarction 19 months after stenting. Jpn Heart J 2004;45(1):147–52.
31. Ong A, McFadden E, Regar E et al. Late Angiographic Stent Thrombosis (LAST) events with drug-eluting stents. J Am Coll Cardiol 2005;45:2088–92.
32. Karvouni R, Korovesis S, Katritsis DG. Very late thrombosis after implantation of sirolimus eluting stent. Heart 2005;91(6):e45.
33. Wang F, Stouffer GA, Waxman S, Uretsky BF. Late coronary stent thrombosis: early vs. late stent thrombosis in the stent era. Cathet Cardiovasc Intervent 2002;55:142–7.
34. Wenaweser P, Rey C, Eberli F et al. Stent thrombosis following bare-metal stent implantation: success of emergency percutaneous coronary intervention and predictors of adverse outcome. Eur Heart J 2005;26(12):1180–7.
35. Fujii K, Carlier SG, Mintz GS et al. Stent underexpansion and residual reference segment stenosis are related to stent thrombosis after sirolimus-eluting stent implantation: an intravascular ultrasound study. J Am Coll Cardiol 2005;45(7):995–8.
36. Cheneau E, Leborgne L, Mintz GS et al. Predictors of subacute stent thrombosis: results of a systematic intravascular ultrasound study. Circulation 2003;108(1):43–7.
37. Virmani R, Guagliumi G, Farb A et al. Localized hypersensitivity and late coronary thrombosis secondary to a sirolimus-eluting stent: should we be cautious? Circulation 2004;109:701–5.
38. Feres F, Costa JR Jr, Abizaid A. Very late thrombosis after drug-eluting stents. Cathet Cardiovasc Intervent (in press).
39. Cutlip DE, Baim DS, Ho KK et al. Stent thrombosis in the modern era: a pooled analysis of multicenter coronary stent trials. Circulation 2001;103:1967–71.
40. Malenka DJ, O'Rourke D, Miller MA et al. Cause of in-hospital death in 13,232 consecutive patients undergoing percutaneous transluminal coronary angioplasty. Am Heart J 1999;137:632–8.
41. Lemos PA, Serruys PW, van Domburg RT et al. Unrestricted utilization of sirolimus-eluting stents compared with conventional bare stent implantation in the 'real world': the Rapamycin-Eluting Stent Evaluated At Rotterdam Cardiology Hospital (RESEARCH) registry. Circulation 2004;109(2):190–5.
42. Fajadet J, Morice MC, Bode C et al. Maintenance of long-term clinical benefit with sirolimus-eluting coronary stents. Three-year results of the RAVEL trial. Circulation 2005;111:1040–4.
43. Sousa JE, Costa MA, Abizaid A et al. Four-year angiographic and intravascular ultrasound follow-up of patients treated with sirolimus-eluting stents. Circulation 2005;111(18): 2326–9.
44. Lefevre T, Ormiston J, Guagliumi G et al. The Frontier stent registry: safety and feasibility of a novel dedicated stent for the treatment of bifurcation coronary artery lesions. J Am Coll Cardiol 2005;46(4):592–8.

Section F
General issues

17

The ABC and D of cardiac resuscitation in the cath lab

Pascal Vranckx and Edouard Benit

The integrated cardiac emergency response system • **Initial stabilization of the high-risk cardiac patient: a 'goal-oriented' approach** • **The ABC and D of cardiac resuscitation (specific) in the cath lab** • **Conclusion**

'If anything can go wrong, fix it!'

With increasing operator experience, refinement of angioplasty hardware and technique, and adjunctive pharmacologic treatment, the morphologic and clinical profile of patients acceptable for coronary angioplasty has widened considerably. The timing of this chapter falls at a fascinating point in the history of therapeutics of symptomatic coronary artery disease in general and acute coronary syndromes (ACS) in particular.

- Percutaneous coronary intervention (PCI) is now considered the treatment of choice even for high-risk subgroups in which PCI was previously contraindicated. Many of these procedures are elective (see Chapter 1).
- For patients with acute myocardial infarction accompanied with elevation of the ST segment (STEMI), mechanical revascularization has triumphed over fibrinolytic therapy, provided the procedure can be done promptly by a competent team (see Chapter 2).[1,2]

However, even in the acute setting, the benefits of a specific (percutaneous) procedure should be weighed against the risks involved, taking into account alternative treatment strategies, the individual operator's and overall institution's (interventional and intensive care team) experience.[3] In such circumstances, transfer to a 'center of excellence' that routinely performs complex PCI may be the most effective and efficient course of action. Several elements of a myocardial intervention center (MIC) would improve patient care and outcomes: state-of-the-art facilities for (primary) PCI including experienced senior operators available on a 24-hour basis, written care protocols, and an integrated cardiac emergency medical system (CEMS).

Management of the complex cardiac patient with (potential) hemodynamic compromise has become a special dimension for specialized MIC. Safe transport of the high-risk cardiac patient requires accurate assessment and stabilization before transport. Clinical management during transport must aim to at least equal management at the point of referral and must prepare the patient for admission to the receiving service. In this chapter we will:

- define the role of an integrated CEMS and emphasize the importance of a systematic, organized, and co-ordinated effort to deal with the high- risk/complex cardiac patient
- introduce the principle of 'goal-oriented' therapy to guide initial stabilization (resuscitation end-points) for the acute cardiac patient
- elaborate on the 'chain of survival' during resuscitation in the cath lab.

THE INTEGRATED CARDIAC EMERGENCY RESPONSE SYSTEM

The CEMS provides a framework for prehospital, interhospital, and intrafacility care for the complex and high-risk cardiac patient. The rationale behind this approach is that early intervention in response to physiologic instability might prevent further deterioration in many patients.

This approach requires an increased awareness of the dangers of physiologic instability, written care protocols and immediate 24-hour availability of a cardiac emergency response team (CERT). The CERT quickly responds to abnormalities in patients' vital signs, specific conditions, and staff concerns in much the same way as a cardiac arrest team would, but at an earlier stage of physiologic instability. The CERT should include a senior (cardiac) critical care physician or equivalent, experienced in all aspects of diagnosing and treating complex cardiac patients. For preference, this should be a senior staff physician of the intensive cardiac care unit who is authorized to admit patients, to describe the patient's condition, and to obtain advice about stabilization and transport. The CERT should have well-established lines of communication with the cath lab personnel and the emergency department.

Pre-cath lab care: intrafacility and interfacility transfer of patients

Intrafacility and interfacility movement of high-risk acute cardiac patients is often challenging. It not only exemplifies the multidisciplinary ethos of a CEMS but also demands a high degree of investment of financial and human resources, requires interaction of many departments in the organization of regional health affairs, and emphasizes the importance of crew resource management, immediacy of mission, need for constant updating of improvization and technology, and the integral requirement for assurance of quality and accountability.

The intrafacility and interhospital transport is co-ordinated with the receiving unit to ensure that the patient is safely delivered to a MIC (cath lab) in stable or improved condition. Referring and tertiary institutions should develop contingency plans in close collaboration, using locally available resources adapted to the patient's clinical needs. Hospital- and nonhospital-based transport organizations may develop a multitiered response capability in terms of team crew composition and resource utilization. The severity of patient illness, level of physiologic support required, and hemodynamic stability should guide the staffing of the transport team and time commitment. Choices need to be balanced between the need for rapid transport and the need to provide adequate levels of care. The sending physician must decide if the benefit of waiting for the expertise of a specialized cardiac retrieval team outweighs the risk of sending the patient quickly but with 'potentially' less qualified personnel. Such a strategy strongly depends on a reliable and expert pretransport information gathering and risk assessment.

Pre-transport co-ordination and communication in the receiving center should be the joint responsibility of a senior staff member trained in (cardiac) critical care (CERT physician) and the receiving hospital specialist to whose care the patient is referred. Ideally, the referring hospital staff should only need to make one single telephone call to activate the CERT (key role of a dedicated cardiac emergency telephone number). Using a script based on written protocols for cardiac emergencies, the receiving physician can question callers, rapidly assess the condition of the patient, and activate the necessary emergency service to prepare for the patient's arrival. This single contact point can also be utilized as a source for immediate clinical advice from the accepting physician.

In some instances (e.g. when a receiving institution provides the transport team), the receiving physician may determine the mode of transport. However, the mode of transportation (ground or air) usually is determined by the transferring physician, in consultation with the receiving physician, based on the urgency of the medical condition (stability of the patient), time savings anticipated with air transport, weather conditions, medical interventions necessary for ongoing life support during transfer, and the availability of personnel and resources.

It is important that referral process guidelines for patient transport be established (Table 17.1). To reduce the likelihood of complications during transport, the transport team members preferably should receive training and experience in the care of critically ill (cardiac) patients and should be supervised by a physician with experience and training in emergency medicine or (cardiac) critical care. It is strongly recommended that a minimum of two people accompany a high-risk cardiac patient. Unstable critically ill (cardiac) patients should be accompanied by a physician with training in airway management and advanced cardiac life support (ACLS). If there will not be a physician in attendance, the referring and accepting physicians also should agree as to who will assume responsibility for on-line medical control during the transport.

Risk stratification: forewarned is forearmed

Careful risk assessment for each patient informs decisions regarding therapeutic interventions, triage among alternative levels of hospital care, and allocation of clinical resources. Clinical and angiographic characteristics are proven to be equally important in determining procedural risk with PCI.[2,4–7] This subject is discussed in detail in Chapters 2 and 13. A rapid, effective triage, based on simple clinical criteria, is integral to the emergency cardiac care of patients referred for primary PCI. It should trigger decisions concerning initial stabilization therapy and the level of care needed to assure a safe medical transport and to allow for the index PCI procedure. Important items to decide upon are the need for mechanical ventilatory and/or hemodynamic support.

Patients with left ventricular pump failure in the setting of acute ischemic syndromes may go through a period of 'pre-shock' with nonhypotensive peripheral hypoperfusion before they develop cardiogenic shock.[8] Early recognition and treatment may prevent the onset of hypotension and tissue hypoperfusion. Determining which patients are high risk for severe hemodynamic compromise and death from myocardial infarction can quickly be ascertained by simple and readily available clinical criteria.[9–15] Age, heart rate, systolic blood pressure (SBP) and KILLIP class at presentation have consistently been among the strongest independent prognostic variables. The more extensive the regional dysfunction, the greater the

Table 17.1   Checklist for safe intrafacility and interfacility movement of high-risk acute cardiac patients

- *All critically ill patients need **secure intravenous access** before transport.* If peripheral venous access is unavailable, central venous access is established. If needed, fluid resuscitation and inotropic support are initiated, with all intravenous fluids and medications maintained in plastic (not glass) containers.
- A patient should not be transported before ***airway stabilization*** if it is judged likely that airway intervention will be needed en route (a process made more difficult in a moving vehicle). With mechanically ventilated patients, endotracheal tube position is noted and secured before transport, and the adequacy of oxygenation and ventilation is reconfirmed. A nasogastric tube is inserted in those patients requiring mechanical ventilation.
- A ***Foley catheter*** is inserted in patients requiring strict fluid management, for transports of extended duration, and for patients receiving diuretics.
- Soft ***wrist and/or leg restraints are applied when agitation*** could compromise the safety of the patient or transport crew, especially with air transport. If the patient is combative or unco-operative, the use of sedative and/or neuromuscular blocking agents may be indicated. A neuromuscular blocking agent should not be used without sedation and analgesia.
- ***Minimal equipment***: a blood pressure monitor (or standard blood pressure cuff), pulse oximeter, and cardiac monitor/defibrillator accompany every patient without exception. All critically ill patients undergoing transport receive *the same level of basic physiologic monitoring* during transport as they had in the intensive care unit. Equipment for airway management, sized appropriately for each patient, is also transported with each patient, as is an oxygen source of ample supply to provide for projected needs plus a 30-minute reserve. All battery-operated equipment is fully charged and capable of functioning for the duration of the transport.
- ***Basic resuscitation drugs***, including epinephrine and antiarrhythmic agents, are transported with each patient in sudden cardiac arrest or arrhythmia. Supplemental medications, such as sedatives and narcotic analgesics, are considered in each specific case. An ample supply of appropriate intravenous fluids and continuous drip medications (regulated by battery-operated infusion pumps) is ensured.
- ***Standing orders:*** if a physician will not be accompanying the patient during transport, protocols must be in place to permit the administration of these medications and fluids by appropriately trained personnel under emergency circumstances.
- ***History/handover:*** the patient's medical record and relevant laboratory and radiographic studies are copied for the receiving facility. The preparation of records should not delay patient transport, however, as these records can be forwarded separately (by facsimile, courier, or internet) if and when the urgency of transfer precludes their assemblage beforehand.

adverse affect on global left ventricular (LV) function. A single measurement of plasma N-terminal pro-brain natriuretic peptide (or BNP) and left ventricular ejection fraction, assessed by either echocardiography or angiography, is a complementary independent predictor of major adverse events on follow-up after myocardial infarction.[16–19] A limited and focused transthoracic echocardiography may be of additional help in diagnosing mechanical complications of an acute myocardial infarction (ventricular septal rupture, left ventricular free wall rupture, acute mitral regurgitation).

INITIAL STABILIZATION OF THE HIGH-RISK CARDIAC PATIENT: A 'GOAL-ORIENTED' APPROACH

The primary physiologic task of the cardiovascular system is to deliver enough oxygen (O_2) to meet the metabolic demands of the body. Shock and tissue hypoxia occur when the cardiorespiratory system is unable to cover metabolic demand adequately. Therefore determining the adequacy of tissue oxygenation is central to determining the health of the patient.

Early hemodynamic assessment of the critically ill patient on the basis of physical findings, vital signs, central venous pressure, and urinary output fails to detect persistent global tissue hypoxia.[20] Hence, in addition to standard clinical evaluation, repeated measurements of blood lactate and SvO_2 may be helpful (Tables 17.2, 17.3).[21]

Table 17.2   Limits of mixed venous oxygen saturation

SvO_2 >75%	Normal extraction
	O_2 supply >O_2 demand
75% >SvO_2 >50%	Compensatory extraction
	Increasing O_2 demand or decreasing O_2 supply
50% >SvO_2 >30%	Exhaustion of extraction
	Beginning of lactic acidosis, O_2 supply <O_2 demand
30% >SvO_2 >25%	Severe lactic acidosis
SvO_2 <25%	Cellular death

Table 17.3   Physiology of mixed venous and central venous oxygen saturation

- **O_2 delivery (DO_2)** describes whole-body oxygen supply according to the following formula:

$$DO_2 = CO \times CaO_2 \tag{1}$$
$$CaO_2 = (Hb \times 1.36 \times SaO_2) + (PaO_2 \times 0.0031) \tag{2}$$

  – CO is cardiac output and
  – CaO_2 is arterial oxygen content: oxygen bound to hemoglobin (product of hemoglobin concentration (Hb) and arterial O_2 saturation (SaO_2)) + physically dissolved oxygen (arterial PO_2 (PaO_2)).

- **Oxygen demand** can be summarized in the whole-body oxygen consumption (**VO_2**), which is expressed mathematically by the Fick principle as the product of CO and arteriovenous O_2 content difference (CaO_2–CvO_2):

$$VO_2 = CaO_2 - CvO_2 \tag{3}$$
$$CvO_2 = (Hb \times 1.36 \times SvO_2) + (PvO_2 \times 0.0031) \tag{4}$$

  – (CvO_2) is mixed venous O_2 content.

- **Oxygen extraction (O_2ER):**

$$VO_2/DO_2 = (CaO_2 - CvO_2)/CaO_2$$

  Equation 3 may be transposed to:

$$CvO_2 = CaO_2 - VO_2/CO \tag{5}$$

  As physically dissolved oxygen can be neglected, Equation 5 may be written as:

$$Hb \times 1.36 \times SvO_2 \approx (Hb \times 1.36 \times SaO_2) - VO_2/CO \leftrightarrow (SvO_2 \sim VO_2/CO)$$

  This equation demonstrates that SvO_2 is directly proportional to the ratio of VO_2 to CO. Thus SvO_2 reflects the relationship between whole-body O_2 consumption and cardiac output. Indeed, it has been shown that the SvO_2 is well correlated with the ratio of O_2 supply to demand.

Mixed venous oxygen saturation has been shown to be a surrogate for the cardiac index as a target for hemodynamic therapy.[22] Pulmonary artery catheterization measures true mixed venous oxygen saturation (SvO_2), while measuring central venous saturation ($ScvO_2$) via a central venous catheter in the superior vena cava reflects principally the degree of oxygen extraction from the brain and the upper part of the body. $ScvO_2$ values may differ from SvO_2 values, and this difference varies in direction and magnitude with cardiovascular insufficiency. However, despite the variable difference between the two variables, changes in SvO_2 are closely mirrored by changes in $ScvO_2$ under experimental[23] and clinical conditions.[24] $ScvO_2$ may be a valuable alternative to SvO_2 when a PA catheter is not available. Reaching the critical DO_2, ensuring that VO_2 needs are met, is a crucial objective whether these two variables are calculated or intuitively estimated.

In the acute cardiac patient, the cardio-circulatory system is mainly challenged by two different conditions. Firstly, a drop in DO_2 can be induced by anemia, hypoxia, hypovolemia or heart failure. Secondly, fever, pain, stress, and/or respiratory failure, etc. may also decrease SvO_2 or $ScvO_2$ by increasing whole-body VO_2. Understanding these basic principles, every high-risk cardiac patient becomes a 'VIP'. In the early stabilization, three items should be addressed.

1. The need for sedation and ventilatory support. (*Ventilation*)
2. The need for inotropic/vasopressor support. Do we need central venous access? (*Infuse*)
3. The need for mechanical cardiac support. (*Pump*)

A multifaceted strategy

A more definitive resuscitation strategy involves goal-oriented manipulation of cardiac preload, afterload, and contractility to achieve a balance between whole-body oxygen supply and oxygen demand (see Table 17.3).[25] To decrease oxygen consumption in patients in whom hemodynamic optimization cannot be achieved, mechanical ventilation and sedatives need to be considered.

Drugs used to maintain cardiac output

The following section provides general information on the use of vasoactive and inotropic agents to maintain cardiac output and blood pressure in patients with compromised hemodynamics at risk of cardiac arrest or in the postarrest period. After cardiac arrest or resuscitation from shock, the victim may have ongoing hemodynamic compromise secondary to a combination of inadequate cardiac pumping function, excessively increased systemic or pulmonary vascular resistance or very low systemic vascular resistance.

Dopamine and dobutamine are the most commonly used inotropic agents. They have different effects on systemic hemodynamics, cardiac output, and systemic vascular resistance (Table 17.4). Dobutamine is the first-choice inotrope for patients with measured or suspected low cardiac output in the presence of adequate left ventricular filling pressure (or clinical assessment of adequate fluid resuscitation) and adequate mean arterial pressure. Norepinephrine and dopamine both exert a combined inotrope/vasopressor effect and may be used in case of hypotension. However, in the high-risk cardiac patient, especially when the capability exists for

Table 17.4 Inotropes and vasopressors

		Heart rate	Blood pressure	Cardiac output	Systemic vascular resistance
Dopamine	2–10 µg/kg per minute	↑	↑→	↑	↑→↓
Dobutamine	2–20 µg/kg per minute	↑	↑→	↑	↑
Norepinephrine	0.1–2 µg/kg per minute	↑	↑	↑→	↑
Milrinone	0.375–0.75 µg/kg per minute	↑	↓→	↑	↓→

monitoring cardiac output in addition to blood pressure, a vasopressor such as norepinephrine and an inotrope such as dobutamine may be used separately to target specific levels of mean arterial pressure and cardiac output.

Inotropes and vasopressors should be infused through a secure vascular line, preferably one that is placed centrally. Vascular access sites must be evaluated and, when necessary, central venous access obtained, if possible from the neck.

Mechanical hemodynamic support (see also Chapter 12)

This includes not only the use of an intra-aortic balloon pump (IABP), but also immediate triage to more sophisticated percutaneous (or implantable) ventricular cardiopulmonary support (CPS) modalities. Patient selection is the single most crucial factor in determining a successful outcome in patients who receive temporary mechanical circulatory support.

Elective high-risk PCI can be performed safely without IABP or CPS in most circumstances. Emergency high-risk PCI such as direct PCI for acute MI can usually be performed without IABP or CPS. CPS for high-risk PCI should be reserved only for patients at the extreme end of the spectrum of hemodynamic compromise, such as those with extremely depressed LV function (EF <25%) and patients in cardiogenic shock. However, it should be noted that in patients with borderline hemodynamics, ongoing ischemia or cardiogenic shock, insertion of an IABP just prior to coronary instrumentation has been associated with improved outcomes and reduced inotropic use. Furthermore, it is reasonable to obtain vascular access in the contralateral femoral artery prior to the procedure in patients in whom the risk of hemodynamic compromise is high, thereby facilitating IABP insertion, if necessary.

Oxygenation and ventilation

Following the formula to calculate DO_2 (see Table 17.3), tissue oxygen delivery could be increased by administering supplemental oxygen to increase the arterial oxygen tension (PaO_2). In patients breathing spontaneously, oxygen supplements may be administered by nasal cannula, simple facemasks, and nonrebreathing masks. With these so-called low-flow devices, the concentration of oxygen delivered (FIO_2) is dependent on:

1. the flow of oxygen into the device
2. the size of the equipment reservoir (e.g. the volume of the facemask)
3. the size of the anatomic reservoir (volume of the oral and nasal pharynx)

4. the capability of the filling reservoir during the transition between expiration and inspiration and the ventilatory pattern of the patient.

Because of all these factors, it is nearly impossible to predict the FIO_2 that a patient is receiving with a low-flow system. In general, FIO_2 and minute ventilation are inversely related (Table 17.5).

In patients with severe cardiopulmonary distress for whom the effort of breathing is intolerable, mechanical ventilation substitutes for the action of the respiratory muscles. The objectives of mechanical ventilation are primarily to decrease the work of breathing and reverse life-threatening hypoxemia or acute progressive respiratory acidosis. The inspiratory effort expended by patients with acute respiratory failure is about four times the normal value, and it can be increased to six times the normal value in individual patients.[26,27]

The need for mechanical ventilation and artificial airways can also be reduced by substituting noninvasive ventilatory support when appropriate. Noninvasive mechanical ventilation (NIV), delivered through tight-fitting facemasks, has been shown to maintain adequate gas exchange and to limit the need for endotracheal intubation in patients with acute respiratory failure due to acute pulmonary edema,

---

Table 17.5 Estimate FIO_2 with low-flow oxygen delivery systems*

Nasal cannulas
A nasal cannula is used to provide supplemental oxygen to a patient who is breathing spontaneously. Nasal cannulas are often better tolerated than a facemask and are suitable for patients who require modest oxygen supplementation. Nasal cannula flow rates >4 L/min for prolonged periods are often poorly tolerated because of the drying effect on the nasal mucosa.

System	Flow (L/min)	FIO_2 (fraction of inspired oxygen)
Nasal cannula	1	0.24
	2	0.28
	3	0.32
	4	0.36
	5	**0.40**
	6	0.44

Masks
If the patient demonstrates effective spontaneous ventilation, use a simple facemask to provide oxygen at a concentration of 30–50%. If a higher concentration of oxygen is desired, it may be administered through a nonrebreathing mask, typically at a flow of 15 L/min. Masks should be available in a selection of sizes. To provide a consistent concentration of oxygen, the mask of appropriate size should provide an airtight seal without pressure on the eyes. A small under-mask volume is desirable to minimize rebreathing of exhaled gases.

System	Flow (L/min)	FIO_2 (fraction of inspired oxygen)
Simple mask	≥5	0.40–0.60
Partial rebreathing mask	≥8	≥0.60
Nonrebreathing mask	≥10	≥0.80

*Values are estimated based on a tidal volume of 500 mL, a respiratory rate of 20 breaths per minute, an inspiratory time of 1 second, and an anatomic reservoir of 50 mL.

status asthmaticus or chronic obstructive pulmonary disease.[28-31] NIV can be safely used outside the ICU by experienced nurses, respiratory therapists, and physicians. However, relative hemodynamic stability and full patient co-operation are two important prerequisites when choosing a NIV mode.

THE ABC AND D OF CARDIAC RESUSCITATION (SPECIFIC) IN THE CATH LAB

The chain of survival, first conceptualized for out-of-hospital sudden cardiac arrest, applies to in-hospital arrest as well.[32] The outcome of cardiac arrest and cardiopulmonary resuscitation (CPR) is dependent on critical interventions, particularly early recognition of cardiopulmonary arrest, early activation of trained responders, early defibrillation when indicated, effective chest compressions, assisted ventilation, and early advanced life support (ALS).[33] These elements will be projected on the specific patient setting of the cath lab. Minimal requirements for equipment, architecture, and organization may become evident (Table 17.6).

Patients in the cath lab are highly monitored and nearly all cardiac arrests are 'witnessed' by trained physicians and/or nurses. Basic life support, including (automated) external defibrillation, can be provided within seconds. As the 'response time' is nearly zero and most arrests are confronted in the electrical phase (which lasts ≈5 minutes),[34] the key intervention in most cases is indeed prompt defibrillation. The cath lab personnel will act as first responders in case of a cardiac arrest. There is a clear need for regular refresher training to maintain their training in basic life support and in the use of (automated) external defibrillators.

In case of sustained cardiac arrest, a cardiac arrest team (CAT) should be alarmed by a simple push on the (alarm) button. Ideally, the CAT (CERT or equivalent) should consist of a group of experts in ACLS who are familiar with the specific cath lab environment and organization. They should consider potential radiation exposure and respect the aseptic aspect of the PCI procedure.

Even in expert hands, the quality of CPR remains a concern.[35-37] There are several potential practical solutions for helping to improve poor CPR quality. The first involves mechanical devices that can provide chest compressions reliably at a set rate and depth.[36,38] These 'hands free' devices have the potential to generate better hemodynamic characteristics than manual chest compressions[39] and could allow for ongoing PCI and instrumentation during active CPR. However, their application in the cath lab setting has still to be proved. Another solution is to improve monitoring and feedback to reduce human error during manual CPR, by using devices such as end-tidal CO_2 monitors[40] and 'smart defibrillators', which can measure CPR characteristics and provide audio feedback to alert the rescuers to errors such as incorrect chest compression or ventilation rate.

Resuscitation challenges care providers to make decisions quickly and under pressure. Providers must occasionally limit their focus for a brief time to a specific aspect of the resuscitative attempt: getting the IV infusion line started, placing the tracheal tube, identifying the rhythm, or remembering the 'right' medication to order. But, as suggested in the title, rescuers constantly must return to an overall view of each resuscitative attempt.

- *A=Airway control with endotracheal intubation*
- *B=Breathing effectively: verify with primary and secondary confirmation of proper tube placement*

Table 17.6 Minimal requirements for equipment, architecture and training

Architecture
The basic ground plan for a room is rectangular, with at least 2.0–2.5 meter traffic area beyond the working area. Adequate access to the head of the bed should also be provided to allow for endotracheal intubation, resuscitation and central venous catheterization in emergency situations.
The following services should be provided in the patient area:

- Electricity (220 V single phase electrical supply): 9–12 grounded sockets. The patient areas should be served by a maintained stand-by power source which is activated after a maximum of 5 seconds interruption of the normal electrical current.
- Central medical vacuum source capable of generating a subatmospheric pressure of 500 mmHg (66.6 Kpa) and maintaining 40 liter/min of air flow: 2–3 outlets, type low vacuum with keyed plug-in connections.
- Medical oxygen 100% at a pressure of 5 bar (500 Kpa). This pressure should remain constant when the flow is 20 litre/min at each outlet when all are in use: 2–3 outlets with flow meter.
- Compressed air: a supply of respirable medical air (free from particles, oil and droplets) should be available at a pressure of 5 bar (500 Kpa). This pressure should remain constant when the flow is 20 litre/min at each outlet when all are in use: 2–3 outlets.
- High intensity lighting.

Communication: Provision should be made for easy and rapid communication.

- Telephone: an emergency phone bypassing the central hospital phone is desirable.
- Alarm calls: an emergency code alarm button must be provided per room.

Monitoring
Modular systems are preferred to maintain necessary flexibility. Uniformity with other areas such as operating theater, ICU is recommended. The monitors should be placed in such a way to permit unobstructed comfortable viewing. Physiologic monitoring should be available for:

- ECG.
- Arterial pressure.
- Pulse oxymetry/respiration monitoring.

Additional equipment

- Volumetric pump/automatic syringe: four to six/room.
- Manual resuscitation/ventilation system (Ambu, Laerdal type) and airway maintenance material.
- Defibrillator (preferably biphasic), adult/pediatric paddles, rechargeable.
- Pacemakers.
- Emergency trolley with extended drug and resuscitation equipment.
- Transport:
  • Case for emergency drugs and transport of IC patients.
  • Transport monitor (ECG, invasive, noninvasive blood pressure monitoring, pulse oxymetry, respiration monitoring).
  • Transport ventilator (readily available).
- Mobile echocardiography machine (readily available).
- 12-lead ECG (readily available).
- Intra-aortic balloon pump (readily available).

Training
All members of the catheterization team (physicians, nurses, and technologists) should complete a course in basic CPR. Certification in advance cardiac life support is also strongly urged for all members of the cardiac catheterization team. Yearly recertification is recommended.

- *C=Circulation, which incorporates vital signs, ECG monitoring, access to the circulation via IV lines, and then administration of rhythm-appropriate medications*
- *D=Differential diagnosis*

A directive to 'consider the differential diagnoses' improves the resuscitation protocols, because this is a recommendation to stop and think: What caused this arrest?

CONCLUSION

We underscore the basic principle: 'Prevention is better than cure'! The ABC and D of cardiac resuscitation in the cath lab starts at the time a patient is planned for PCI: in the emergency department, at the referring or satellite center. Published estimates of risk for an individual patient inform decisions regarding therapeutic interventions, triage among alternative levels of hospital care, and allocation of clinical resources. The concept of networking for co-ordination among tertiary centers, community hospitals, emergency rooms, and transportation is an important aspect in this setting. There is a clear need for highly trained (cardiac) critical care physicians and nurses to support the cath lab team in 'the cure' of the cardiac patient.

REFERENCES

1. Topol EJ. Current status and future prospect for acute myocardial intervention therapy. Circulation 2003;108(Suppl):III 6–III 13.
2. Grines CL, Serruys P, O'Neil WW. Fibrinolytic therapy. Is it the treatment of the past? Circulation 2003;107:2338–42.
3. de Feyter PJ, McFadden E. Risk score for percutaneous coronary intervention: forewarned is forearmed. J Am Coll Cardiol 2003;42:1729–30.
4. Singh M, Lennon RJ, Holmes DR et al. Correlations of procedural complications and a simple integer risk score for percutaneous coronary intervention. J Am Coll Cardiol 2002;40:387–93.
5. Singh M, Rihal CS, Selzer F et al. Validation of Mayo Clinic risk adjustment model for in hospital complications after percutaneous coronary interventions, using the National Heart Lung, and Blood Institute dynamic registry. J Am Coll Cardiol 2003;42:1722–8.
6. Teirstein PS, Vogel RA, Dorros G et al. Prophylactic versus standby cardiopulmonary support for high risk percutaneous transluminal angioplasty. J Am Coll Cardiol 1993;21:590–6.
7. Halkin A, Singh M, Nikolsky E et al. Prediction of mortality after primary percutaneous coronary intervention for acute myocardial infarction. The CADILLAC risk score. J Am Coll Cardiol 2005;45:1397–405.
8. Menon V, Slater JN, White HD et al. Acute myocardial infarction complicated by systemic hypoperfusion without hypotension: report of the SHOCK Trial Registry. Am J Med 2000;108:374–80.
9. Lee KL, Woodlief LH, Topol EJ et al. Predictors for 30 day mortality in the era of reperfusion for acute myocardial infarction. Circulation 1995;91:1659–68.
10. Hunter AM, Weaver WD. Task force 2: acute coronary syndromes: section 2A-prehospital issues. J Am Coll Cardiol 2000;35:846–53.
11. Hands ME, Rutherford JD, Muller JE et al. The in hospital development of cardiogenic shock after myocardial infarction: incidence, predictors of occurrence, outcome and prognostic factors. The Milis study group. J Am Coll Cardiol 1989;14:40–6.
12. Hasdai D, Calif RM, Thompson TD et al. Predictors of cardiogenic shock after thrombolytic therapy for acute myocardial infarction. J Am Coll Cardiol 2000;35:136–43.

13. Morrow DA, Antman EM, Charlesworth A et al. TIMI risk score for ST-elevation myocardial infarction: a convenient, bedside, clinical score for risk assessment at presentation: an InTIME II trial substudy. Circulation 2000;102:2031–7.
14. Normand ST, Glickman ME, Sharma RG, McNeil BJ. Using admission characteristics to predict short-term mortality from myocardial infarction in elderly patients: results from the Cooperative Cardiovascular Project. JAMA 1996;275:1322–8.
15. Morrow DA, Antman EM, Giugliano RP et al. A simple risk index for rapid initial triage of patients with ST-elevation myocardial infarction: an In TIME II substudy. Lancet 2001,258:1571–5.
16. Arakawa N, Nakamura M, Aoki H et al. Relationship between plasma level of brain natriuretic peptide and the myocardial infarct size. Cardiology 1994;85:334–40.
17. Negaya N, Nishikimi T, Goto Y et al. Plasma brain natriuretic peptide is a biochemical marker for the prediction of progressive remodeling after acute myocardial infarction. Am Heart J 1998;135:21–8.
18. Richards AM, Nicholls MG, Espiner EA et al. B-type natriuretic peptides and ejection fraction for prognosis after myocardial infarction. Circulation 2003;107:2786–92.
19. Picard MH, Davidoff R, Sleeper LA et al, for the SHOCK Trial. Echocardiographic predictors of survival and response to early revascularization in cardiogenic shock. Circulation 2003;107:279–84.
20. Rady MY, Rivers EP, Nowak RM. Resuscitation of the critically ill in the ED: responses of blood pressure, heart rate, shock index, central venous oxygen saturation, and lactate. Am J Emerg Med 1996;14:218–25.
21. Vincent JL, De Backer D. Oxygen transport – the oxygen delivery controversy. Intens Care Med 2004;30:1990–6.
22. Gattinoni L, Brazzi L, Pelosi P et al. A trial of goal-oriented hemodynamic therapy in critically ill patients. N Engl J Med 1995;333:1025–32.
23. Reinhart K, Rudolph T, Bredle DL et al. Comparison of central venous to mixed venous oxygen saturation during changes in oxygen supply/demand. Chest 1989,95:1216–21.
24. Reinhart K, Kuhn HJ, Hartog C et al. Continuous central venous and pulmonary artery oxygen saturation monitoring in the critically ill. Intens Care Med 2004,30:1572–8.
25. Beal AL, Cerra FB. Multiple organ failure syndrome in the 1990s: systemic inflammatory response and organ dysfunction. JAMA 1994;271:226–33.
26. Jubran A, Tobin JM. Pathophysiologic basis of acute respiratory distress in patients who fail a trial of weaning from mechanical ventilation. Am J Respir Crit Care Med 1997;155:906–15.
27. Field S, Kelly SM, Macklem PT. The oxygen cost of breathing in patients with cardiorespiratory disease. Am Rev Respir Dis 1982;126:9–13.
28. Bersten AD, Holt AW, Vedig AE, Skowronski GA, Baggoley CJ. Treatment of severe cardiogenic pulmonary edema with continuous positive airway pressure delivered by face mask. N Engl J Med 1991;325:1825–30.
29. Masip J, Betbese AJ, Paez J et al. Non-invasive pressure support ventilation versus conventional oxygen therapy in acute pulmonary oedema. Lancet 2000;356:2126–32.
30. Meduri GU, Cook TR, Turner RE, Cohen M, Leeper KV. Noninvasive positive pressure ventilation in status asthmaticus. Chest 1996;110:767–74.
31. Brochard L, Mancebo J, Wysocki M et al. Noninvasive ventilation for acute exacerbations of chronic obstructive pulmonary disease. N Engl J Med 1995;333:817–22.
32. Kaye W, Mancini ME, Giuliano KK et al. Strengthening the in-hospital chain of survival with rapid defibrillation by first responders using automated external defibrillators: training and retention issues. Ann Emerg Med 1995;25:163–8.
33. Kern KB, Hilwig RW, Berg RA, Sanders AB, Ewy GA. Importance of continuous chest compression during cardiopulmonary resuscitation: improved outcome during a simulated single lay-rescuer scenario. Circulation 2002;105:645–9.
34. Weisfeldt ML, Becker LB. Resuscitation after cardiac arrest: a 3-phase time-sensitive model. JAMA 2002;288:3035–8.

35. Wik L, Kramer-Johansen J, Myklebust H et al. Quality of cardiopulmonary resuscitation during out-of-hospital cardiac arrest. JAMA 2005;293:299–304.
36. Abella BS, Alvarado JP, Myklebust H et al. Quality of cardiopulmonary resuscitation during in-hospital cardiac arrest. JAMA 2005,293:305–10.
37. Pitts S, Kellermann AL. Hyperventilation during cardiac arrest. Lancet 2004;364:313–5.
38. Steen S, Liao Q, Pierre L et al. Evaluation of LUCAS, a new device for automatic mechanical compression and active decompression resuscitation. Resuscitation 2002;55:285–99.
39. Halperin HR, Tsitlik JE, Gelfand M et al. A preliminary study of cardiopulmonary resuscitation by circumferential compression of the chest with use of a pneumatic vest. N Engl J Med 1993;329:762–8.
40. White RD, Asplin BR. Out-of-hospital quantitative monitoring of end-tidal carbon dioxide pressure during CPR. Ann Emerg Med 1994;23:25–30.

18

Cardiac arrhythmias complicating percutaneous coronary interventions: management and prevention

Georgios Kourgiannidis, Peter Geelen and Pedro Brugada

Electrophysiology of coronary interventions • **Clinical arrhythmias** • **Prevention**
• **Conclusion**

Arrhythmias that occur during percutaneous coronary interventions (PCIs) may range from innocent and well-tolerated rhythms, such as accelerated idioventricular rhythm, to life-threatening tachycardias requiring emergent and prompt treatment upon occurrence, like ventricular fibrillation. All these arrhythmias can occur in the setting of primary or rescue PCI, or during an elective intervention, being far more frequent in the former setting. They can be either tachycardias or bradycardias and they are mainly related to ischemia, reperfusion, and vasovagal reactions. Table 18.1 gives an overview of the mechanisms and the triggers of these arrhythmias during PCI.

Table 18.1 Overview of mechanism and trigger events for arrhythmias during percutaneous coronary interventions

Mechanism	Trigger event
Ischemia	• Balloon inflation • Dissection (obstructive) • Spasm • Coronary air emboli • Wedged infusions • Cannulation of the conus artery • Distal embolization • Ostial stenoses
Reperfusion	• Restoration of coronary blood flow
Vasovagal reaction	• Pain (puncture, sheath removal) • Fear • Dehydration, diuretics, nitrates • RCA intervention
Other	• Contrast agent infusion • Pharmacologic agents for coronary blood flow reserve measurement

A combination of mechanisms can exist. This is often seen with Bezold–Jarisch reflex activation during PCI and reperfusion of RCA stenoses.

Although sustained arrhythmias related to PCI may need urgent treatment to prevent an acute negative outcome, they bear no prognostic significance, in contrast to ventricular tachyarrhythmias seen remotely after an acute myocardial infarction.

ELECTROPHYSIOLOGY OF CORONARY INTERVENTIONS

Ischemia and reperfusion

Coronary flow cessation has well-established consequences for the electrophysiologic properties of the myocardium. These include changes in action potential amplitude and duration, a rise in extracellular K concentration, and diminished cell-to-cell coupling through gap junctions. The net effects of all these changes are areas of tissue – especially in the epicardial border zone of ischemia – with inhomogeneous cellular refractoriness and slowed conduction. These effects are the substrate for re-entry tachycardias. Enhanced ventricular automaticity and triggered activity as a result of catecholamine-induced afterdepolarizations are also implicated in both ischemia and myocardial reperfusion.[1,2]

Ongoing ischemia, as in acute myocardial infarction, makes PCI-related arrhythmias more frequent than during elective procedures. The presence of intracoronary thrombus is a well-established arrhythmogenic factor during interventions.[3,4] Balloon inflation *per se* has been shown to increase QT dispersion which is an index of repolarization abnormality and thus an index of arrhythmia susceptibility.[5,6] Prolonged balloon inflations as performed before the widespread use of stents are a known adverse factor. PCI-related arrhythmias occur less frequently, however, in patients with chronic severe lesions due to the presence of collateral circulation and preconditioned myocardium.[7] Ischemia can also be the initiating factor for bradycardias instead of tachycardias. This is particularly true for sinus bradycardia and atrioventricular (AV) block occurring during ischemia involving sinus node and AV node arteries.[8,9]

During reperfusion, restoration of blood flow after a period of ischemia in still viable tissue results in gradual normalization of the action potential. Potassium along with metabolites derived from anaerobic metabolism is washed out whereas intracellular calcium accumulates. Heterogeneous recovery of the refractory period may result in intramural re-entry. Reperfusion arrhythmias, along with stunning, microvascular dysfunction and lethal injury, are collectively described as reperfusion injury.

Ventricular arrhythmias, like ventricular tachycardia (usually fast and polymorphic) and ventricular fibrillation, may occur during the intended (balloon inflation) or unintended (dissection, spasm, air embolization) cessation of blood flow and also during reperfusion. In general, reperfusion tachyarrhythmias typically have sudden onset and progress quickly into ventricular fibrillation (VF), in contrast to arrhythmias due to coronary occlusion which show a more gradual course with less common progression to ventricular fibrillation.[10] Ventricular fibrillation may indeed be more frequent during reperfusion than coronary artery occlusion.[11]

Clinically, reperfusion arrhythmias are dependent on ischemia duration and severity. Patients with more extensive myocardial damage present more frequently with these arrhythmias. In human percutaneous transluminal coronary angiography (PTCA) studies, reperfusion arrhythmias correlate well with elevated creatine phosphokinase (CPK), Troponin-T (TnT) levels,[12,13] and further worsening of left ventricular (LV) function after the acute phase of ST elevation myocardial infarction (STEMI).[14] Timely restoration of blood flow (<3 hours) increases their incidence as more myocardial tissue is salvaged. Hypertrophic hearts are also more prone to ischemia and reperfusion arrhythmias than normal ones.[15]

Clinical and experimental evidence is available of the proarrhythmic effect of angiotensin in ischemia-reperfusion injury (especially in carriers of the DD allele).[16,17] Administration of an angiotensin II blocker may be beneficial against reperfusion arrhythmias. The preconditioning effect of the first balloon inflation also protects against the occurrence of arrhythmias during the following inflations.[18]

At the atrial level, PTCA-induced ischemia has also been found to prolong the signal-averaged P-wave duration by increasing the ventricular and left atrial end-diastolic pressures.[19] Successful PTCA of the right coronary artery is correlated with elimination of atrial afterpotentials.[20] These observations may correlate with the occasional appearance of atrial fibrillation in the catheterization laboratory.

Contrast agents and drugs

The administration of contrast agents during a coronary intervention has prominent electrophysiologic effects. Sinus bradycardia, PR prolongation due to AV conduction delay, and repolarization changes have been observed. Occasionally, sinus arrest, high-degree AV block, premature ventricular contractions (PVCs), and ventricular fibrillation occur. Prolonged coronary infusions or infusions with the catheter tip wedged to the coronary orifice can facilitate the appearance of these arrhythmias. The presence of ischemia as well as inherent contrast agent properties (specific molecule, osmolality and ionic composition, especially sodium and calcium concentration) can lower the ventricular fibrillation threshold.[21] High osmolar (ionic) contrast agents are considered more likely to induce VF in comparison with newer nonionic compounds.[22]

Prolongation of QRS duration and repolarization abnormalities, like QT prolongation and T-wave amplitude changes, can occur during brief intracoronary flushes of saline. Standard saline flushes have more pronounced ECG effects compared with infusions of lactated Ringer's solution (LR) or LR with 5% dextrose (D5LR).[23]

Papaverine infusions used for coronary flow reserve assessment can cause striking QT interval prolongation and induction of ventricular tachycardia (torsade de pointes) (Figure 18.1). Intracoronary adenosine injection can cause asystole and transient AV block – especially during right coronary artery (RCA) infusions – and occasionally, ventricular fibrillation.

Vasovagal reactions

Periprocedural bradycardia and hypotension due to the activation of Bezold–Jarisch reflex is a common event in the catheterization laboratory. Its genesis is multifactorial. Pain, fear, lack of adequate hydration, extreme fasting, use of diuretics or nitrates can be risk factors for vagal reactions. Inferoposterior ischemia or infarction is associated with vagal reactions due to the activation of inhibitory cardiac receptors with vagal afferents that are located predominantly in the inferoposterior wall of the left ventricle.

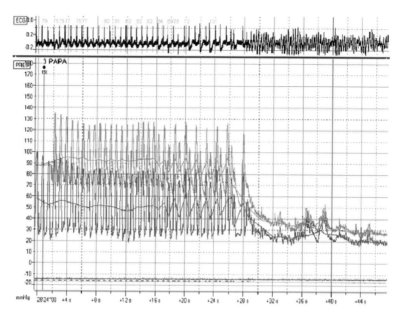

Figure 18.1 Polymorphic ventricular tachycardia induced during intracoronary infusion of papaverine for coronary flow reserve measurement.

CLINICAL ARRHYTHMIAS (Table 18.2)

Incidence

Most of the data concerning the incidence of PCI-related arrhythmias are derived from primary PTCA studies. Altogether, reperfusion arrhythmias can occur as frequently as in 78% of PCIs.[12] A twofold increase in ventricular extrasystolic activity is the most commonly encountered arrhythmia after reperfusion (occurring in 48% of PTCAs). Accelerated idioventricular rhythm appears in 39% of cases.[12] Bradycardia after balloon inflation (especially in inferoposterior infarctions) is reported to occur in 2–16% of cases.[12,24] Atrial fibrillation is estimated at about 5% and transient AV block at 9% of procedures.[24]

Table 18.2 Arrhythmias associated with PCI
Bradyarrhythmias Sinus bradycardia AV block Asystole
Tachyarrhythmias Ventricular extrasystoles Accelerated idioventricular rhythm VT (sustained and nonsustained)/VF Atrial fibrillation

Sustained ventricular tachycardia or fibrillation are relatively rare events in the modern transcatheter reperfusion era. Their frequency is reported to be 4.3% in a large series which particularly studied the occurrence of these two arrhythmias in the setting of acute myocardial infarction.[25]

In elective PTCA, symptomatic bradycardia and hypotension was reported to occur in 14% of cases post PCI and to appear more commonly in patients having LAD angioplasty or being on therapy with beta or calcium blockers.[26]

Sustained ventricular tachycardia and ventricular fibrillation

Sustained ventricular tachycardia (VT) and ventricular fibrillation are two life-threatening arrhythmias which may complicate PCIs (Figure 18.2). The cardiologist should therefore be ready for fast and adequate treatment. Both tachycardias can be the result of ongoing ischemia or reperfusion of myocardial tissue. In a large study of 3065 primary PCIs in the modern era, sustained VT and VF correlated with smoking, lack of periprocedural beta blockers, time from symptoms to cath lab less than three hours, thrombolysis in myocardial infarction (TIMI) flow 0 and RCA-related infarct.[25] A small orifice caliber has been suggested as a reason for this RCA predilection in the appearance of VF.[27] Importantly, those malignant arrhythmias which appeared in the laboratory did not influence one-year outcome. This is in contrast to the unfavorable prognosis of ventricular arrhythmias occurring more than 48 hours after acute myocardial infarction. This is explained by the fact that the former arrhythmias reflect ongoing ischemia or reperfusion whilst the late ventricular tachycardias are related to irreversibly diseased myocardium as an arrhythmogenic substrate. Consistent results were seen in a smaller study which found no VF recurrence in the next 24 hours after its occurrence in the laboratory during reperfusion. RCA infarcts were again associated with a higher incidence of VF.[24]

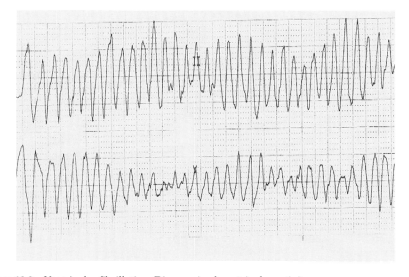

Figure 18.2   Ventricular fibrillation. Disorganized ventricular activity.

Immediate management with DC shock (200 joules increased to 300 and if necessary to 360 if previous shocks are not successful), synchronized for VT or nonsynchronized for VF, is the therapy of choice. In patients who tolerate ventricular arrhythmias hemodynamically well, a single bolus of 0.1–0.25 mg intracoronary verapamil can be tried in case of arrhythmias which occur after reperfusion.[28] In cases refractory to external cardioversion, intravenous bolus treatment with amiodarone before shock delivery can increase efficiency. It should be kept in mind that arrhythmias are the result of ischemia and reperfusion and not the primary disease. Immediate efforts to restore coronary blood flow are mandatory. Antiarrhythmic treatment after the catheterization laboratory is not necessary.

Accelerated idioventricular rhythm/ventricular extrasystoles/nonsustained VT

Accelerated idioventricular rhythm is an accelerated broad QRS rhythm of ventricular origin with a rate less than 100 beats per minute. It is considered the archetype of reperfusion arrhythmias. The origin of the ventricular complexes lies in the Purkinje fibers which display enhanced automaticity during the period of reperfusion. In thrombolysis studies it has been used as a noninvasive, although inaccurate, marker of reperfusion. In a PCI study which compared electrocardiographic changes in STEMI patients 10 minutes after complete reperfusion achieved either by thrombolysis, primary PTCA or rescue PTCA, the overall incidence of accelerated idioventricular rhythm was only 42%. Interestingly, 13% of patients did not show any type of reperfusion arrhythmia although complete reperfusion was established. Moreover, TIMI 2 or 3 flow had no impact on reperfusion arrhythmias. The occurrence of accelerated idioventricular rhythm did not correlate with the severity of infarction as assessed by TnT status in another study.[13]

An increase in the number of PVCs is a commonly occurring reperfusion arrhythmia after the balloon deflation, without having clinical consequences. Nonsustained ventricular tachycardia (defined as ≥3 ventricular complexes with heart rate >100 beats per minute) is seen in 5% and 9% of primary and rescue PCIs respectively.[12]

All of these reperfusion arrhythmias are regarded as benign arrhythmias and do not need additional therapeutic measures as long as they do not result in hemodynamic compromise. Their peak incidence is within two hours of the inflation and they last for less than 24 hours,[13] with ventricular premature beats (isolated as well as runs) being the last to resolve.

Supraventricular tachycardias

Supraventricular arrhythmias as atrial premature beats or atrial fibrillation can occur in the catheterization laboratory. The appearance of atrial fibrillation is multifactorial. It can be the result of increased atrial stretch due to raised left ventricular end-diastolic pressures, increased sympathetic stimulation, AV valvular insufficiency, atrial infarction or pericarditis.[29] Atrial fibrillation can occur also after restoration of blood flow as a reperfusion arrhythmia. In this setting its frequency is estimated as 5–10% in the immediate post balloon inflation period.[12,24] Pharmacologic (amiodarone) or electrical therapy should be used for conversion of new-onset atrial fibrillation to sinus rhythm. Rate control can be achieved with digitalis. Treatment for atrial premature beats is not necessary.

Bradycardias

Bradycardias can be the result of ischemia and reperfusion injury of impulse propagating and conducting tissue or the result of vagal stimulation. Sinus bradycardia and various degrees of AV block (first-degree to complete AV block) and even asystole can occur. Ischemia can be the mechanism for all of these arrhythmias. RCA-related PCIs and infarctions are often associated with sinus bradycardia and/or AV block. These bradycardias are often benign and reversible as they are often vagally mediated, involving the sinus node and the proximal AV conduction system, and are related to less extensive myocardial damage. The opposite is true for anteroseptal infarctions where AV conduction disturbances indicate large anteroseptal necrosis involving the distal His–Purkinje system.

Bradycardia can also occur as a result of reperfusion. The incidence can be as high as 16% during the first ten minutes after balloon deflation and blood flow restoration.[12] The incidence of transient complete AV block was reported to be 9%.[24] All cases of AV block resolved in the laboratory and no recurrence was noticed during 24 hours of rhythm monitoring. PCI of the right coronary artery was also significantly related to reperfusion-induced AV block.

Sinus bradycardia does not need treatment unless it causes hemodynamic compromise due to extremely low rate or ventricular dysfunction. Atropine 1–2 mg can be given. In case of complete AV block, temporary pacing may be necessary. Temporary pacing through the guidewire has been used for the treatment of bradycardia as well as for the treatment of VT (overdrive pacing)[30] or asystole. Adequate hydration, pain control, and reassurance are helpful for periprocedural vasovagal reactions.

PREVENTION

Optimal anti-ischemic treatment before starting PCI is of paramount importance for the prevention of sustained ventricular tachyarrhythmias occurring in the catheterization laboratory. Beta blockers seem to be particularly effective in the prevention of VF/VT as it has been shown that lack of beta blocker treatment is a strong risk factor for sustained ventricular tachyarrhythmias during PCI.[25] Angiotensin enzyme inhibitors may also reduce the incidence of reperfusion arrhythmias. Dipyridamole 0.5 mg/kg intravenously before balloon inflation has been shown to protect against reperfusion arrhythmias.[31] Optimizing electrolyte balance and arterial oxygenation is also essential.

CONCLUSION

Although interventional techniques for treating coronary artery disease have improved significantly during recent years, cardiac arrhythmias may still complicate PCIs. These arrhythmias range from innocent extrasystoles to sustained ventricular tachycardia and fibrillation necessitating immediate treatment. Primary PTCA is a risk factor for their occurrence as ischemia-reperfusion injury (more frequently the latter) is the usual underlying pathophysiologic mechanism. Right coronary intervention and lack of beta blocker pretreatment are clear risk factors for the occurrence of sustained ventricular arrhythmias. In general, cardiac arrhythmias which occur during PCI are usually limited to the catheterization laboratory. They lack prognostic significance, in contrast to ventricular tachycardias occurring more than 48 hours after myocardial infarction, and long-term treatment is not indicated.

REFERENCES

1. Carmeliet E. Cardiac ionic currents and acute ischemia: from channels to arrhythmias. Physiol Rev 1999;79(3):917–1017.
2. Janse MJ, Wit AL. Electrophysiological mechanisms of ventricular arrhythmias resulting from myocardial ischemia and infarction. Physiol Rev 1989;69(4):1049–69.
3. Coronel R, Wilms-Schopman FJG, Janse MJ. Profibrillatory effects of intracoronary thrombus in acute regional ischemia of the in situ porcine heart. Circulation 1997;96:3985–91.
4. Goldstein JA, Butterfield MC, Ohnishi Y et al. Arrhythmogenic influence of intracoronary thrombosis during acute myocardial ischemia. Circulation 1994;90:139–47.
5. Kajiyama A, Saito D, Murakami T et al. Relation of QT-interval variability to ventricular arrhythmias during percutaneous transluminal coronary angioplasty. Jpn Circ J 2001;65: 779–82.
6. Nowinski K, Jensen S, Lundahl G et al. Changes in ventricular repolarization during percutaneous transluminal coronary angioplasty in humans assessed by QT interval, QT dispersion and T vector loop morphology. J Intern Med 2000;248:126–36.
7. Airaksinen KE, Ikaheimo MJ, Huikuri HV. Stenosis severity and the occurrence of ventricular ectopic activity during acute coronary occlusion during balloon angioplasty. Am J Cardiol 1995;76(5):346–9.
8. Ando' G, Gaspardone A, Proietti I. Acute thrombosis of the sinus node artery: arrhythmological implications. Heart 2003;89:e5.
9. Ahrensfield D, Balke CW, Benitez RM et al. Transient sinus node dysfunction in acute myocardial infarction associated with the use of a coronary stent. Cathet Cardiovasc Intervent 2000;50:349–51.
10. Krumholz HM, Golberger AL. Reperfusion arrhythmias after thrombolysis: electrophysiologic tempest, or much ado about nothing. Chest 1991;99(4 Suppl):135S–140S.
11. Wit AL, Janse MJ. Reperfusion arrhythmias and sudden cardiac death. Circ Res 2001;89:741–3.
12. Wehrens XHT, Doevendans PA, Ophuis TJO et al. A comparison of electrocardiographic changes during reperfusion of acute myocardial infarction by thrombolysis or percutaneous transluminal coronary angioplasty. Am Heart J 2000;139:430–6.
13. Bonnemeier H, Wiegand UKH, Giannitsis E et al. Temporal repolarization inhomogeneity and reperfusion arrhythmias in patients undergoing successful primary percutaneous coronary intervention for acute ST-segment elevation myocardial infarction: impact of admission of troponin T. Am Heart J 2003;145:484–92.
14. Engelen DJ, Gressin V, Krucoff MW et al. Usefulness of frequent arrhythmias after epicardial recanalization in anterior wall acute myocardial infarction as a marker of cellular injury leading to poor recovery of left ventricular function. Am J Cardiol 2003;92:1143–9.
15. Shimada Y, Avkiran M. Susceptibility to ischemia and reperfusion arrhythmias in myocardial hypertrophy. Jpn Heart J 2003;44:989–1004.
16. Harada K, Komuro I, Hayashi D et al. Angiotensin II type 1a receptor is involved in the occurrence of reperfusion arrhythmias. Circulation 1998;97:315–17.
17. Takezako T, Zhang B, Serikawa T et al. The D allele of the angiotensin-converting enzyme gene and reperfusion-induced ventricular arrhythmias in patients with acute myocardial infarction. Jpn Circ J 2001;65:603–9.
18. Airaksinen KEJ, Huikuri HV. Antiarrhythmic effect of repeated coronary occlusion during balloon angioplasty. J Am Coll Cardiol 1997;29:1035–8.
19. Batur MK, Yildirir A, Onalan O et al. Angioplasty induced myocardial ischemia prolongs the signal-averaged P-wave duration in single vessel coronary artery disease. Europace 2002;4:289–93.

20. Budeus M, Hennersdorf M, Dierkes S et al. Effects of right coronary artery PTCA on variables of P-wave signal averaged electrocardiogram. Ann NonInvasive Electrocardiol 2003;8:150–6.
21. Hirshfeld JW. Radiographic contrast agents. In: Skorton DJ, Schelbert HR, Wolf GL, Brundage BH, eds. Marcus Cardiac Imaging: A Companion to Braunwald's Heart Disease. (electronic edition). Philadelphia, PA: WB Saunders, 1996: Ch 18.
22. Ritchie JL, Nissen SE, Douglas JS et al. Use of nonionic or low osmolar contrast agents in cardiovascular procedures. J Am Coll Cardiol 1993;21:269–73.
23. Romanelli MF, Meissner MD, Fromm BS et al. Prominent ECG repolarization changes associated with intracoronary infusion of normal saline: comparisons with alternate coronary catheter flush solutions. Cathet Cardiovasc Intervent 1999;48:359–64.
24. Giglioli C, Margheri M, Valente S et al. The incidence and timing of major arrhythmias following successful primary angioplasty for acute myocardial infarction. Ital Heart J 2005;6:28–34.
25. Mehta RH, Harjai KJ, Grines L. Sustained ventricular tachycardia or fibrillation in the cardiac catheterization laboratory among patients receiving primary percutaneous coronary intervention: incidence, predictors, and outcomes. J Am Coll Cardiol 2004;43:1765–72.
26. Mager A, Strasberg B, Rechavia E et al. Clinical significance and predisposing factors to symptomatic bradycardia and hypotension after percutaneous transluminal coronary angioplasty. Am J Cardiol 1994;74:1085–8.
27. Huang JL, Ting CT, Chen YT et al. Mechanisms of ventricular fibrillation during coronary angioplasty: increased incidence for the small orifice caliber of the right coronary artery. Int J Cardiol 2002;82:221–8.
28. Kato M, Dote K, Sasaki S et al. Intracoronary verapamil rapidly terminates reperfusion tachyarrhythmias in acute myocardial infarction. Chest 2004;126:702–8.
29. Antman EM, Anbe DT, Armstrong PW et al. ACC/AHA guidelines for the management of patients with ST-elevation myocardial infarction. Circulation 2000;110:e82–292.
30. Goode G, Bennett D. Successful coronary pace-termination of ventricular tachycardia during coronary angioplasty. Cathet Cardiovasc Diagn 1997;42:31–2.
31. Yoshida Y, Hirai M, Yamada T et al. Antiarrhythmic efficacy of dipyridamole in treatment of reperfusion arrhythmias. Circulation 2000;101:624–30.

19

Renal complications after percutaneous intervention: cholesterol embolism and contrast nephropathy

Patricia JM Best, Roxanna Mehran and Charanjit S Rihal

Cholesterol embolization syndrome • **Contrast-induced nephropathy**

Renal complications after a percutaneous coronary intervention (PCI) are one of the most common complications associated with the procedure. The primary causes of renal failure after PCI are cholesterol emboli syndrome and, more commonly, contrast-induced nephropathy (CIN). Understanding the differential diagnosis of renal failure after PCI, the implications, prognosis, and treatment modalities is essential for all interventionalists.

CHOLESTEROL EMBOLIZATION SYNDROME

Cholesterol embolization or systemic atheroemboli are an uncommon but important cause of renal failure after cardiac catheterization and PCI. Cholesterol emboli can affect all organs and may present as progressive renal failure up to four weeks after an invasive procedure. Renal involvement is found in approximately 65% of cases of cholesterol embolization and clinically occurs in approximately 1% of patients after cardiac catheterization when evaluated prospectively.[1] The diagnosis of cholesterol embolism can be made clinically by the appearance of livido reticularis or other peripheral stigmata of embolization, by elevated blood eosinophils, and by a pathologic diagnosis from a renal biopsy. Renal biopsy may demonstrate cells and other material in the vascular lumen and the so-called 'ghost' artifact due to extraction of cholesterol during tissue processing.[2,3] At autopsy, renal involvement can be confirmed pathologically in 75% of patients who have cholesterol emboli. However, the lack of renal pathologic findings does not exclude the diagnosis of cholesterol emboli.

Risk factors for the development of cholesterol emboli include male gender, advanced age, use of large-caliber catheters, and anticoagulant and thrombolytic therapy. Approximately 85% of patients with cholesterol emboli have had an invasive procedure within the preceding three months, making direct vascular trauma of an atherosclerotic vessel the most common mechanism for the development of cholesterol emboli.[4] Because atherosclerosis is a requirement for the development of cholesterol emboli, it is not surprising that these patients more frequently have cardiovascular risk factors. Another mechanism involved in the development of cholesterol emboli syndrome is activation of the complement system which is seen in over half of these patients. Additionally, recent anticoagulant and thrombolytic therapy use is found in 13–22% of patients with cholesterol emboli. This finding may be due to the loss of superficial clots which are stabilizing plaque and their dissolution may allow for the plaque embolization. In a recent study by Fukumoto and colleagues, independent predictors of cholesterol embolization were the patient presenting with an acute coronary syndrome, diffuse atherosclerosis (multivessel coronary disease, cerebrovascular disease, and abdominal aortic aneurysms), hypertension, smoking, a baseline serum creatinine ≥2.0 mg/dL, and a C-reactive protein ≥1.0 mg/dL.[1] Importantly, patients may also present with accelerating hypertension, which is difficult to control because of activation of the renin–angiotensin system.

Treatment of cholesterol emboli-induced renal failure is mainly supportive but responses to high-dose corticosteroids with or without plasma exchange, low-density lipoprotein apheresis, and statin therapy have been reported.[4-6] Avoidance or discontinuation of anticoagulation is necessary because it can worsen the condition by increasing further embolization. Mortality after cholesterol embolization has been reported to be as high as 81%, with over half the survivors progressing to require dialysis. Once patients are stable on dialysis, their outcomes were not different from those of the general dialysis population.[4] The paucity of treatment options in these patients and the marked morbidity and mortality associated with cholesterol emboli warrant future studies. Keen clinical awareness is needed to accurately diagnose this rare but significant cause of renal failure after PCI.

CONTRAST-INDUCED NEPHROPATHY

Contrast-induced nephropathy (CIN) is by far the most common cause of acute renal failure following PCI, and is the third most common cause of in-hospital acute renal failure.[7] CIN is most typically defined as an increase in serum creatinine of 0.5 mg/dL but multiple definitions have been used, including an increase in serum creatinine of 1 mg/dL or a 25% increase or decrease in the creatinine clearance. Typically with CIN, the creatinine starts to rise 24–48 hours after contrast exposure and peaks between three and seven days. The reported incidence of CIN has varied widely, in part because of methodologic differences between studies. For example, reports have varied in the timing of creatinine measurements after contrast exposure and differ in how meticulously the creatinine was followed.

The true frequency of CIN is likely underestimated.[8] In most patient populations, between 5% and 20% of patients develop CIN after coronary angiography or a PCI, but this number varies depending on the risk of the population being studied.[9-12] Further studies evaluating the incidence of CIN requiring dialysis after PCI found that it was present in only 6.6–7.7/1000 patients, but that these patients had an even higher mortality than those with CIN not requiring dialysis.[13,14]

Thus, CIN is a frequent complication after a PCI, characterized by a rise in serum creatinine shortly after PCI, and infrequently requires dialysis.

Mechanisms

The exact mechanism of CIN is unknown but multiple potential mechanisms exist and are being investigated. Contrast agents initially act as renal vasodilators, but subsequently have a potent vasoconstrictor effect.[15,16] Reduction in renal blood flow is partially mediated through stimulation of the renin–angiotensin system and by inhibiting the production of vasodilating substances such as prostacyclin.[17,18] During the reduction in renal blood flow, creatinine clearance is reduced and the thick ascending limb of the loop of Henle in the medulla becomes hypoxic. Contrast agents also may alter glomerular permeability and cause proximal tubular injury. An osmotic diuresis ensues and increases the metabolic demand of the already hypoxic medulla. Thus, medications that increase renal blood flow may decrease the likelihood of acute and persistent renal dysfunction.

Clinical implications

CIN is a significant source of morbidity and mortality. The development of CIN after coronary angiography is associated with a risk of death of 6.6–13 times that of patients who do not develop CIN.[13,19,20] If dialysis is required, the likelihood of death increases to 8.5–13.5 times the mortality of those with CIN but without the need for dialysis.[13,14] In a study by Gruberg and colleagues, one-year mortality in patients with CIN requiring dialysis was 54.5%[14] and in the study by McCullough and colleagues the mortality at two years was 81%.[13] Additionally, CIN markedly prolongs hospitalization among patients who survive and is associated with increased procedural complications including cardiac arrest, shock, intra-aortic balloon pump use, stroke and vascular complications (Table 19.1).[19] Some patients experience a permanent rise in serum creatinine after contrast exposure. Even if the creatinine returns to baseline, there is evidence that renal dysfunction may persist.[21,22] Thus, CIN is an important complication after a PCI because it is strongly associated with procedural complications, in-hospital complications and death, and long-term morbidity and mortality. When CIN requires dialysis, the morbidity and mortality associated with it is even higher.

Multiple CIN risk factors, including both patient factors (Table 19.2) and procedural factors (Table 19.3), have been identified.

The main predictor of CIN is baseline renal function, primarily a creatinine clearance <60 mL/min, although the presence of diabetes and the type and amount of

Table 19.1   Procedural complications comparing patients who developed CIN after a PCI with those who did not (modified from Rihal et al[19])

Variable, %	CIN (n=254)	No CIN (n=7332)	*P*-value
Procedural success	72.8	94.0	<0.0001
Death	22.0	1.4	<0.0001
Q-wave myocardial infarction	3.9	0.9	<0.0001
Creatinine kinase rise	16.9	6.1	<0.0001
Shock	13.0	3.1	<0.0001
Cardiac arrest	11.4	1.5	<0.0001
Intra-aortic balloon pump use	11.4	3.1	<0.0001
Femoral bleeding	3.1	1.4	0.03
Stroke	1.2	0.03	0.05
Adult respiratory distress syndrome	9.4	0.7	<0.0001
Gastrointestinal bleeding	4.3	1.2	<0.0001

Table 19.2 Patient factors associated with CIN

- Baseline creatinine or creatinine clearance
- Diabetes mellitus
- Female gender
- Advanced age (>70 years)
- Nephrotoxic medications
- Anemia
- Acute coronary syndrome
- Volume depletion, hypotension, and hypovolemia
- Intra-aortic balloon pump use
- Low cardiac output
- Congestive heart failure
- Renal transplant patient
- Hypoalbuminemia
- Multiple myeloma

Table 19.3 Procedural factors associated with CIN

- Contrast amount
- Osmolality of contrast
- Multiple contrast media injections within 72 hours

contrast are also strong risk factors.[8,23,24] Other factors such as age and female gender may be risk factors because of their association with renal function. Procedural factors are important to identify as these factors are controllable by the interventionalist. High osmolar contrast agents are associated with a greater incidence of CIN, particularly in the highest risk patients with diabetes and chronic kidney disease defined as a baseline serum creatinine >1.5 mg/dL (47.7% vs 33.3%).[25] In the recent NEPHRIC study, 129 diabetics with a baseline creatinine 1.5–3.5 mg/dL undergoing angiography were randomized to the iso-osmolar contrast agent iodixanol or the low-osmolar contrast agent iohexanol (Figure 19.1).[26] The iso-osmolar contrast agent was associated with a lower incidence of CIN (3% vs 26%, P=0.002). Other procedural

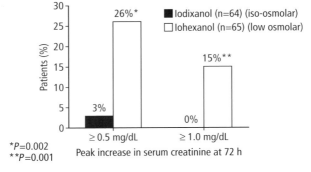

*P=0.002
**P=0.001

Figure 19.1 Differences in the peak serum creatinine at 72 hours based on the use of iodixanol or iohexnol in the randomized NEPHRIC Study.[26]

factors, such as the amount of contrast used, are important predictors of CIN and in a study by McCullough and colleagues, no patient who received <100 mL of contrast developed CIN requiring dialysis.[13] Techniques such as short bolus contrast injections, minimizing tests during the intervention, and the use of biplane fluoroscopy can all aid in lowering the contrast amount used and help to prevent CIN.

Using these patient and procedural risk factors, predictive risk scores for CIN have been developed.[27,28] Mehran and colleagues (Tables 19.4, 19.5) developed a simple and reliable estimate of CIN, and CIN requiring dialysis. Using a risk score to predict the development of CIN may aid in targeting prevention strategies to the highest risk patients.

Prevention

Treatments to prevent CIN have focused primarily on mechanisms that prevent the reduction in renal blood flow and hypoxia to the renal medulla caused by the contrast. Multiple agents have been studied (Table 19.6), but in large studies few have actually been associated with benefit (Table 19.7).

Hydration is the mainstay of preventive therapy and has consistently resulted in a reduction in CIN.[29] Additionally, in a prospective study by Mueller and colleagues of

Table 19.4   Risk factor scores for a predictive score for CIN (modified from Mehran et al[27])

Risk factor	Score
Hypotension (systolic blood pressure <80 mmHg for 1 h requiring inotropic support)	5
Intra-aortic balloon pump (within 24 h periprocedurally)	6
Congestive heart failure, NYHA Class III/IV	5
Age >75 years	4
Anemia (hematocrit <39% for men and <36% for women)	3
Diabetes	3
Contrast media volume	1 for each 100 mL
Serum creatinine >1.5 mg/dL Or Estimated glomerular filtration rate < 60 mL/min/1.73 m^2	4 Or 2 for 40–60 mL/min/1.73 m^2 4 for 20–40 mL/min/1.73 m^2 6 for <20 mL/min/1.73 m^2

Table 19.5   Risk scores for CIN and outcomes (modified from Mehran et al[27])

Risk score	Risk of CIN	Risk of dialysis
≤5	7.5%	0.04%
6–10	14.0%	0.12%
11–16	26.1%	1.09%
≥16	57.3%	12.6%

Table 19.6   Agents that do NOT prevent contrast nephropathy
• Mannitol • Furosemide • Theophylline • Larginine • Dopamine • Atrial natriuretic peptide • Mixed endothelin antagonists • Calcium channel blockers • Fenoldopam

Table 19.7   Agents that may prevent contrast nephropathy

Definite
  • Hydration
  • Low osmotic contrast agents
Possible
  • N-acetylcysteine
  • Bicarbonate
  • Hemofiltration
  • Use of alternate contrast agents (gadolinium)
  • Statins

1620 patients undergoing PCI, hydration with normal saline compared with half-isotonic saline on the day of the procedure was associated with more than a 50% reduction in the incidence of CIN (2.0% vs 0.7%).[30] Other strategies such as forced diuresis with an infusion of mannitol or with furosemide administration are no longer recommended due to lack of efficacy or worsened renal function with their use (Figure 19.2).[31-33]

Low-dose dopamine increases renal medullary blood flow through the dopaminergic receptors, and was thought to be a promising agent for the prevention

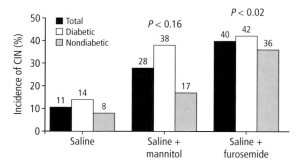

Figure 19.2   Effects of saline, mannitol, and furosemide on the prevention of contrast-induced nephropathy.[33]

of CIN. Despite its theoretical benefits, low-dose dopamine had little or no effect on the incidence of CIN in small randomized trials.[31,34–36] One possible reason why dopamine was ineffective was that, although at low doses it should have effects primarily at the DA_1 dopamine receptor subtype which increases renal blood flow in the medulla and inner cortex, it may also stimulate the DA_2 dopamine receptor which reduces renal blood flow. Fenoldopam, a DA_1 dopamine receptor agonist that has no effect on the DA_2 dopamine receptors, seemed like an ideal agent and in small studies, appeared to protect against CIN in high-risk patients.[37,38] However, in the prospective randomized controlled CONTRAST study by Stone and colleagues of 283 patients, no benefit was demonstrated and the drug is no longer used (Figure 19.3).[39]

Several agents are being investigated that may have a role in the prevention of CIN. One of the most controversial is N-acetylcysteine (NAC). The initial enthusiasm for a therapeutic role of NAC came from the study by Tepel and colleagues.[40] In this prospective randomized study of 83 patients undergoing a CT scan, patients were given 600 mg of NAC twice on the day before the procedure and twice on the day of the procedure. This resulted in a marked reduction of CIN from 12% to 2% ($P=0.01$). Multiple studies of NAC use followed, primarily with oral dosing similar to that of Tepel's study but also including IV studies. Additionally, mechanistic studies have been performed that suggest the benefit of N-acetylcysteine may be due to the prevention of increases in oxidative stress that occur with contrast exposure.[41] Furthermore, serum creatinine levels can be lowered with administration of NAC in normal volunteers without altering cystatin C levels, another marker of renal function.[42] This suggests that NAC alters creatinine metabolism but may not actually alter true CIN. Ten meta-analyses of available trials have been performed. These suggest a small benefit when N-acetylcysteine is used in conjunction with hydration for the prevention of CIN, but the significant heterogeneity of the studies precludes drawing definitive conclusions.[43–50] A large multicenter randomized clinical trial with end-points other than serum creatinine or estimated creatinine clearance will be necessary in order to fully ascertain the benefits of N-acetylcysteine.

Another agent possibly helpful for the prevention of CIN is bicarbonate. In a prospective study by Merten and colleagues of 119 patients who received a bolus of 3 mL/kg/h of 154 mEq/L of sodium bicarbonate or sodium chloride for one hour

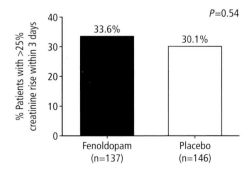

Figure 19.3 The effects of fenoldopam on the prevention of contrast-induced nephropathy in the CONTRAST trial.[39]

before cardiac catheterization and then 1 mL/kg/h for six hours after the procedure, a significant reduction in CIN at two days was seen (Figure 19.4).[51] Larger trials are necessary to confirm this finding before widespread application is warranted.

Hemofiltration may also be a strategy for the prevention of CIN. In a study by Marenzi and colleagues of 114 patients with 58 randomized to continuous venovenous hemofiltration for 4–6 hours before angiography and 18–24 hours after, a significant reduction in CIN was seen with hemofiltration (Figure 19.5).[52] However, alterations in the incidence of CIN by the definition of creatinine to determine renal dysfunction may be misleading given that the hemofiltration decreases the creatinine. Furthermore, other studies of hemodialysis have shown no benefit in prevention of CIN.[53–56] Even if with large studies there is benefit in preventing CIN with hemofiltration, because of the vascular access risk and intensive care unit requirements, this prevention strategy would be limited to very select, high-risk patients.

Other alternatives to prevent CIN include the use of gadolinium as a contrast agent in isolated case reports.[57,58] Although gadolinium does not delineate fine detail of the coronary vessels to the same extent that our standard contrast agents do, it generally provides adequate visualization and therefore could be an acceptable alternative contrast agent. However, in a retrospective study, CIN was found to be

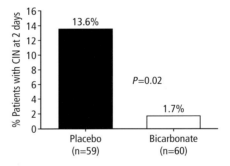

Figure 19.4 Prevention of contrast-induced nephropathy by bicarbonate.[51]

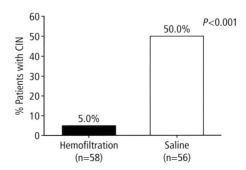

Figure 19.5 The use of continuous venovenous hemofiltration for the prevention of contrast-induced nephropathy.[52]

3.5% after gadolinium studies.[59] Further prospective studies are under investigation to determine if gadolinium is safer than standard contrast agents.

In summary, renal complications after PCI are common and are associated with significant morbidity and mortality. Careful prevention and identification of these complications are needed in a good interventional practice.

REFERENCES

1. Fukumoto Y, Tsutsui H, Tsuchihashi M, Masumoto A, Takeshita A. Cholesterol Embolism Study (CHEST) Investigators. The incidence and risk factors of cholesterol embolization syndrome, a complication of cardiac catheterization: a prospective study. J Am Coll Cardiol 2003;42:211–16.
2. Bashore TM, Gehrig T. Cholesterol emboli after invasive cardiac procedures. J Am Coll Cardiol 2003;42:217–18.
3. Vidt DG. Cholesterol emboli: a common cause of renal failure. Ann Rev Med 1997;48:375–85.
4. Modi KS, Rao VK. Atheroembolic renal disease. J Am Soc Nephrol 2001;12:1781–7.
5. Hasegawa M, Kawashima S, Shikano M et al. The evaluation of corticosteroid therapy in conjunction with plasma exchange in the treatment of renal cholesterol embolic disease. A report of 5 cases. Am J Nephrol 2000;20:263–7.
6. Cabili S, Hochman I, Goor Y. Reversal of gangrenous lesions in the blue toe syndrome with lovastatin – a case report. Angiology 1993;44:821–5.
7. Hou SH, Bushinsky DA, Wish JB, Cohen JJ, Harrington JT. Hospital-acquired renal insufficiency: a prospective study. Am J Med 1983;72:243–8.
8. Berns AS. Nephrotoxicity of contrast media. Kidney Int 1989;36:730–40.
9. D'Elia JA, Gleason RE, Alday M et al. Nephrotoxicity from angiographic contrast material. A prospective study. Am J Med 1982;72:719–25.
10. Parfrey PS, Griffiths SM, Barrett BJ et al. Contrast material-induced renal failure in patients with diabetes mellitus, renal insufficiency, or both. A prospective controlled study. N Engl J Med 1989;320:143–9.
11. Manske CL, Sprafka JM, Strony JT, Wang Y. Contrast nephropathy in azotemic diabetic patients undergoing coronary angiography. Am J Med 1990;89:615–20.
12. Mason RA, Arbeit LA, Giron F. Renal dysfunction after arteriography. JAMA 1985;253:1001–4.
13. McCullough PA, Wolyn R, Rocher LL, Levin RN, O'Neill WW. Acute renal failure after coronary intervention: incidence, risk factors, and relationship to mortality. Am J Med 1997;103:368–75.
14. Gruberg L, Mehran R, Dangas G et al. Acute renal failure requiring dialysis after percutaneous coronary interventions. Cathet Cardiovasc Intervent 2001;52:409–16.
15. Nygren A, Ulfendahl HR. Effects of high- and low-osmolar contrast media on renal plasma flow and glomerular filtration rate in euvolaemic and dehydrated rats. A comparison between ioxithalamate, iopamidol, iohexol and ioxaglate. Acta Radiol 1989;30:383–9.
16. Weisberg LS, Kurnik PB, Kurnik BR. Radiocontrast-induced nephropathy in humans: role of renal vasoconstriction. Kidney Int 1992;41:1408–15.
17. Katzberg RW, Morris TW, Burgener FA, Kamm DE, Fischer HW. Renal renin and hemodynamic responses to selective renal artery catheterization and angiography. Invest Radiol 1977;12:381–8.
18. Workman RJ, Shaff MI, Jackson RV, Diggs J, Frazer MG, Briscoe C. Relationship of renal hemodynamic and functional changes following intravascular contrast to the renin-angiotensin system and renal prostacyclin in the dog. Invest Radiol 1983;18:160–6.
19. Rihal CS, Textor SC, Grill DE et al. Incidence and prognostic importance of acute renal failure after percutaneous coronary intervention. Circulation 2002;105:2259–64.
20. Sadeghi HM, Stone GW, Grines CL et al. Impact of renal insufficiency in patients undergoing primary angioplasty for acute myocardial infarction. Circulation 2003;108:2769–75.

21. Finn WF. Enhanced recovery from postischemic acute renal failure. Micropuncture studies in the rat. Circ Res 1980;46:440–8.

22. Oken DE, DiBona GF, McDonald FD. Micropuncture studies of the recovery phase of myohemoglobinuric acute renal failure in the rat. J Clin Invest 1970;49:730–7.

23. Davidson CJ, Hlatky M, Morris KG et al. Cardiovascular and renal toxicity of a nonionic radiographic contrast agent after cardiac catheterization. A prospective trial. Ann Intern Med 1989;110:557–60.

24. Rich MW, Crecelius CA. Incidence, risk factors, and clinical course of acute renal insufficiency after cardiac catheterization in patients 70 years of age or older. A prospective study. Arch Intern Med 1990;150:1237–42.

25. Rudnick MR, Goldfarb S, Wexler L et al. Nephrotoxicity of ionic and nonionic contrast media in 1196 patients: a randomized trial. The Iohexol Cooperative Study. Kidney Int 1995;47:254–61.

26. Aspelin P, Aubry P, Fransson SG, Strasser R, Willenbrock R, Berg KJ. Nephrotoxicity in High-Risk Patients Study of Iso-Osmolar and Low-Osmolar Non-Ionic Contrast Media Study Investigators. Nephrotoxic effects in high-risk patients undergoing angiography. N Engl J Med 2003;348:491–9.

27. Mehran R, Aymong ED, Nikolsky E et al. A simple risk score for prediction of contrast-induced nephropathy after percutaneous coronary intervention: development and initial validation. J Am Coll Cardiol 2004;44:1391–9.

28. Bartholomew BA, Harjai KJ, Dukkipati S et al. Impact of nephropathy after percutaneous coronary intervention and a method for risk stratification. Am J Cardiol 2004;93:1515–19.

29. Eisenberg RL, Bank WO, Hedgock MW. Renal failure after major angiography can be avoided with hydration. AJR Am J Roentgenol 1981;136:859–61.

30. Mueller C, Buerkle G, Buettner HJ et al. Prevention of contrast media-associated nephropathy: randomized comparison of 2 hydration regimens in 1620 patients undergoing coronary angioplasty. Arch Intern Med 2002;162:329–36.

31. Stevens MA, McCullough PA, Tobin KJ et al. A prospective randomized trial of prevention measures in patients at high risk for contrast nephropathy: results of the P.R.I.N.C.E. Study. Prevention of Radiocontrast Induced Nephropathy Clinical Evaluation. J Am Coll Cardiol 1999;33:403–11.

32. Weisberg LS, Kurnik PB. Risk of radiocontrast nephropathy in patients with and without diabetes mellitus. Kidney Int 1994;45:259–65.

33. Solomon R, Werner C, Mann D, D'Elia J, Silva P. Effects of saline, mannitol, and furosemide to prevent acute decreases in renal function induced by radiocontrast agents. N Engl J Med 1994;331:1416–20.

34. Gare M, Haviv YS, Ben-Yehuda A et al. The renal effect of low-dose dopamine in high-risk patients undergoing coronary angiography. J Am Coll Cardiol 1999;34:1682–8.

35. Hall KA, Wong RW, Hunter GC et al. Contrast-induced nephrotoxicity: the effects of vasodilator therapy. J Surg Res 1992;53:317–20.

36. Hans B, Hans SS, Mittal VK, Khan TA, Patel N, Dahn MS. Renal functional response to dopamine during and after arteriography in patients with chronic renal insufficiency. Radiology 1990;176:651–4.

37. Lepor N. Radiocontrast nephropathy: the dye is not cast. Rev Cardiovasc Med 2000;1:43–54.

38. Tumlin JA, Wang A, Murray PT, Mathur VS. Fenoldopam mesylate blocks reductions in renal plasma flow after radiocontrast dye infusion: a pilot trial in the prevention of contrast nephropathy. Am Heart J 2002;143:894–903.

39. Stone GW, McCullough PA, Tumlin JA et al. CONTRAST Investigators. Fenoldopam mesylate for the prevention of contrast-induced nephropathy: a randomized controlled trial. JAMA 2003;290:2284–91.

40. Tepel M, van der Giet M, Schwartzfeld C, Laufer U, Liermann D, Zidek W. Prevention of radiographic-contrast-agent induced reductions in renal function by acetylcysteine. N Engl J Med 2000;343:180–4.

41. Drager LF, Andrade L, Barros de Toledo JF, Laurindo FR, Machado Cesar LA, Seguro AC.

Renal effects of N-acetylcysteine in patients at risk for contrast nephropathy: decrease in oxidant stress-mediated renal tubular injury. Nephrol Dial Transplant 2004;19:1803–7.

42. Hoffmann U, Fischereder M, Kruger B, Drobnik W, Kramer BK. The value of N-acetylcysteine in the prevention of radiocontrast agent-induced nephropathy seems questionable. J Am Soc Nephrol 2004;15:407–10.

43. Misra D, Leibowitz K, Gowda RM, Shapiro M, Khan IA. Role of N-acetylcysteine in prevention of contrast-induced nephropathy after cardiovascular procedures: a meta-analysis. Clin Cardiol 2004;27:607–10.

44. Nallamothu BK, Shojania KG, Saint S et al. Is acetylcysteine effective in preventing contrast-related nephropathy? A meta-analysis. Am J Med 2004;117:938–47.

45. Pannu N, Manns B, Lee H, Tonelli M. Systematic review of the impact of N-acetylcysteine on contrast nephropathy. Kidney Int 2004;65:1366–74.

46. Kshirsagar AV, Poole C, Mottl A et al. N-acetylcysteine for the prevention of radiocontrast induced nephropathy: a meta-analysis of prospective controlled trials. J Am Soc Nephrol 2004;15:761–9.

47. Alonso A, Lau J, Jaber BL, Weintraub A, Sarnak MJ. Prevention of radiocontrast nephropathy with N-acetylcysteine in patients with chronic kidney disease: a meta-analysis of randomized, controlled trials. Am J Kidney Dis 2004;43:1–9.

48. Birck R, Krzossok S, Markowetz F, Schnulle P, van der Woude FJ, Braun C. Acetylcysteine for prevention of contrast nephropathy: meta-analysis. Lancet 2003;362:598–603.

49. Bagshaw SM, Ghali WA. Acetylcysteine for prevention of contrast-induced nephropathy after intravascular angiography: a systematic review and meta-analysis. BMC Med 2004;2:38.

50. Duong MH, MacKenzie TA, Malenka DJ. N-acetylcysteine prophylaxis significantly reduces the risk of radiocontrast-induced nephropathy: comprehensive meta-analysis. Cathet Cardiovasc Intervent 2005;64:471–9.

51. Merten GJ, Burgess WP, Gray LV et al. Prevention of contrast-induced nephropathy with sodium bicarbonate: a randomized controlled trial. JAMA 2004;291:2328.

52. Marenzi G, Marana I, Lauri G et al. The prevention of radiocontrast-agent-induced nephropathy by hemofiltration. N Engl J Med 2003;349:1333–40.

53. Ferrari P, Vogt B. Hemofiltration and the prevention of radiocontrast-agent-induced nephropathy. N Engl J Med 2004;350:836–8.

54. Hsieh YC, Ting CT, Liu TJ, Wang CL, Chen YT, Lee WL. Short- and long-term renal outcomes of immediate prophylactic hemodialysis after cardiovascular catheterizations in patients with severe renal insufficiency. Int J Cardiol 2005;101:407–13.

55. Huber W, Jeschke B, Kreymann B et al. Haemodialysis for the prevention of contrast-induced nephropathy: outcome of 31 patients with severely impaired renal function, comparison with patients at similar risk and review. Invest Radiol 2002;37:471–81.

56. Vogt B, Ferrari P, Schonholzer C et al. Prophylactic hemodialysis after radiocontrast media in patients with renal insufficiency is potentially harmful. Am J Med 2001;111:692–8.

57. Sarkis A, Badaoui G, Slaba S, Moussalli A, Jebara VA. Gadolinium-based coronarography in a patient with renal failure: first clinical report. Cathet Cardiovasc Intervent 2001;54:68–9.

58. Bokhari SW, Wen YH, Winters RJ. Gadolinium-based percutaneous coronary intervention in a patient with renal insufficiency. Cathet Cardiovasc Intervent 2003;58:358–61.

59. Sam AD 2nd, Morasch MD, Collins J, Song G, Chen R, Pereles FS. Safety of gadolinium contrast angiography in patients with chronic renal insufficiency. J Vasc Surg 2003;38:313–18.

Section G
Noncoronary cardiac interventions

20

Complications of percutaneous valve interventions

Alec Vahanian, Jean-Pierre Bassand, Younes Boudjemline, Alain Cribier, Vasilis Babaliaros, Carla Agatiello and Ted Feldman

Percutaneous mitral commissurotomy • **Percutaneous aortic valvuloplasty**
• **Percutaneous pulmonary valvuloplasty** • **New percutaneous valve interventions**
• **Percutaneous mitral valve repair** • **Conclusion**

Interventional cardiology was introduced by Andreas Grüntzig in the 1970s and since then it has become a major player in the treatment of coronary disease, and peripheral, congenital, and acquired valve diseases. This review will cover the complications of the current percutaneous valve procedures: mitral commissurotomy, aortic valvuloplasty, pulmonary valvuloplasty, and the new developments of percutaneous aortic and pulmonary valve replacement, and mitral valve repair.

PERCUTANEOUS MITRAL COMMISSUROTOMY

Percutaneous mitral commissurotomy (PMC) has been in use since 1984. The good immediate and mid-term results obtained since then have led to its widespread dissemination. The several thousand procedures performed in patients with different clinical conditions and valve anatomy have allowed us to accurately assess the risk involved (Table 20.1).[1–10]

Table 20.1 Major complications of percutaneous mitral commissurotomy

Study	Number	Mortality (%)	Hemopericardium (%)	Embolism (%)	Severe mitral regurgitation (%)
Tuzcu et al[1]	311	1.7	–	–	8.7 (>2+ increase)
Ben Farhat et al[2]	463	0.4	0.7	2	4.6
Chen et al[3]	4832	0.12	0.8	0.5	1.4
NHLBI[4]	738	3	4	3	3
Iung et al[5]	2773	0.4	0.2	0.4	4.1
Stefanadis et al[6]	893	0.3	0	0	3.1
Cribier et al[7]	882	NA	1.4	NA	2.1

NA, not available; NHLBI, National Heart, Lung, and Blood Institute.

Procedural mortality ranges from 0% to 3%. The main causes of death are massive hemopericardium or the poor condition of the patient, often a factor in end-stage patients.

The incidence of *hemopericardium* varies from 0.5% to 12%. It may be related to transseptal catheterization or to left ventricular perforation by the guidewires or the balloon itself.

Hemopericardium usually has immediate clinical consequences resulting in tamponade and should always be suspected when hypotension occurs during PMC. In this situation echocardiography should be performed urgently before deterioration occurs (Figure 20.1). Hemopericardium requires pericardiocentesis performed under echocardiographic guidance after reversal of anticoagulation. If this is successful, PMC can be reattempted and the patient should be closely monitored. If pericardiocentesis fails, surgery is necessary. According to circumstances this could be drainage of the pericardial effusion alone or could also include valve surgery. Hemopericardium related to the transseptal puncture mostly occurs when the operator is less experienced.[1,5,8] Unfavorable patient characteristics such as severe atrial enlargement or moderate thoracic deformity also increase risk. In such cases echocardiographic monitoring using either transesophageal or intracardiac approaches could be helpful. In teams experienced in transseptal catheterization, echocardiographic guidance is restricted to cases where unexpected difficulties occur. Finally, extreme cardiothoracic deformity can, in very rare cases, be a contraindication to the technique. Furthermore, the occurrence of hemopericardium may be technique dependent. The performance of 'over-the-wire' techniques, such as the double balloon technique and its variant the multitrack technique[10] or the metallic commissurotome,[7] carries a higher risk of hemopericardium and requires the balloons to be carefully positioned and guidewires with a soft, precurved tip to be used. With a non-'over-the-wire' technique, such as Inoue's, the risk of left ventricular perforation is virtually eliminated.[9]

To minimize the risk of hemopericardium, PMC should not be performed in patients with high anticoagulation (INR >2). In such patients, who are otherwise at

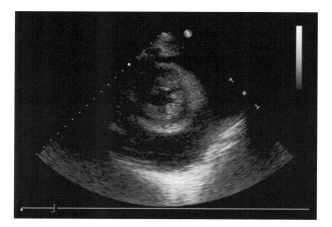

Figure 20.1   Massive pericardial effusion after PMC. Transthoracic echocardiography shows the pericardial effusion. Parasternal short-axis view (courtesy of Dr D Messika-Zeitoun).

high risk for left atrial thrombosis, vitamin K should not be given before the procedure and PMC should be delayed until a satisfactory level of coagulability is reached.

Embolism is encountered in 0.5–5% of cases. It may be due to a thrombus that was pre-existing or that developed during the procedure, to air leaking from the balloon, and, very rarely, to calcium. Cerebral embolism usually results in a stroke and treatment should be in collaboration with a stroke center. Cerebral imaging should be performed on an emergency basis to rule out hemorrhage, then fibrinolytic therapy should be administered early in the absence of contraindication. Coronary embolism most often leads to transient ST segment elevation in inferior leads, which is well tolerated when it is due to micro-bubbles of air that can occur when using the Inoue balloon and will resolve spontaneously. If it is due to embolization of a large quantity of air, such as when the balloon ruptures with the double balloon technique, it may lead to vagal reaction. In the case of persistent ST segment elevation coronary angiography should be performed. If a coronary occlusion is present, coronary angioplasty can be performed, while thromboaspiration could be an appealing alternative.

Although the incidence of embolism is low, its potential consequences are severe and all possible precautions should be taken to prevent it. PMC is contraindicated in patients with a thrombus floating in the left atrial cavity or located on the atrial septum so transesophageal echocardiography should be performed a few days prior to intervention to rule out the presence of such thrombi. No consensus has been reached regarding indication of PMC in patients with thrombosis in the left atrial appendage.[9,11] In such cases, the indications for PMC are limited to patients with contraindications to surgery or those without urgent need for intervention when oral anticoagulation can be given for at least two months and a new transesophageal echocardiographic examination shows the disappearance of the thrombus.

During PMC, heparin should be given as a bolus at a dose of around 3–5000 iu after the transseptal catheterization.

Severe mitral regurgitation is rare but represents an ever-present risk; its frequency ranges from 2% to 19%[1–10,12,13] (Figure 20.2). Surgical findings[13] have shown that it is related to noncommissural leaflet tearing, which could be associated with chordal rupture. In these cases, one or both commissures are often too tightly fused to be split (Figure 20.3). Severe mitral regurgitation may also be due to excessive commissural splitting or, in very rare cases, rupture of a papillary muscle. The majority of cases of

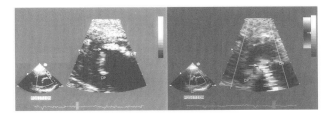

Figure 20.2   Severe mitral regurgitation after PMC. Periprocedural echocardiography shows a tear in the anterior leaflet (left) from which originates severe regurgitation (right). CA = anterior commissure. CP = posterior commissure (courtesy of Dr B Cormier).

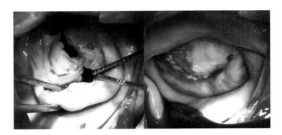

Figure 20.3   Severe mitral regurgitation. Operative view showing a median tear of the anterior leaflet (left) and the subsequent repair using a pericardial patch (right) (courtesy of Prof. C Acar).

severe mitral regurgitation occur in patients with unfavorable anatomy. In rare cases (<1%) a poor hemodynamic tolerance leading to hemodynamic collapse or refractory pulmonary edema may necessitate the support of an intra-aortic balloon pump en route to emergency surgery. As mitral regurgitation is usually initially well tolerated, surgery can be performed on a scheduled basis. In most cases, valve replacement is required because of the severity of the underlying valve disease. Conservative surgery has been successfully performed in cases of less severe valve deformity.[13]

At the present stage, the occurrence of severe mitral regurgitation remains largely unpredictable for a given patient[5,12] and its development depends more on the distribution of morphologic changes than on their severity. Patients with severe subvalvular impairment while the valves, *per se*, remain pliable also seem to be at higher risk. Scores that take into account the uneven distribution of anatomic deformities of the leaflets or commissural area have been developed.[14] Preliminary results for their use are promising but disputed.

The stepwise Inoue technique combined with echocardiographic monitoring is likely to decrease the incidence of severe regurgitation, even if it does not eliminate it. The balloon should be properly sized and the procedure should be stopped if the degree of regurgitation increases by more than 1+, especially if the regurgitation is located in a commissural area and if its mechanism is leaflet tear or chordal rupture.

The frequency of *interatrial shunts* due to tears of the septum reported after PMC varies from 10% to 90% depending on the technique used for detection.[1–10,15] They are usually small and without consequences since most of them will disappear on follow-up after successful PMC. If PMC is not successful, septal tears require closure at the time of subsequent surgery.

The incidence of transient, *complete heart block* is rare (<1%) and exceptionally requires implantation of a permanent pacemaker. *Atrial fibrillation* rarely occurs during the procedure. When it does, it is usually transient and resolves within a few hours under medical treatment. In rare cases, it requires electric countershock a few days after.

After the transvenous approach, *vascular complications* are the exception when using the antegrade approach but are more frequently seen with the retrograde approach.[6] In teams experienced in transseptal catheterization, left heart catheterization may be avoided to simplify the procedure and further reduce the incidence of vascular complication as well as shorten the duration of hospital stay.[16]

Endocarditis is extremely rare and does not justify prophylaxis before the procedure.

Overall, the considerable simplification resulting from use of the Inoue balloon could lead to a false sense of security and must not overshadow the importance of training. PMC should only be performed by groups whose experience with transseptal catheterization has been positive and who have been able to carry out an adequate number of procedures. This is particularly true for patients who have minimal symptoms, are pregnant or display cardiothoracic deformity.

PERCUTANEOUS AORTIC VALVULOPLASTY

The percutaneous treatment of inoperable aortic stenosis was first introduced in 1986.[17] This technique was largely abandoned by the mid 1990s because of the associated complications and the problem of valve restenosis.

The incidence of complications in historical registries and recent monocentric series is shown in Table 20.2.[17-21]

Death may result from progressive heart failure, hemopericardium, disruption of the aortic valve or severe arrhythmias, as well as other procedural complications. It may also be due to the poor cardiac and extracardiac condition of the patients, such as cardiogenic shock or severe co-morbidity.

Vascular injury at the access site has traditionally been the most common complication reported with percutaneous aortic valvuloplasty (PAV). Currently, it is unusual for vascular injury to require surgical repair thanks to the use of the following technical improvements: 12 F femoral sheath, which is compatible with a 23 mm ZMED II balloon (NuMED Inc., Hopkinton, NY) and other smaller balloons that can be used to perform valvuloplasty; and the 10 F Prostar XL arterial closure device (Abbott Vascular Devices, Redwood City, CA)[20] with no need for preclosure. Reversal of heparin with protamine is also helpful. The use of an antegrade approach decreases the incidence of such complications but carries the risks inherent to transseptal catheterization and is much more demanding.[21]

Table 20.2 Comparison of complications between historical and contemporary registry of patients after percutaneous aortic valvuloplasty

Complication	Mansfield Scientific Aortic Valvuloplasty Registry 1986–8 (492 patients)	Charles Nicolle Hospital experience, University of Rouen, France 2002–5 (141 patients)
Procedural death (within 24 hours)	24 (4.9%)	3 (2.1%)
Additional death (within 7 days)	13 (2.6%)	3 (2.1%)
Embolic events	11 (2.2%)	2 (1.4%)
Permanent neurologic sequelae	5 (1.1%)	0 (0%)
Left ventricular perforation resulting in tamponade	8 (1.6%)	0 (0%)
Massive aortic regurgitation	5 (1.1%)	2 (1.4%)
Vascular injury	52 (11%)	8 (5.7%)
Need for surgical repair	27 (5.5%)	0 (0%)
Nonfatal arrhythmias	5 (1.1%)	5 (3.5%)
Other	8 (1.6%)	1 (1%)
Patients with complications	101 (20.5%)	15 (10.6%)

Massive aortic regurgitation after PAV is rare. In patients with small stature or heavily calcified valves, dilatations can begin with a 20 mm balloon and advance to a 23 mm balloon if initial results are insufficient, balloon size appears small or there is no notable waist during inflation. If massive aortic regurgitation occurs, surgical valve replacement is necessary and its timing depends on clinical tolerance.

Hemopericardium is currently unusual and mostly the consequence of left ventricular perforation by the guidewire, crossing catheter or valvuloplasty balloon. If hypotension occurs during the procedure, this etiology should be checked for immediately. Hemopericardium can be avoided by crossing the valve with a diagnostic catheter and straight guidewire that is quickly exchanged, under fluoroscopic visualization, for a long wire with a preshaped, curved or 'ribboned' tip. In very rare cases massive hemopericardium is due to rupture of the aorta, which has a very poor prognosis even when operated immediately (Figure 20.4).

As with retrograde catheterization, clinically apparent *cerebral embolic events* are rare with PAV.[22] To help prevent these events, 5000 iu of heparin can be administered intravenously at the beginning of the procedure and the valve should be crossed with the minimum number of guidewire passes. An Amplatz 1 or 2 (according to the size of the aorta) or Sones catheter can be used to direct a straight guidewire across the valve in the left anterior oblique projection. The development of neurologic changes should prompt urgent imaging and a neurologist should be consulted.

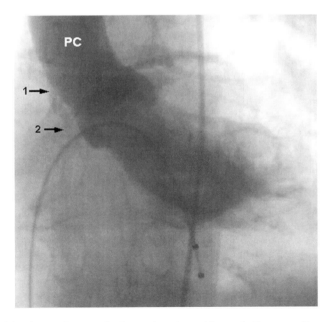

Figure 20.4   Massive aortic regurgitation and rupture of the aorta. Supra-aortic angiogram after PAV with a 23 mm balloon catheter in an elderly female reveals massive aortic regurgitation and rupture of the aorta. 1=origin of rupture. 2=continued extravasation of contrast dye. PC=pigtail catheter (courtesy of Prof. A Cribier).

High-degree atrioventricular block is rare and can occur in patients with previous conduction abnormalities. Often, it will resolve within 24–48 hours; otherwise permanent pacing is necessary. Valvuloplasty can be performed with a right ventricular pacing lead in place, which also allows pacing of the heart at a rate of 200–220 beats/minute, preventing balloon migration and allowing more complete inflation without potential damage from balloon movement in the ventricle or aorta.[23]

Overall, comparison of the early and recent results obtained with PAV in expert centers shows clear improvement. However, complications are a concern in common practice due to the lack of experience in performing this technique, which either has been abandoned or is very seldom used in most centers.

PERCUTANEOUS PULMONARY VALVULOPLASTY

Since the first description of balloon dilatation of a valvular pulmonic stenosis, percutaneous pulmonary valvuloplasty (PPV) has gained in popularity and is now considered to be the first-line treatment. The efficacy of this technique in terms of gradient relief has been well documented in a large number of series (Figure 20.5).

Complication and mortality rates are very low, reported to be respectively around 2.6% and 0.2%.[24,25] The incidence of complications is inversely related to age, with a higher incidence in infants.

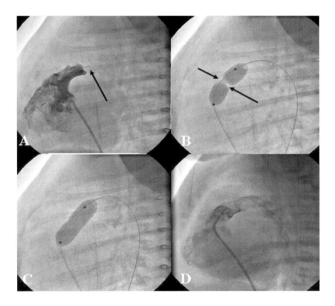

Figure 20.5 Balloon dilatation of a critical valve stenosis in a neonate. A. Angiogram in lateral view in the right ventricular infundibulum showing a tiny passage of dye contrast from the right ventricle to the pulmonary artery. B. After the advancement of a guidewire in the pulmonary artery through the stenosis, a balloon catheter is inflated in the area of the critical stenosis. C. Full opening of the stenosis is obtained after complete inflation of the balloon catheter. D. Angiogram at the end of the procedure showing a perfect opening of the right ventricular outflow tract (courtesy of Dr Y Boudjemline).

Vessel rupture is usually fatal, in particular in small patients in whom covered stents could not be used for repair. However, it can be avoided by careful sizing of the balloon according to measurements of the annulus using echocardiography and angiograms. A balloon-to-annulus ratio of around 1.3 is usually recommended.

Dynamic infundibular stenosis frequently occurs after this procedure; however, it usually disappears spontaneously after a few hours or after the prescription of oral beta blockers. Three particular groups will be discussed separately.

In patients with old pulmonary valve stenosis occurrence, possible complications depend on the presence or absence of atrial septal defect and/or right heart failure. If there is interatrial shunting, blood desaturation may increase during the procedure. Complications related to blood hyperviscosity should be prevented by correct hydration of the patient prior to the procedure, avoidance of contrast dye, and preliminary blood exchange. If a right heart failure is present with no atrial shunt, there is a high risk of low cardiac output and cardiac arrest during the procedure, in particular during valvular crossing. In this case, the procedure should use a stepwise dilatation technique and be completed as quickly as possible.

Newborns with critical stenosis or valve atresia are usually treated with a prostaglandin infusion to maintain the patency of the ductus arteriosus. To perforate the atretic valve, careful assessment using various fluoroscopic projections needs to ascertain that the wire is in the pulmonary artery or in the descending aorta before the balloon is advanced over the guidewire and inflated.[26] The prostaglandin infusion can be continued a few days, or even weeks, after the procedure to allow right ventricle compliance to recover. In some patients, a surgical shunt needs to be added later if saturation remains low.

The increased pulmonary blood flow created by this procedure can improve cyanosis in patients with pulmonary stenosis and a ventricular septal defect in the context of a complex heart defect. Because full opening of the valve would lead to pulmonary hypertension, special care should be taken to avoid over-opening the outflow tract and exposing the pulmonary artery bed to high pressure, which would rule out a later partial cavopulmonary connection.

NEW PERCUTANEOUS VALVE INTERVENTIONS

Percutaneous valve replacement and repair is an extremely young field. At the time of writing, fewer than 200 patients worldwide have been treated with any form of percutaneous valve intervention beyond balloon valvuloplasty.

Most of the complications related to these procedures have been fundamentally complications of cardiac catheterization. In addition to the complications of arterial catheterization, the specific problems related to transseptal catheterization will remain a baseline part of the complication rate of several of these procedures. Furthermore, the analysis of the results should take into account the fact that surgery was contraindicated or at very high risk in most patients. Finally, all of these procedures have been performed with first-generation, often prototype, equipment.

Percutaneous aortic valve replacement

After the failure of PAV, the rationale behind percutaneous aortic valve replacement (PAVR) was to find a percutaneous treatment for the large number of patients suffering from aortic stenosis who have a contraindication to or are very high risk for surgery.

The Percutaneous Valve Technologies/Edwards LifeSciences valve was the first device to be used for PAVR and the only one for which experience is reported so far. Forty patients have been enrolled for implantation based on a compassionate basis[23,27] (Table 20.3).

Most valves have been implanted using an antegrade transseptal approach. This allows a 24 F access sheath to be placed in a femoral vein, obviating arterial complications. However, this requires transseptal placement of a wire loop through the circulation, with the wire passing from the inferior vena cava to the right atrium, atrial septum, left atrium, left ventricle, and into the aorta, and then snared in the descending aorta.

Periprocedural mortality (within 24 hours) has been 10% in the patients enrolled for this study. Mortality at 30 days has been significantly higher, frequently due to pre-existing co-morbid conditions.

Intraprocedural transient hemodynamic collapse can lead to cardiac arrest and subsequent death if not managed promptly. It can occur in patients with depressed left ventricular function, cardiogenic shock or even small hypercontractile ventricles if antegrade implantation is attempted. In this situation, the guidewire loop (Figure 20.6) can exert traction on the anterior mitral leaflet, causing massive mitral regurgitation. A Sones catheter introduced from the contralateral femoral artery can remedy this problem by maintaining the shape of the guidewire loop within the left ventricular cavity. If this maneuver does not work, the guidewire should be withdrawn into the left atrium. Proceeding to valve implantation during a shock state can be catastrophic.

Vascular injury is a major concern in patients with underlying vascular disease and retrograde valve implantation (requiring a 24 F sheath in the femoral artery) is higher risk. Use of the antegrade method or closure devices in patients undergoing retrograde implantation has reduced this complication.[20] Patients with a femoral artery that is ≤7 mm should not be considered for retrograde implantation.

Stroke has been previously discussed in the PAV section and does not differ for prosthetic implantation.

Pericardial tamponade can be due to a complication of transseptal catheterization or ventricular perforation by the guidewire or the right ventricular pacing lead.

Table 20.3   Comparison of complications between the initial and current registry of patients undergoing percutaneous aortic valve replacement

	Pilot and I-REVIVE Trial (2002–4) 20 patients	RECAST Trial (2004–5) 20 patients
Procedural death (within 24 hours)	3	1
Additional death (within 7 days)	0	0
Transient hemodynamic collapse intraprocedure	8	1
Acute percutaneous heart valve migration	1	2
Moderate to severe paravalvular insufficiency	4	1
Tamponade	1	1
Stroke	1	0
Vascular injury requiring surgery	5	1
Renal failure requiring hemodialysis post procedure	3	0

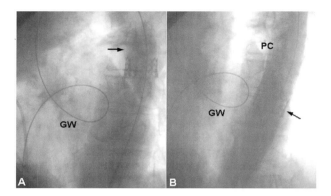

Figure 20.6   Damage to the mitral valve during PAVR. A. The PHV is deployed with a good guidewire loop (GW) configuration and stable hemodynamics. B. The PHV is deployed with a small guidewire loop (GW) which resulted in traction on the anterior mitral valve leaflet and subsequent hemodynamic collapse. C. As the PHV passes from the left atrium into the left ventricle, the guidewire loop (GW) is maintained with the help of a Sones catheter (SC) which is deep-seated in the left ventricle (courtesy of Prof. A Cribier).

Damage to the mitral valve and the atrial septum is seen exclusively with the antegrade approach where the anterior leaflet of the mitral valve can be transected during guidewire placement. This complication can be prevented by performing all guidewire maneuvers, such as removal or externalization to the arterial system, through a pigtail catheter. The atrial septum can be damaged after antegrade PAV prior to deployment of the prosthesis. In this situation, the edges of the deflated dilatation balloon may cause significant damage during removal. This can be avoided by using the retrograde approach whenever possible to perform PAV before prosthesis deployment. Persistent atrial septal defects after antegrade approach are not seen in the series from Rouen.[27]

The risk of *paravalvular leaks* is increased in patients with heavy valve calcification that can prevent full apposition of the prosthesis in the irregular orifice (Figure 20.7).

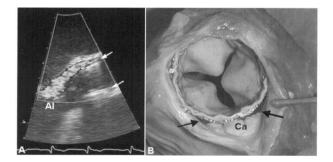

Figure 20.7   Paravalvular aortic insufficiency. A. Transesophageal image showing the stent frame of the aortic prosthesis (PHV) (arrows) and significant paravalvular aortic insufficiency (AI). B. Autopsy specimen showing malapposition of PHV (arrows) because of a large nodule of calcium (Ca) (courtesy of Prof. A Cribier).

Paravalvular leaks have been common as a result, though most are not severe, and are far better tolerated than the aortic stenosis they supplant. A notable waist in the 23 mm predilatation balloon during inflation should preclude these patients from valve implantation. Currently, new techniques such as use of larger devices (26 mm in place of the original 23 mm) are being developed to remedy this problem.

Valve migration can occur if the prosthesis is undersized or placed too high. Patients with a large aortic annulus (>23 mm) and mild valvular calcification are at risk for this complication. Once it has occurred, the valve can be moved distally into the descending aorta and deployed without clinical sequelae (Figure 20.8). Rapid right ventricular pacing (200–220 beats/minute) electrically arrests the motion of the heart during implantation and reduces the risk of migration.

Renal failure requiring hemodialysis post procedure is rare.

Obstruction of the coronaries by this percutaneous aortic valve prosthesis has not been an important problem.

Bearing in mind the high complication rate and technical difficulties of the antegrade approach, the current trend is to favor, whenever possible, the retrograde approach. This approach is much simpler and seems to have fewer complications because of technical improvements in catheter profiles, delivery systems, and the use of closure devices.

Pulmonary valve stenting and replacement

Right ventricle (RV) to pulmonary artery (PA) conduits have been widely used to surgically re-establish the continuity between the RV and PA. Their life span is limited by the development of progressive but inevitable obstruction. Surgical replacement of obstructed conduits is associated with increased morbidity. Successful

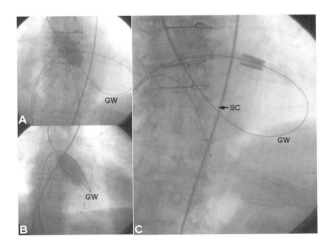

Figure 20.8 Migration of PAV prosthesis. A. LAO projection of a migrated PHV that has been moved into the descending aorta with the help of a partially inflated balloon catheter (arrow). GW=guidewire loop in left ventricle. B. Angiogram in the descending aorta shows a patent PHV (arrow) without obstruction to flow. GW=guidewire loop in left ventricle. PC=pigtail catheter (courtesy of Prof. A Cribier).

balloon angioplasty of those lesions has been described. However, the incidence of early and late failure is extremely high.

Stent implantation resulted in significant immediate hemodynamic and angiographic improvement.[28] Despite good mid-term results, several complications have been reported, namely misplacement, embolization or malposition of stent, balloon rupture during inflation, vascular damage, and/or hemodynamic disturbance. Long Mullins sheaths are used to avoid stent slippage and misplacement. A balloon-in-balloon catheter can be used to limit the risk of stent flaring and misplacement by allowing dye injection between the two balloon inflations and repositioning of valved stent before final deployment. Premounted stents, avoiding the need for large sheaths, limit risks of hemodynamic disturbance in infants and stent slippage.

Stent implantation by applying the valve of the conduit against its wall creates a pulmonary insufficiency that is deleterious for the RV.[29] This was the rationale for mounting a biologic valve into a stent (Numed, Medtronic Inc), the valved stent being deployed using a custom-made delivery system.[30] The current experience is in 78 patients, who have a mean of over three prior open heart surgical procedures, and shows good results in terms of clinical improvement, hemodynamics, and valvular competency.

There was no procedural mortality.

Urgent surgery was needed in four patients: in three because of device embolization, and in one because of homograft rupture (Figure 20.9). Most embolizations encountered were preventable. Patient selection is crucial to the success of the procedure. The valve is available up to 22 mm in diameter, making percutaneous valve insertion impossible in patients with a larger RV outflow tract (RVOT). Therefore, analysis of previous surgeries and noninvasive assessment of RVOT anatomy using MRI with 3D reconstruction or angiograms in multiple

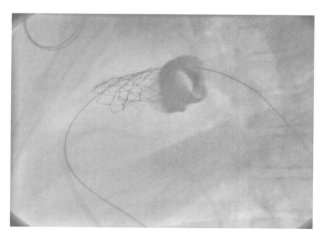

Figure 20.9 Angiogram showing homograft rupture after pulmonary valved stent implantation. The patient had a hemothorax. Surgical exploration did not find active bleeding. Patient was therefore treated conservatively and the valved stent was left in place (courtesy of Prof. P Bonhoeffer).

projections is mandatory. Devices and approaches for extending present indications to patients with large RVOT are currently being developed.[31]

Residual obstruction after stent deployment is related either to incomplete opening of the stent or to in-stent stenosis. In-stent stenosis was found in seven patients. Angiography showed the wall of the valve encroaching into the lumen of the stent. This was the result of suturing only the ends of the venous wall to the ends of the stent. It was treated by implantation of an additional valved stent inside the first stent (n=5) or by surgical removal of devices (n=2) (Figure 20.10). The device design was modified to prevent this latter by suturing the whole length of the venous segment to the entire length of the stent. So far, no further in-stent stenosis has been encountered. Incomplete opening of stent can be seen in heavily calcified lesions. This can be treated by further dilatation with high-pressure balloons.

Misplacement of valved stent can result from difficulties in maneuvering the delivery catheter due to the tortuous course to the lesion site, which emphasizes the need for a strong support (obtained by using a super-stiff guidewire) and excellent wire position. Valve misplacement can easily be avoided by using conduit calcification as a marker and dye injection through the sheath during device deployment. Stent migration and damage to cardiac structures during advancement of valved stents are prevented by the use of a front-loading long sheath, premounted catheter with a balloon inside based on a balloon-in-balloon technology.

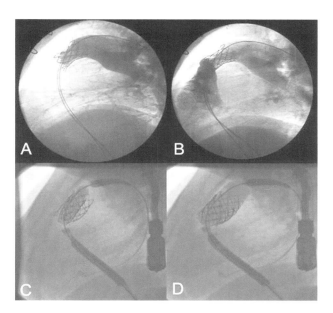

Figure 20.10 Angiograms performed in a patient with in-stent stenosis. A. Lateral view showing a perfectly functioning valve. B. Proximal injection showing a space between the stent and the contrast column (wall of the valve encroaching into the lumen of the stent). C, D. The in-stent stenosis is treated by the insertion of a second valved stent with a modified design where the whole length of the venous segment was sutured to the entire length of the stent (courtesy of Prof. P Bonhoeffer).

Endocarditis required late operation in one patient. As with any surgical implant, patients should also undergo prevention of endocarditis.

PERCUTANEOUS MITRAL VALVE REPAIR

Mitral regurgitation is the second most frequent valve disease and conservative surgical techniques are increasingly performed. The percutaneous approach attempts to reproduce two surgical techniques: ring annuloplasty and edge-to-edge valve repair.

A variety of ring annuloplasty technologies using a coronary sinus approach are in development. There is insufficient human experience in any of these to understand what the likely complications might be. The potential for obstruction, thrombosis, and perforation of the coronary sinus all seem to be minimal in the preclinical animal experience.

Mitral valve leaflet repair using the Evalve Mitra-clip (Figures 20.11, 20.12) has the largest experience in a clinical trial,[32] which included 27 patients who were all surgical candidates. Besides potential complications related to transseptal catheterization, the most important complication to date has been detachment of the clip from one of the two mitral leaflets in two patients. This has not resulted in embolization in any patients. The mechanism of clip detachment from a single leaflet appears to be related to placement of the clip when it is not perpendicular enough to the line of mitral coaptation, so that an insufficient amount is inserted in one of the two clip arms. Prior to gaining clinical trial experience, there was some concern that having a large-caliber device interfering with the mitral apparatus during device delivery would not be well tolerated. Remarkably, this 24 F guide catheter system is well tolerated during

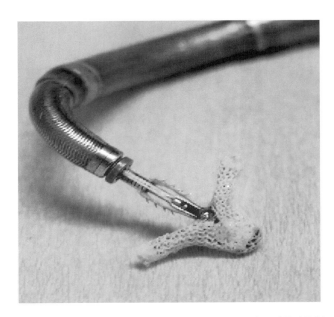

Figure 20.11 Evalve Mitra-clip and delivery catheter (courtesy of Prof. Ted Feldman).

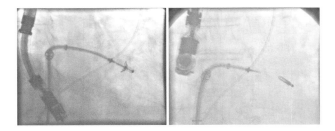

Figure 20.12 Percutaneous mitral valve repair using the Evalve Mitra-clip. The procedure is performed under transesophageal guidance. RAO view. On the left, the clip is open. On the right, it is closed and released (courtesy of Prof. Ted Feldman).

clip maneuvering and placement, and did not result in hemodynamic instability during the procedures.

A wide variety of additional devices are still at the experimental stage, such as another design for edge-to-edge repair involving the use of one or more sutures deployed via a catheter-based device, or anchoring devices placed through the left ventricular cavitary side of the mitral annulus for a more direct annuloplasty than the coronary sinus approach. The potential for complications will be defined as these devices are used in humans.

CONCLUSION

After nearly 20 years of extensive clinical evaluation, the technique of percutaneous valve dilatation is now here to stay. PMC is an effective procedure that carries a small but definite risk. In order to decrease risk and optimize patient selection, it is recommended to limit the performance of the procedure to experienced centers. Finally, the use of a stepwise Inoue technique under echographic monitoring is likely to make the procedure even safer.

PAV probably has a very limited role in isolation but may find new applications as the first step in the performance of PAVR. It carries a significant risk, which is due to the technique and even more to the patient's condition. However, the incidence of complications has decreased through technical improvement and continuous efforts to be vigilant to all medical conditions.

Percutaneous pulmonary dilatation is the preferred treatment in pulmonary valvular stenosis.

The new techniques of percutaneous valve intervention are at an early stage but they have opened a very exciting field of investigation. The preliminary results show us that these techniques are feasible. Refinements in both technique and technology are occurring rapidly, but the specific data regarding the most prevalent and common complications will be absent until large enough numbers of patients have been treated to gain an appreciation of real complication rates in both the short and long term.

REFERENCES

1. Tuzcu EM, Block PC, Palacios IF et al. Comparison of early versus late experience with percutaneous mitral balloon valvuloplasty. J Am Coll Cardiol 1991;17:1121–4.

2. Ben Farhat M, Betbout F, Gamra H et al. Results of percutaneous double-balloon mitral commissurotomy in one medical center in Tunisia. Am J Cardiol 1995;76:1266–70.
3. Chen CR, Cheng TO. Percutaneous balloon mitral valvuloplasty by the Inoue technique: a multicenter study of 4832 patients in China. Am Heart J 1995;129:1197–202.
4. National Heart, Lung, and Blood Institute Balloon Valvuloplasty Registry. Complications and mortality of percutaneous balloon mitral commissurotomy. Circulation 1992;85:2014–24.
5. Iung B, Nicoud-Houel A, Fondard O et al. Temporal trends in percutaneous mitral commissurotomy over a 15-year period. Eur Heart J 2004;25:702–8.
6. Stefanadis CI, Stratos CG, Lambrou SG et al. Accomplishments and perspectives with retrograde nontransseptal balloon mitral valvuloplasty. J Interv Cardiol 2000;13:269–80.
7. Cribier A, Eltchaninoff H, Carlot R. Percutaneous mechanical mitral commissurotomy with the metallic valvotome: detailed technical aspect and overview of the results of the multicenter registry 882 patients. J Interv Cardiol 2000;13:255–62.
8. Harrison KJ, Wilson JS, Hearne SE et al. Complications related to percutaneous transvenous mitral commissurotomy. Cathet Cardiovasc Diagn 1994;2:52–60.
9. Vahanian A, Cormier B, Iung B. Percutaneous transvenous mitral commissurotomy using the Inoue balloon: international experience. Cathet Cardiovasc Diagn 1994;2:8–15.
10. Bonhoeffer P, Hausse A, Yonga G. Technique and results of percutaneous mitral valvuloplasty with the multi-track system. J Interv Cardiol 2000:13:263–9.
11. Chen WJ, Chen MF, Liau CS et al. Safety of percutaneous transvenous balloon mitral commissurotomy in patients with mitral stenosis and thrombus in the left atrial appendage. Am J Cardiol 1992;70:117–19.
12. Herrmann HC, Lima JAC, Feldman T et al. Mechanisms and outcome of severe mitral regurgitation after Inoue balloon valvuloplasty. J Am Coll Cardiol 1993;27:783–9.
13. Acar C, Jebara VA, Grare PH et al. Traumatic mitral insufficiency following percutaneous mitral dilation: anatomic lesions and surgical implications. Eur J Cardiothorac Surg 1992;6:660–4.
14. Padial LR, Abascal VM, Moreno PR et al. Echocardiography can predict the development of severe mitral regurgitation after percutaneous mitral valvuloplasty by the Inoue technique. Am J Cardiol 1999;83:1210–13.
15. Cequier A, Bonan R, Dyrda I et al. Atrial shunting after percutaneous mitral valvuloplasty. Circulation 1990;81:1190–7.
16. Gupta S, Schiele F, Xu C et al. Simplified percutaneous mitral valvuloplasty with the Inoue balloon. Eur Heart J 1998;19:610–66.
17. Cribier A, Savin T, Saoudi N et al. Percutaneous transluminal valvuloplasty of acquired aortic stenosis in elderly patients: an alternative to valve replacement? Lancet 1986;1:63–7.
18. McKay RG. The Mansfield Scientific Aortic Valvuloplasty Registry: overview of acute hemodynamic results and procedural complications. J Am Coll Cardiol 1991;17:485–91.
19. Isner JM. Acute catastrophic complications of balloon aortic valvuloplasty. The Mansfield Scientific Aortic Valvuloplasty Registry Investigators. J Am Coll Cardiol 1991;17:1436–44.
20. Solomon LW, Fusman B, Jolly N et al. Percutaneous suture closure for management of large French size arterial puncture in aortic valvuloplasty. J Invasive Cardiol 2001;13:592–6.
21. Sakata Y, Sayed Z, Salinger MH, Feldman T. Percutaneous balloon aortic valvuloplasty: antegrade transseptal vs. conventional retrograde transarterial approach. Cathet Cardiovasc Intervent 2005;64:314–21.
22. Omran H, Schmidt H, Hackenbroch M et al. Silent and apparent cerebral embolism after retrograde catheterisation of the aortic valve in valvular stenosis: a prospective, randomised study. Lancet 2003;361:1241–6.
23. Cribier A, Eltchaninoff H, Bash A et al. Percutaneous transcatheter implantation of an aortic valve prosthesis for calcific aortic stenosis: first human case description. Circulation 2002;106:3006–8.
24. McCrindle BW. Independent predictors of long-term results after balloon pulmonary valvuloplasty. Valvuloplasty and Angioplasty of Congenital Anomalies (VACA) Registry Investigators. Circulation 1994;89:1751–9.

25. Stanger P, Cassidy SC, Girod DA et al. Balloon pulmonary valvuloplasty: results of the Valvuloplasty and Angioplasty of Congenital Anomalies Registry. Am J Cardiol 1990;65:775–83.
26. Agnoletti G, Piechaud JF, Bonhoeffer P et al. Perforation of the atretic pulmonary valve. Long-term follow-up. J Am Coll Cardiol 2003;41:1399–403.
27. Cribier A, Eltchaninoff H, Tron C et al. Early experience with percutaneous transcatheter implantation of heart valve prosthesis for the treatment of end-stage inoperable patients with calcific aortic stenosis. J Am Coll Cardiol 2004;43:698–703.
28. Powell AJ, Lock JE, Keane JF. Prolongation of right ventricular to pulmonary artery conduit life span by percutaneous stent implantation intermediate-term results. Circulation 1995;92:3282–8.
29. Matzoulis MA, Balaji S, Webber SA. Risk factors for arrhythmia and sudden cardiac death late after repair of tetralogy of Fallot: a multicentre study. Lancet 2000;356:975–81.
30. Bonhoeffer P, Boudjemline Y, Qureshi SA et al. Percutaneous insertion of the pulmonary valve. J Am Coll Cardiol 2002;39:1664–9.
31. Boudjemline Y, Agnoletti G, Piechaud JF et al. Percutaneous pulmonary valve replacement: towards a modification of the prosthesis. Arch Mal Coeur Vaiss 2003;96:461–6.
32. Feldman T, Wasserman HS, Herrmann HC et al. Percutaneous mitral valve repair using the edge-to-edge technique: six month results of the EVEREST Phase I clinical trial. J Am Coll Cardiol 2005;46:2134–40.

21

Complications during percutaneous closure of patent foramen ovale, atrial and ventricular septum defects

Guy S Reeder, Eric Eeckhout and Horst Sievert

Devices for atrial septal defect/patent foramen ovale closure • Device implantation
 • Malposition and device embolization • Device malfunction • Cardiac perforation
 • Air embolism • Arrhythmia • Vascular complications • Patent foramen ovale
 • Residual shunt • Thrombus formation • Transient ischemic attack or stroke
 • Device erosion • Percutaneous closure of ventricular septal defect • Conclusion

Percutaneous closure of an atrial septal defect was first described in 1976 by King et al.[1] Since then, it is estimated that more than 30,000 percutaneous closure procedures have been performed in patients with patent foramen ovale (PFO) and atrial septal defects (ASD). Continued evolution of device design and operator experience have resulted in remarkably low complication rates for these procedures. As a result, percutaneous closure is considered a first-line therapy in carefully selected patients; nonetheless, significant early and late complications have been documented and will be reviewed in this chapter.

DEVICES FOR ATRIAL SEPTAL DEFECT/PATENT FORAMEN OVALE CLOSURE

The attributes of nine commonly used devices for closure of the atrial septum/patent foramen ovale are shown in Table 21.1. Of these, the largest number of procedures has been performed with the CardioSEAL and Amplatzer systems. The CardioSEAL and related STARFlex devices use a double umbrella made of Dacron fabric supported by a metallic framework and, in the case of the latter, a self-centering mechanism using nitinol microsprings. The Amplatzer atrial septal occluder and patent foramen ovale device utilize a nitinol wire-frame mesh with enclosed polyester disks. The differences in device designs are readily apparent in Figure 21.1. Nonetheless, all devices share in common some type of metallic supporting structure with a fabric portion to occlude interatrial blood flow, and can be collapsed in some fashion to allow catheter deployment. By far the most experience has been gained with the STARFlex and Amplatzer devices.

DEVICE IMPLANTATION

Excellent descriptions of devices and implantation methodology have been published.[2] Common features include establishing the size and location of the

Table 21.1 Comparative summary of percutaneous ASD and PFO occlusion devices (modified from reference 19)

Device	Design and construction
Rashkind-PDA-Umbrella	Double umbrella made of polyurethane foam, each disk consists of a 4-arm framework. Device sizes: 11 and 17 mm
Sideris Buttoned Device (3rd and 4th generation)	1) square occluder button; 2) rhomboid counter occluder. Device sizes: 25–50 mm
ASDOS	Two self-opening umbrellas (5-arm nitinol wire skeleton) with polyurethane membranes. Device sizes: 25–60 mm
Angel Wings	Two interconnected square nitinol wire frames covered with Dacron fabric with a central conjoint ring. Device sizes: 18–40 mm
CardioSEAL	Noncentering double umbrella device modified from the Clamshell device with a 4-arm metallic framework covered with Dacron. Device sizes: 17–40 mm
STARFlex	CardioSEAL modification with a self-centering mechanism achieved by nitinol microsprings. Device sizes: 23–40 mm
Amplatzer	Self-centering double disk with a short connecting waist made from nitinol wire frame filled with polyester fabric. Device sizes: (ASD) 4–40 mm; (PFO) 25–35 mm
Helex	Nitinol wire with ultrathin expanded polytetrafluoroethylene formed into two equal-size opposing disks that bridge the septal defect. Device sizes: 15–35 mm
PFO Star (1st and 2nd generation)	Two Ivalon square disks, each umbrella is expanded by 4 nitinol arms – 1st generation: 2 mm center posts; 2nd generation: 3 and 5 mm center posts. Device sizes: 18–30 mm

ASD=atrial septal defect; PFO=patent foramen ovale.

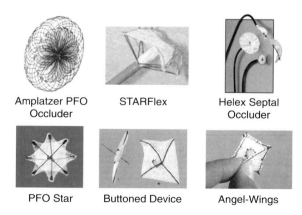

Amplatzer PFO Occluder	STARFlex	Helex Septal Occluder
PFO Star	Buttoned Device	Angel-Wings

Figure 21.1 Various devices used for percutaneous catheter-based patent foramen ovale (PFO) closure. Reproduced with permission.[2]

interatrial defect, usually with prior transesophageal echocardiography, use of transesophageal or intracardiac echocardiography to monitor device deployment, crossing of the defect with a catheter or guidewire, positioning of the delivery system, and deployment first of the left atrial side of the device followed by the right atrial side. Opportunities exist for inadvertent trauma or complications related to establishing femoral venous access, cardiac perforation with catheter or guidewire, inadvertent trauma from positioning of the delivery system and/or the device, thrombus formation with subsequent embolism or introduction of air into the right or left heart chambers, and cardiac arrhythmias. Additionally, the device may fail to engage the atrial septum properly, become detached prematurely with embolization, or embolize from its position in the atrial septum following deployment. Fortunately, with evolution of devices and improved operator experience, the occurrence of these complications has become very low. A summary of these complications may be found in Table 21.2.

MALPOSITION AND DEVICE EMBOLIZATION

This was described in up to 3.5% of cases in a review of 1417 procedures published in 2002.[3] This complication is almost exclusively limited now to patients with large atrial septal defects (stretched sizes greater than 25 mm) or where there is a markedly deficient rim, especially superiorly. In either case, the left atrial side of the device may not grasp the atrial septum and can subsequently prolapse into the right atrium during deployment. Transesophageal or intracardiac echocardiographic monitoring will help the operator appreciate this situation immediately and avoid premature device detachment. Variations in positioning of the delivery system (right versus left superior pulmonary vein) and modest oversizing of the device have been used to reduce this problem.[4–7]

Device embolizations tend to occur early, usually during the procedure, but may rarely occur up to one week after implantation.[8] Most devices will embolize within the right heart and can often be retrieved with a gooseneck snare and pulled into the delivery sheath and removed. In the case of the Amplatzer device, a technique for stabilizing the device with a guidewire and then snaring the right atrial screw pin has been described for removal of embolized devices within the right heart.[9] In our experience with over 500 Amplatzer devices for ASD and PFO closure, we had one embolization. In this patient, premature release of the device occurred in the left atrium. The device embolized through the left heart and came to rest in the iliac artery

Table 21.2 Complications reported during ASD/PFO closure		
Complication	Frequency (%)	Remedy
Malposition/device embolization	0–3.5	Snare and replace, rarely surgery
Device fracture	0–14	Usually observe, replace if large shunt
Cardiac perforation	0.5	Pericardiocentesis; rule out erosion
Air embolism	0–1	None, avoid with careful technique
Arrhythmia	2.6–3.1	Cardioversion, observation, rarely antiarrhythmics
Vascular complications	<1	Usually none needed

bifurcation. The device was snared and extracted through the femoral artery and a second, successful device placement was subsequently performed. There were no long-term sequelae. Surgical removal has been reported if percutaneous removal of the embolized device is not possible.[10]

DEVICE MALFUNCTION

Fracture of one of the metallic arms has been reported in 6–14% of implanted CardioSEAL or STARFlex devices.[11,12] No such complication is possible with the Amplatzer device. Arm fractures may or may not be associated with residual leak, and do not require revision unless associated with malposition or large residual shunt.

CARDIAC PERFORATION

This complication presents with clinical features of cardiac tamponade. Twenty-four cases of documented or presumed cardiac perforation involving the Amplatzer device have been described.[13] Most of these events occurred within the first day following implantation though one occurred as late as three years after the procedure. Guidewire perforation as well as late erosion of the device were implicated. Unexplained hypotension during the implantation procedure should suggest cardiac perforation with tamponade and can be confirmed immediately with echocardiography. Even small pericardial effusions developing acutely can produce tamponade. In our institution, echo-directed pericardiocentesis is the procedure of choice. Cardiac surgery may be required if significant device erosion is responsible or if pericardial effusion recurs.

AIR EMBOLISM

Clinically apparent air embolism is uncommon, probably occurring in less than 1% of cases. This complication is suggested by ST segment elevation in the inferior leads during or immediately post procedure. Entrainment of air into the delivery system may occur during removal of a large central dilating stylet. Embolized air may cross the atrial septum and obtain access to the most superior coronary sinus and subsequently embolize into the right coronary artery. Myocardial infarction has not been reported nor are there known long-term sequelae. This complication may be minimized by slowly withdrawing the dilator from the delivery sheath, and holding the Luer lock end of the catheter as low as possible on the table during guidewire exchanges and catheter aspiration, to avoid development of an air/fluid meniscus within the catheter.

ARRHYTHMIA

Atrial arrhythmias have been reported in 2–3% of patients following device closure of ASD or PFO.[14,15] This is usually self-terminating within the first few weeks to months after the procedure though it can exceptionally require temporary antiarrhythmic therapy. Heart block has occasionally been reported and we have observed one case in our practice possibly related to the use of the Amplatzer device.

VASCULAR COMPLICATIONS

Typically, both femoral veins and often a femoral artery are cannulated. The need for femoral artery cannulation in routine cases is doubtful. The incidence of vascular complications can be expected to be similar to that for right heart catheterization. With the use of intracardiac echocardiography, a 10 F sheath has been required; a recent reduction in size to 8 F will lessen the potential risk of vascular trauma due to larger sheath sizes in young patients.

PATENT FORAMEN OVALE

The above discussion relates primarily to atrial septal defect closure procedures. In a systematic review, Khairy et al published data from ten studies of transcatheter PFO closure involving 1355 patients.[16] The authors documented a 1.5% incidence of major complications defined as death, hemorrhage requiring blood transfusion, cardiac tamponade, need for surgical intervention, and massive fatal pulmonary emboli. There was a 7.9% incidence of minor complications including bleeding, atrial arrhythmias, transient AV nodal block, device arm fractures, device embolization with successful catheter retrieval, asymptomatic device thrombosis, air embolism, arteriovenous fistula formation, and femoral hematoma.

Late complications occurring after ASD/PFO closure are summarized in Table 21.3.

RESIDUAL SHUNT

If residual shunt can be considered a complication, it is by far the most common, occurring in up to 20% of patients with the CardioSEAL/STARFlex device in early series, and as little as 1–4% for the Amplatzer device more recently.[17,18] At present, comparable closure rates above 90% can be achieved with both devices.

THROMBUS FORMATION

The prevalence of device-related thrombus was investigated in a prospective follow-up of 1000 patients undergoing device closure with a variety of devices, by transesophageal echocardiography at four weeks and six months or as clinically indicated.[19] Thrombus was found in 1.2% of patients who had undergone ASD

Table 21.3 Late complications after ASD/PFO closure		
Complication	Frequency (%)	Remedy
Residual shunt	1–20	Observe, 2nd device?
Thrombus	1.2–2.5	Anticoagulate, ?thrombolysis
TIA or stroke	0.2–4.9	Transesophageal echocardiogram for device thrombus, residual shunt
Device erosion	0.1	Surgical removal
Late device embolization	Rare	Snare or surgery
Infection	Rare	Remove if needed
Atrial arrhythmia	Rare	Observation usually

closure, and in 2.5% of patients undergoing PFO closure. Incidence of thrombus was device related, highest in the CardioSEAL/STARFlex/PFO Star devices and lowest in the Amplatzer device group. Risk factors for device thrombus included postprocedure atrial fibrillation and persistent atrial septal aneurysm. A prothrombotic disorder could be identified in only two patients with device-related thrombus and pre-existing PFO device placement. In 17 of the 20 patients with device thrombus, anticoagulation was successful in thrombus resolution; in three patients surgical thrombus removal was performed. Two patients suffered minor strokes and one a transient ischemic attack (TIA) in this group of 20 patients with device-related thrombus. Residual atrial septum aneurysm was not a risk factor for development of thromboembolic events. There was no correlation between postprocedure treatment with warfarin versus aspirin versus aspirin plus clopidogrel and subsequent development of thrombus.

TRANSIENT ISCHEMIC ATTACK OR STROKE

The incidence of TIA or stroke post procedure is highly related to the characteristics of the patient population, especially past history of stroke or TIA. Thus, in 442 patients undergoing ASD device closure for atrial septal defect, one TIA occurred during follow-up (0.2%); patients were treated with aspirin alone following device closure.[17] Similarly, in 1000 patients undergoing ASD and PFO closure reported above, three neurologic events occurred (0.3%).[19] On the other hand, in a population of patients with pre-existing cryptogenic stroke undergoing PFO closure for presumed paradoxical thromboemboli, a systematic review of ten studies showed a wide range of recurrent neurologic events, from 0% to 4.9%.[16] The higher incidence of events in some of these studies suggests that nondevice (and non-PFO)-related causes are the most likely explanation.

DEVICE EROSION

Whereas cardiac perforation has been described during the implantation of a number of different devices, late erosion of the device through a cardiac wall resulting in pericardial tamponade has been described only for the Amplatzer device and is included here in late complications.[20–23]

In a review published in 2004, Amin et al[23] described a total of 28 cases of device erosion, out of an estimated 30,000 implanted devices, yielding an incidence of 0.1%. A third of these developed symptoms within one day, another third within three days, but the remainder presented between 20 days and three years from device implantation. Erosions occurred at the superior aspect of either the right or left atrium and sometimes also involved erosion of the aorta with fistula to the left or right atria. Deficiency of the aortic rim of the atrial septal defect was described in 89% and it is likely that deficiency of the superior rim was also present, allowing contact between the left or right atrial flange of the Amplatzer device and the superior left or right atrial wall. It is suspected that repetitive cardiac motion causes tissue erosion by the device. Recommendations for avoidance of this complication include avoidance of device oversizing (in particular not to choose a device size >1.5 larger than the static diameter of the defect), an awareness of potential risk in patients with deficient aortic and superior rims, and aggressive evaluation of patients who developed unexplained pericardial effusion at any time following the procedure. Additionally, it seems logical that careful intracardiac echocardiographic inspection of the device flanges and avoidance of contact with the superior atrial walls prior to device release would be useful.

We have not observed this complication in over 500 Amplatzer device placements. Other late complications such as embolization, infection or persistent atrial arrhythmias or heart block are exceedingly rare.

PERCUTANEOUS CLOSURE OF VENTRICULAR SEPTAL DEFECT

Whereas most atrial septal defects are of the secundum variety and lend themselves to device closure, the opposite is true for ventricular septal defects (VSD). At the present time, attempts at closure of VSDs have been mostly limited to defects in the muscular ventricular septum. The number of cases reported in the literature is somewhat under 500 to date. Impingement on the atrioventricular and semilunar valves, as well as the conduction system, has limited treatment of inflow and membranous ventricular septal defects, though devices are under development for the latter.

Devices used for VSD closure have included the Rashkind double umbrella device, the Sideris button device, and more recently the CardioSEAL/STARFlex system and the Amplatzer muscular VSD occluder device. The technique for implantation of these devices is more complicated than for ASD or PFO. Most operators have used an arteriovenous loop as described by Lock et al.[24] This allows the VSD to be initially crossed from the less trabeculated left ventricular side and the device implanted from the right ventricular side, and provides necessary stabilization of the guidewire and delivery system during deployment.

Knauth et al described a 13-year experience in closing unrepaired congenital or postoperative residual muscular ventricular septal defects in 170 patients using the CardioSEAL/STARFlex family of devices.[25] The population was highly selected and included patients with one or more VSDs producing hemodynamic derangement that were considered technically difficult to close surgically or in patients with high surgical risks. A total of 332 adverse events occurred in 153 of the 170 patients (90%) and nearly half of these were graded as moderately serious or serious (Table 21.4). Device arm fractures occurred in 10–18% of devices, and 11% of patients had at least one device explanted. During follow-up, there were 14 deaths with an all-cause mortality of 8.2%; in at least one patient, the cause of death was directly related to the device. While 90% of patients had some reduction of shunt flow, 60% had residual shunting, and device embolization and malposition were major problems.

Holzer et al[26] reported a registry of device closure of congenital muscular ventricular septal defects using the Amplatzer VSD occluder device. Seventy-five patients with a median age of 1.4 years underwent 83 procedures and were followed a median of 211 days post procedure. A total of 20.5% of procedures involved multiple device implantations. Complications are shown in Table 21.5. A total of 59 adverse events or complications occurred in 34 (45%) patients, and included death in two patients, device embolization retrieved successfully in three of 75 patients, two retrieved percutaneously, and one at surgery. Other significant complications included arrhythmia, hypotension, stroke or TIA in three patients and stroke at follow-up in one patient. Moderate or large residual shunts were present in 7% of cases at follow-up.

Table 21.4 Complications of muscular VSD closure (n=170 patients) using the CardioSEAL/STARFlex devices (modified from reference 25)

Event	No.
Related to device	
New-onset valvar regurgitation	9
Device malposition	9
Delivery system malfunction	6
Device embolism	5
Vascular access	2
Arrhythmia	6
Perforation of the heart	1
Congestive heart failure	1
Related to catheterization	
Vascular access	20
Valve injury	2
Perforation of the heart	1
Arrhythmia	42
Blood loss requiring transfusion	92
Fluoroscopy time >150 min per device	4
Contrast >6.0 mL/kg	2
Hemodynamic	29
Fever >38.5°C	17
Pulmonary/respiratory	13
Infectious	4
Neurologic	9
Gastrointestinal	6
Device explant	18
Death	14

Table 21.5 Adverse events after device closure of muscular VSD (n=75 patients) with Amplatzer device (from reference 26)

Event	No.
Procedure-related complications	28/75 (37.3%)
Arrhythmia/conduction anomalies	15/75 (20.0%)
Hypotension/cardiac arrest	9/75 (12.0%)
Hematoma/pseudoaneurysm/TX	5/75 (6.7%)
CVA/TIA	3/75 (4.0%)
Equipment/technical issues	3/75 (4.0%)
Device embolization	2/75 (2.7%)
Cardiac perforation	1/75 (1.3%)
Other	5/75 (6.7%)
Death	3/75 (4.0%)
Procedure related	2/75 (2.7%)
Unrelated/unknown	1/75 (1.3%)
Unresolved complications (alive)	6/75 (7.89%)
RBBB	2/75 (2.63%)
LVOT gradient	2/75 (2.63%)
Stroke	1/75 (1.31%)

CVA=cerebrovascular accident; LVOT=left ventricular outflow tract; RBBB=right bundle branch block; TIA=transient ischemic attack; TX=transfusion.

Percutaneous closure of postinfarction muscular ventricular septal defect has been attempted.[25,27,28] Holzer et al[27] reported outcomes of 18 patients, eight undergoing primary closure of postinfarct VSD and ten following attempted surgical closure. Complications are shown in Table 21.6 in this small group of patients. In two patients, the device could not be successfully deployed but in patients in whom deployment was possible, there was substantial reduction of shunt. Two of eight patients presenting for primary closure survived to median follow-up of 332 days. There were no procedure-related deaths; overall mortality was 41%. The periprocedural complications were relatively minimal given the high morbidity of this patient population. No early or late device embolizations were noted. Given the small number of patients reported in the literature, conclusions regarding efficacy and occurrence of potential complications cannot be definitely drawn.

CONCLUSION

For closure of secundum atrial septal defect and patent foramen ovale, percutaneous catheter-based therapies are possible with a low incidence of complications, though some, such as device erosion or thrombus formation, can be potentially serious. Complications are higher for closure of ventricular septal defect and many fewer such patients are likely candidates for device closure to begin with. Further development of devices and operator experience is anticipated. Knowledge of complications, especially those occurring late, is essential for all care providers who evaluate these patients early and at late follow-up.

Table 21.6 Complications and residual shunts after attempted percutaneous device closure in postinfarction VSD in 18 patients (from reference 27)

Event	No.
Device released successfully	16 (89%)
Procedure-related complications	4 (22%)
Blood loss/transfusion	2 (11%)
Bradycardia	2 (11%)
LV dysfunction	1 (6%)
Technical complications	0
Death	7 (41%)
Procedure related	0
Unrelated/unknown	7 (41%)
Residual shunt: immediate result	n=16
Closed	2 (12.5%)
Trivial or small	13 (81.3%)
Moderate or large	1 (6.3%)
Residual shunt: 24-h results	n=16
Closed	2 (12.5%)
Trivial or small	10 (62.5%)
Moderate or large	4 (25%)
Residual shunt: outpatient follow-up	n=10
Closed	2 (20%)
Trivial or small	6 (60%)
Moderate or large	2 (20%)

REFERENCES

1. King TD, Thompson SL, Steiner C, Mills NL. Secundum atrial septal defect. Nonoperative closure during cardiac catheterization. JAMA 1976;235:2506–9.
2. Meier B. Closure of patent foramen ovale: technique, pitfalls, complications, and follow up. Heart 2005;91:444–8.
3. Chessa M, Carminati M, Butera G et al. Early and late complications associated with transcatheter occlusion of secundum atrial septal defect. J Am Coll Cardiol 2002;39:1061–5.
4. Harper RW, Mottram PM, McGaw DJ. Closure of secundum atrial septal defects with the Amplatzer septal occluder device: techniques and problems. Cathet Cardiovasc Intervent 2002;57:508–24.
5. Du ZD, Koenig P, Cao GL, Waight D, Heitschmidt M, Hijazi ZM. Comparison of transcatheter closure of secundum atrial septal defect using the Amplatzer septal occluder associated with deficient versus sufficient rims. Am J Cardiol 2002;90:865–9.
6. Kannan BRJ, Francis E, Sivakumar K, Anil SR, Kumar RK. Transcatheter closure of very large (≥ 25 mm) atrial septal defects using the Amplatzer septal occluder. Cathet Cardiovasc Intervent 2003;59:522–7.
7. Du ZD, Cao QL, Rhodes J, Heitschmidt M, Hijazi ZM. Choice of device size and results of transcatheter closure of atrial septal defect using the Amplatzer septal occluder. J Intervent Cardiol 2002;15:287–92.
8. Verma PK, Thingnam SK, Sharma A, Taneja JS, Varma JS, Grover A. Delayed embolization of Amplatzer septal occluder device: an unknown entity. A case report. Angiology 2003;54:115–18.
9. Peuster M, Boekenkamp R, Kaulitz R, Fink C, Hausdorf G. Transcatheter retrieval and repositioning of an Amplatzer device embolized into the left atrium. Cathet Cardiovasc Intervent 2000;51:297–300.
10. Berdat PA, Chatterjee T, Pfammatter JP, Windecker S, Meier B, Carrel T. Surgical management of complications after transcatheter closure of an atrial septal defect or patent foramen ovale. J Thorac Cardiovasc Surg 2000;120:1034–9.
11. Carminati M, Giusti S, Hausdorf G et al. A European multicentric experience using the CardioSEAL and STARFlex double umbrella devices to close interatrial communications holes within the oval fossa. Cardiol Young 2000;10:519–26.
12. Pedra CA, Pihkala J, Lee KJ et al. Transcatheter closure of atrial septal defects using the CardioSEAL implant. Heart 2000;84:320–6.
13. Divekar A, Gaamangwe T, Shaikh N, Raabe M, Ducas J. Cardiac perforation after device closure of atrial septal defects with the Amplatzer septal occluder. J Am Coll Cardiol 2005;45:1213–18.
14. Billinger K, Trepels T, Reschke M, Ostermayer S, Sievert H. Short term complications within 6 months following transcatheter closure of patent foramen ovale (PFO) in 703 consecutive patients. Abstract presented at 6th International Workshop Catheter Interventions in Congenital Heart Disease and Other Non-Coronary Procedures with Live Case Demonstrations, June 19–21, 2003, Frankfurt, Germany.
15. Fischer G, Stieh J, Uebing A, Hoffmann U, Morf G, Kramer HH. Experience with transcatheter closure of secundum atrial septal defects using the Amplatzer septal occluder: a single centre study in 236 consecutive patients. Heart 2003;89:199–204.
16. Khairy P, O'Donnell CP, Landzberg MJ. Transcatheter closure versus medical therapy of patent foramen ovale and presumed paradoxical thromboemboli. A systematic review. Ann Intern Med 2003;139:753–60.
17. Du ZD, Hijazi ZM, Kleinman CS, Silverman NH, Larntz K, for the Amplatzer Investigators. Comparison between transcatheter and surgical closure of secundum atrial septal defect in children and adults. J Am Coll Cardiol 2002;39:1836–44.
18. Masura J, Gavora P, Podnar T. Long-term outcome of transcatheter secundum-type atrial septal defect closure using Amplatzer septal occluders. J Am Coll Cardiol 2005;45:505.
19. Krumsdorf U, Ostermayer S, Billinger K et al. Incidence and clinical course of thrombus

formation on atrial septal defect and patent foramen ovale closure devices in 1,000 consecutive patients. J Am Coll Cardiol 2004;43:302–9.

20. Trepels T, Zeplin H, Sievert H et al. Cardiac perforation following transcatheter PFO closure. Cathet Cardiovasc Intervent 2003;58:111–13.

21. Chun DS, Turrentine MW, Moustapha A, Hoyer MH. Development of aorta-to-right atrial fistula following closure of secundum atrial septal defect using the Amplatzer septal occluder. Cathet Cardiovasc Intervent 2003;58:246–51.

22. Preventza O, Sampath-Kumar S, Wasnick J, Gold JP. Late cardiac perforation following transcatheter atrial septal defect closure. Ann Thorac Surg 2004;77:1435–7.

23. Amin Z, Hijazi ZM, Bass JL, Cheatham JP, Hellenbrand WE, Kleinman CS. Erosion of Amplatzer septal occluder device after closure of secundum atrial septal defects: review of registry of complications and recommendations to minimize future risk. Cathet Cardiovasc Intervent 2004;63:496–502.

24. Lock JE, Block PC, McKay RG, Baim DS, Keane JF. Transcatheter closure of ventricular septal defects. Circulation 1988;78:361–8.

25. Knauth AL, Lock JE, Perry SB et al. Transcatheter device closure of congenital and postoperative residual ventricular septal defects. Circulation 2004;110:501–7.

26. Holzer R, Balzer D, Cao QL, Lock K, Hijazi ZM, for the Amplatzer Muscular Ventricular Septal Defect Investigators. Device closure of muscular ventricular septal defects using the Amplatzer muscular ventricular septal defect occluder. J Am Coll Cardiol 2004;43:1257–63.

27. Holzer R, Balzer D, Amin Z et al. Transcatheter closure of postinfarction ventricular septal defects using the new Amplatzer muscular VSD occluder: results of a U.S. registry. Cathet Cardiovas Intervent 2004;61:196–201.

28. Landzberg MJ, Lock JE. Transcatheter management of ventricular septal rupture after myocardial infarction. Semin Thorac Cardiovasc Surg 1998;10:128–32.

Section H
Words of wisdom

22

The Ten Commandments for the young interventional cardiologist

Stéphane Carlier, Koichi Sano and Jeffrey Moses

1. Thou shalt not cut corners • 2. Thou shalt not push • 3. Thou shalt blame thyself
• 4. Thou shalt honor thy protocols • 5. Thou shalt have a perfect access
• 6. Thou shalt always make new mistakes • 7. In doubt, stent thy lesion!
• 8. Heed thy patient! • 9. He who says 'it can't be done' commits blasphemy!
• 10. Every once in a while, thou shalt give the surgeon a case

Large randomized trials that are the foundation of evidence-based medicine are applied every day during percutaneous coronary interventions. Many studies are also reporting on new technologies flourishing in interventional cardiology. While it is mandatory for all of us to catch up with these latest developments, it is too often believed that the newest technology is 'the answer'. This concept can sometimes get a young interventional cardiologist into trouble. We believe that it is equally important to keep in mind some good old wisdom acquired after many years (and many mistakes) in a catheterization laboratory. This knowledge is sometimes difficult to find in research papers and this unique book, with its emphasis on complications, offers a great opportunity to share these thoughts with readers. Let's call them 'The Ten Commandments' that were once presented at a meeting by Professor Moses, director of one of the busiest interventional cardiac catheterization laboratories world-wide.

1. THOU SHALT NOT CUT CORNERS

While it is important to spend the minimum time possible performing a diagnostic or interventional procedure, being quick does not mean cutting corners. We have to simplify procedures but follow well-defined protocols and their completeness must be strictly adhered to.

For example, it is crucial to strive to completely visualize all coronary segments completely and obtain excellent angiograms. New imaging modalities such as IVUS give us helpful information. However, they are additional diagnostic modalities that should be used after obtaining complete views of a coronary tree full of contrast.

Systematically obtaining a left ventricle angiogram at the time of a diagnostic angiogram in patients presenting with an acute myocardial infarction, can yield important information on the LV function, the presence of an interventricular shunt, valvular regurgitation, impeding rupture, etc.

It is crucial to perform a complete hemodynamic assessment for valve diseases. It is not enough to rely only on echo for gradient, or regurgitation severity.

Lack of proficiency is not an excuse and when one cannot cross a valve or find a difficult saphenous vein graft or a coronary ostium with an aberrant origin, a second opinion should be obtained from a more experienced colleague.

Finally, the operator should always ask the surgeon what else he or she needs to be sure that all potential pathologies are completely addressed in one catheterization sitting in order to avoid another diagnostic procedure with its related risks of complications.

2. THOU SHALT NOT PUSH

Nothing should be forced during a diagnostic or interventional procedure. Catheters and wires are meant to glide through the body. They are self-lubricated and when they cease advancing, this suggests a problem and forcing the way can lead to complications. Small movements with orthogonal displacement of friction should be applied. One should only push objects running over a previously placed wire, and its intraluminal location must be double checked, even more cautiously during recanalization of total occlusions.

3. THOU SHALT BLAME THYSELF

When a complication occurs, one must critically consider the important etiologies summarized in Table 22.1. The operator must find the cause of the complication and solve the problem he or she is responsible for. However, the help of other colleagues should also be requested instead of trying to hide the problem or pretend that nothing occurred. Working in a catheterization laboratory involves teamwork and the cause of a complication and the best way to solve it will always be easier to solve with two or more experienced operators reviewing the issues.

4. THOU SHALT HONOR THY PROTOCOLS

Procedures should be standardized as much as possible by writing protocols. It is very important to ensure the quality of care. Standardization offers optimal education to the complete cath lab staff. Moreover, standardization will emphasize special cases as deviation from the protocols and this will better prepare the cath lab staff in unique situations.

5. THOU SHALT HAVE A PERFECT ACCESS

Many complications in the cath lab are related to a problem at the puncture site. If there is bleeding, pain or a hematoma at the puncture site, it must be resolved

Table 22.1 Most common causes of complications	
Hypotension	Occlusion
	Bleed
	Anaphylaxis
	Drug
Arrhythmia	Wire or catheter placement
Chest pain	Occlusion
	No-reflow

before going further and starting the diagnostic or interventional procedure. Overlooking such issues can lead to the case becoming a nightmare sooner or later.

6. THOU SHALT ALWAYS MAKE NEW MISTAKES

We must learn from our old mistakes and review them critically. We must minimize their incidence. Mistakes might well happen, but we should not repeat any made previously, but rather learn from them. We must learn from our own cases and from colleagues. For this, one must systematize data collection and implement a quality assessment process. Setting standards will allow for new, more creative errors and complications that will have to be reviewed in an open forum. Presenting old complications is boring whereas a well-conducted quality assessment review process will always be educational. We have such a meeting once monthly and the presence of all staff from our laboratory is mandatory. They present and review any of their complications and address corrective measures to consider and implement.

7. IN DOUBT, STENT THY LESION!

Stents were initially developed for the life-threatening suboptimal results of balloon angioplasty, in order to avoid cardiac surgery. Since then, their use has expanded drastically, becoming the first choice in the great majority of percutaneous interventions, currently with the drug-eluting stents. So far, no study has demonstrated that stents are inferior to plain balloon angioplasty in any clinical or lesion subset. So, stents must be the first choice when you need to secure a lesion and are first for safety. If in doubt, stent it! Preferably drug eluting stent.

8. HEED THY PATIENT!

Even when an angiogram looks great, serious complications can be hidden. So, if your patient feels bad, you should carefully look over all available information. And look again, in several projections, cautiously. And look, harder! Be careful and think deeply … and digitize! Digitize all records. Do not use paper.

9. HE WHO SAYS 'IT CAN'T BE DONE' COMMITS BLASPHEMY!

Interventional cardiology remains a relatively young cardiology speciality. We started with immature devices and many new tools have only recently been made available. However, there remain a few challenging lesions, including total occlusions, bifurcations, diffuse disease, highly calcified lesions, and lesions containing thrombus. Patients with left main disease or with a poor left ventricular function must also be treated very cautiously and wisely. Although we have overcome many difficult obstacles, there are still very challenging lesions that should not be attempted by all interventional cardiologists. However, when in doubt, a second opinion is always possible. Declaring that a lesion cannot be attempted because one does not dare treat it would be a blasphemy without a second opinion. If in doubt, ask!

10. EVERY ONCE IN A WHILE, THOU SHALT GIVE THE SURGEON A CASE

Surgeons are not our enemies. Development of a good, respectful relationship with them is critical. The most effective way to build a good collaboration is by discussing cases and referring them a patient occasionally. There remain lesion subsets not amenable to full revascularization by percutaneous intervention. Sending a case once in a while is also wise in order to avoid having surgeons wandering in the corridors, second-guessing you and making trouble! Finally, please always remember that 'Better is the Enemy of Good' and that complete revascularization for all patients should always be the primary end-point to secure their long-term prognosis. So, think about the patients and if you cannot fully revascularize all major vessels, do not hesitate to refer. You must first think of the interest of the patient.

23

Ten golden rules for avoiding complications during percutaneous cardiovascular interventions

Malcolm R Bell and Amir Lerman

Rule 1. Select the patient and lesion carefully, plan well, and anticipate problems • **Rule 2. Do not fall victim to the 'oculostenotic reflex'** • **Rule 3. Select a good guide catheter** • **Rule 4. Acquire adequate angiographic views before and after intervention** • **Rule 5. The procedure should be kept as simple as possible** • **Rule 6. You must have excellent knowledge of the equipment** • **Rule 7. Know your own limitations** • **Rule 8. Know when to stop** • **Rule 9. Always maintain the highest level of concentration** • **Rule 10. Learn from your own and others' mistakes and misfortunes**

One of the safest industries today is the aviation industry: thousands of commercial flights and millions of passengers fly daily with negligible risk of serious injury or death. We may speculate that we need to transpose the success of this industry to the practice of interventional cardiology in order to minimize the risks of serious injury and death. The aviation industry has instituted several methods in order to reduce the risks associated with flying, among them routine aircraft maintenance and the pre take-off pilot checklist. Intensive and focused training and experience are essential components of a safe operator – pilot or interventional cardiologist. Commercial pilots follow standard operating procedures but also are trained to avoid taking unnecessary risks or shortcuts in procedures and are aware of the critical importance of avoiding unnecessary distractions and losing their concentration. Operator checklists in the catheterization laboratory are important and have practical and safety benefits. Examples include checking the identity of the patient, knowledge of concurrent drug use, allergies, confirming administration of specific anticoagulants and antiplatelet agents, and knowledge of important baseline laboratory tests. In this chapter, we have compiled a list of 'rules' that are more cognitive and behavioral and serve to emphasize the importance of preparedness, concentration, and teamwork and which, if followed by the operator, should minimize the risk of complications of percutaneous interventional coronary procedures.

It is important for the reader to appreciate that interventional cardiologists may well have their own set of unwritten rules that guide them in their daily practice to maximize their success and minimize their complications. We could envision, as an alternative to 'rules to avoid complications', a list rather of 'rules to maximize success'. It is my belief that these two lists of precepts are closely intertwined although there may be subtle but important differences. However, discussion of avoidance of complications gets to the heart of the Hippocratic precept of *primum non nocere.*

RULE 1. SELECT THE PATIENT AND LESION CAREFULLY, PLAN WELL, AND ANTICIPATE PROBLEMS

The message from this is self-evident: physicians should not rush into any procedure without reviewing the patient's full and complete medical and surgical history, examination findings, and results of all pertinent laboratory tests. The angiogram should be studied carefully, taking into account the coronary anatomy, tortuosity of the target vessel, and lesion characteristics. It is not uncommon for cases to be started with the expectation that the procedure should be relatively straightforward only to discover that the case is in fact far more difficult because of failure to appreciate the angiographic features above. Examples include difficulty with access to the lesion because of severe tortuosity that was not recognized initially or a lesion that is difficult to cross or open because of severe calcification which had not been recognized during a cursory review of the angiogram prior to the procedure.

While many procedures will be relatively straightforward, I find it helpful to ask myself what could potentially go wrong, even if it is unlikely, and how I would approach the problem. Typical issues would be potential loss of side branches, placement of stents at bifurcation segments or treatment of ostial lesions such as ostial left anterior descending (LAD) lesions that may have the potential to compromise the distal left main or circumflex origin. Such preparedness would include ensuring that the right size guide catheter is used and that appropriately sized balloons and stents are immediately available.

RULE 2. DO NOT FALL VICTIM TO THE 'OCULOSTENOTIC REFLEX'

This is an oft-quoted phrase. In my experience, this applies as much to an interventional cardiologist as to a noninvasive cardiologist. The priority in treatment of patients with coronary disease is to perform revascularization of the most important critical lesions. You do not necessarily have to place stents in every vessel or branch that has a stenosis and certainly not in borderline lesions simply 'because you are there'. Percutaneous cardiovascular intervention (PCI) currently is in a relatively advanced stage and the majority of lesions that we are asked to treat can generally be approached with a high expectation of success. Therefore, it is often not a question of whether the PCI can be performed but rather of whether it needs to be performed. In this regard, we should keep in mind the three goals of treatment of patients with coronary artery disease: improving symptoms, reducing risk of subsequent myocardial infarction, and improving survival. It is probably true to say that PCI has never been easier or safer. There is a wide range of easily deliverable balloons and stents along with a wide choice of guidewires. In addition, potent antiplatelet therapy, such as dual therapy with aspirin and clopidogrel, along with intravenously administered glycoprotein IIb/IIIa inhibitors, have all increased the safety of PCI.

The first and probably most important aim is relief of symptoms. PCI is very effective at eliminating or at least improving symptoms of angina. This should be a very realistic expectation for PCI in the majority of our patients. However, particularly in the elective setting, it is unrealistic of us to believe that PCI with stent placement will prevent a future acute myocardial infarction or sudden death. No matter how severe the patient's disease appears to be on a coronary angiogram, we must recognize our current inability to identify future culprit lesions that would lead to plaque rupture and acute myocardial infarction or sudden death. The exception might be in a patient who presents with an acute coronary syndrome with a critical coronary stenosis; successful stent placement might well decrease the chance of a subsequent acute myocardial infarction at this particular site, but certainly not at sites in close proximity. The enormous value of medical therapy, as secondary prevention, cannot be overstated and is arguably more important than the placement of a stent, whether it be drug eluting or non drug eluting. In particular, chronic antiplatelet therapy with aspirin, and clopidogrel in appropriate patients, beta blocker therapy, angiotensin converting enzyme inhibitors in appropriate patients (such as those with diabetes mellitus, heart failure, left ventricular dysfunction or hypertension), and statin therapy all have important roles to play in the prevention of acute myocardial infarction and death.

Finally, it is presumptuous to think that PCI will prolong survival in most patients. The majority of patients treated with PCI have single-vessel disease and normal ejection fraction and thus it is unlikely that survival will be improved in such patients. The exception might be with treatment of isolated LAD coronary artery lesions but this has never been proven in a randomized clinical trial. Improved survival has been documented for patients with multivessel coronary artery disease who undergo coronary artery bypass surgery compared to medical therapy. This survival advantage generally applies to those with two- or three-vessel coronary artery disease, one of which includes the proximal LAD coronary artery, and in those who have decreased left ventricular ejection fraction. The survival advantage of coronary artery bypass surgery over PCI in patients with multivessel disease in whom diabetes mellitus is present should also not be forgotten. There are no contemporary data on the use of drug-eluting stents that would modify this statement currently. It would be speculative to extrapolate the survival advantage of coronary artery bypass surgery over medical therapy to similar patients treated with multiple drug-eluting stents.

RULE 3. SELECT A GOOD GUIDE CATHETER

Placement of current-generation angioplasty balloons and stents is now far easier than it was a decade or so ago. One might be forgiven for thinking that appropriate guide catheter support may be less important than in the past for many lesions simply because most elective procedures for simple lesions appear to proceed so smoothly and easily. It is exactly this type of thinking that can lull one into a false sense of security. While a poorly fitting guide catheter may seem sufficient for a relatively straightforward lesion, it might be totally inadequate a few minutes later when unexpectedly one is faced with a major complication such as an extensive dissection or unexpected difficulty in advancing a stent. A well-fitting guide catheter should always be co-axial in its alignment and without pressure damping. Depending on vessel size, smaller guide catheters such as 5 or 6 F can often be used – smaller guide catheters tend to result in fewer dissections. Another advantage of smaller guide catheters, particularly 5 F, is that their smaller size results in less bleeding and fewer vascular complications.

RULE 4. ACQUIRE ADEQUATE ANGIOGRAPHIC VIEWS BEFORE AND AFTER INTERVENTION

Prior to intervention, at least two angiographic views should be obtained showing the target lesion with adequate visualization of the proximal and distal segments. Following intervention, the same views should be repeated to evaluate the final result. These views should always be obtained without the wire in place as occasionally a wire can conceal the presence of a complication such as a dissection. These views should show the relationship of all important adjacent side branches to avoid unnecessary obstruction of these but also to guide optimal stent placement as they may provide important geographic information. Appropriate vessel–stent sizing is critical for optimal stent placement and all preprocedural angiograms should be performed after the administration of sublingual or preferably intracoronary nitroglycerin to be sure that the vessel is maximally dilated.

Finally, at the conclusion of the procedure, careful scrutiny of the angiogram should be made. Too often, we focus only on the treated segment rather than looking at the angiogram in its entirety. For example, we may miss proximal dissections caused by the guide catheter or guidewire, evidence of coronary perforation (at the treatment site or distal in the vessel) that may result later in pericardial effusion or tamponade, or tell-tale signs of vessel occlusion in a previously treated vessel. I have seen a number of examples during multivessel angioplasty, where the operator did not notice that the first lesion had since occluded because he failed to recognize retrograde filling of the vessel by collaterals simply because he was focused only on the subsequent intervention.

RULE 5. THE PROCEDURE SHOULD BE KEPT AS SIMPLE AS POSSIBLE

While balloon angioplasty and stent placement are fairly straightforward procedures in the majority of patients, other procedures such as directional or rotational atherectomy and laser angioplasty are not so simple. The routine use of such techniques is not generally recommended; their efficacy, compared to simple balloon angioplasty combined with stent placement, is generally unconvincing while their risks, such as procedural myocardial infarction and coronary perforation, are higher.

We should also try to keep the stent procedure as simple as possible. We should resist the urge to place too many stents, particularly if they are too long or too small. Bifurcation lesions remain a major obstacle to interventional cardiologists and despite a multitude of different techniques to deal with them, the efficacy of one over the others is as yet unproven and the frequency of complications, particularly stent thrombosis, and restenosis rates remain higher compared to non-bifurcation lesions.

I firmly believe that the efficacy of what we accomplish in the cath lab during PCI should not necessarily be judged on the immediate results – excellent angiographic outcomes can be expected in the majority of cases. Instead, efficacy should be judged by the early 6–12 month outcomes and later. An excellent early angiographic result with multiple long stents is of little benefit if the patient returns in a few months with severe, diffuse in-stent restenosis, particularly if there is now no 'normal unstented' segment of the vessel available in which arterial or venous grafts can be placed.

RULE 6. YOU MUST HAVE EXCELLENT KNOWLEDGE OF THE EQUIPMENT

This statement is certainly true with respect to the choice of wires, balloons, and stents. It is perhaps even more important when one is using more complex equipment such as the various atherectomy devices, rheolytic devices (for example, AngioJet), brachytherapy, intravascular ultrasound, and distal protection devices, to name but a few. These devices are generally more complicated in their set-up and use. The fact that some of these may be used only infrequently serves to emphasize that the user should be familiar with both these aspects and be able to troubleshoot any problems.

The use of vascular closure devices is also included under this discussion. The efficacy of these devices over a simple manual compression remains unsettled and there are no convincing data to indicate that complication rates have been reduced with the use of these devices. In fact, complications specific to these devices may unfortunately occur occasionally and result in very unusual and dangerous situations, such as embolization of 'collagen plugs' into the distal artery or retention/loss of suture needles in the deeper tissues.

RULE 7. KNOW YOUR OWN LIMITATIONS

The typical interventionalist is a young or middle-aged male. Perhaps there is some truth in the generalization that such individuals rarely doubt their own ability or are reluctant to admit they have any self-doubt or limitations. A useful analogy to remember is that such people rarely stop to ask for directions or help when driving their car. There may also be a tendency for some of these operators to be somewhat cavalier in their approach and they may be somewhat technology orientated rather than viewing the 'whole patient'. On the other hand, older interventionalists should be careful not to become 'set in their ways'. The paucity of female interventional cardiologists does not allow for any generalizations about their approach.

RULE 8. KNOW WHEN TO STOP

While optimal PCI generally requires optimal stent placement and deployment, we need to avoid getting carried away to the point of absolute perfection during an extremely difficult case. This is not meant to imply that one should take short cuts or compromise safety of the procedure. However, memorable quotes from some of my colleagues include 'snatching defeat from the jaws of victory' and 'perfect is the enemy of good'. One needs to maintain a realistic perspective of the patient's risk and the relative risk of the lesion versus the risk of a complication. In particular, we should think carefully before trying to treat every tiny dissection, treating small side branches that may or may not be compromised, treating very small vessels or borderline lesions.

RULE 9. ALWAYS MAINTAIN THE HIGHEST LEVEL OF CONCENTRATION

Each interventional cardiologist will have their own perspective on this. Unlike a surgical operating room, where the majority of patients are being treated under either general anesthesia or heavy sedation, most of our patients are only mildly sedated and are usually quite alert. It is not uncommon for conversations to occur between the patient and the interventional cardiologist but while this may be reassuring to the patient, I personally sometimes find this distracting and I think such conversations should not dominate the procedure and may be better held between the patient and an attendant. Cath labs often become quite noisy with verbal discussions and noisy equipment or monitors, all of which can become distracting. Discussion of matters not directly related to the case between the interventional cardiologist and their assistant, or other team members, should be avoided. Increasingly, procedures are performed as a team: the physician, their immediate assistant, circulating nurse or technician, recording and monitoring technicians, and nurses taking care of sedation and the patient's comfort. Thus there is the potential for misunderstandings or miscommunications if individual team members are too distracted. Alertness of every team member in the room is essential, no matter how easily a procedure appears to be proceeding.

Patients place their trust in us to deal effectively and safely with their heart disease which they often view, quite appropriately, as serious and potentially life threatening. It therefore seems inappropriate for them to be lying there in the room with catheters in their heart, listening to their physician discussing social issues, current events, sporting events or other unrelated matters. Some cath labs routinely play music for the patient and everyone else to listen to. While this might seem progressive and perhaps soothing, we should be careful that this music does not become a focus for discussion and distraction. One simple mistake, either by commission or omission, that occurs because a team member became distracted would be unforgivable. As an analogy, I cannot imagine any of us, while sitting on a commercial airplane, wishing to distract the pilot by engaging him or her in idle conversation during landing or take-off!!

RULE 10. LEARN FROM YOUR OWN AND OTHERS' MISTAKES AND MISFORTUNES

This involves careful analysis and reanalysis of your own complications or near misses as well as those of your colleagues. You should be open and honest about mistakes and recognition of what might have been done to avoid them.

Despite all of the above precautions, we can never always avoid bad luck but at least we should always, in every case, do everything to minimize that chance and be prepared to handle its consequences.

Index

Page references to *figures, tables* are shown in *italics*.